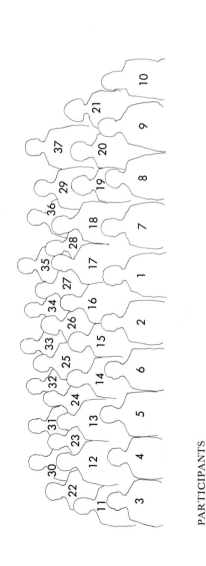

PARTICIPANTS

1. H.I.H. Princess Takamatsu
2. H.I.H. Prince Takamatsu
3. Dr. Weisburger
4. Dr. Farber
5. Dr. Wattenberg
6. Dr. Saffiotti
7. Dr. Magee
8. Dr. Craddock
9. Dr. Maher
10. Dr. Sutherland
11. Dr. Nakahara
12. Dr. Gelboin
13. Dr. Butler
14. Dr. Troll
15. Mrs. Newberne
16. Dr. Newberne
17. Dr. Rajewsky
18. Dr. Laufs
19. Mrs. Lieberman
20. Dr. Lieberman
21. Mrs. Rajewsky
22. Dr. Sugano
23. Dr. Kondo
24. Dr. Williams
25. Dr. McCalla
26. Mrs. Bootsma
27. Dr. Bootsma
28. Mrs. Goldthwait
29. Dr. Goldthwait
30. Dr. Takayama
31. Dr. Sugimura
32. Dr. Matsushima
33. Dr. Takebe
34. Dr. Hashimoto
35. Dr. Okada
36. Dr. Tada
37. Dr. Makino

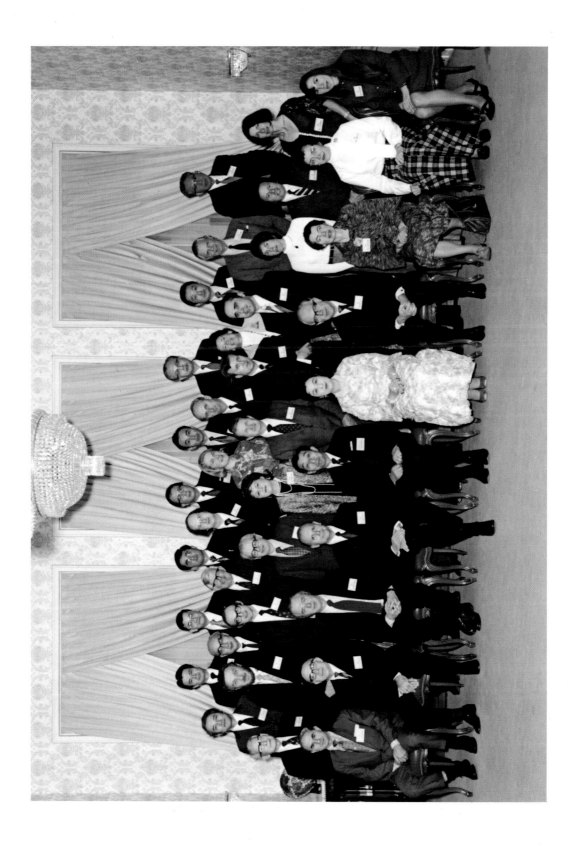

FUNDAMENTALS IN CANCER PREVENTION

Proceedings of the 6th International Symposium of
The Princess Takamatsu Cancer Research Fund, Tokyo, 1975

FUNDAMENTALS IN CANCER PREVENTION

Edited by
PETER N. MAGEE, SHOZO TAKAYAMA,
TAKASHI SUGIMURA, and TAIJIRO MATSUSHIMA

UNIVERSITY PARK PRESS
Baltimore · London · Tokyo

UNIVERSITY PARK PRESS
Baltimore · London · Tokyo

Library of Congress Cataloging in Publication Data
Main entry under title:

Fundamentals in cancer prevention.
  Includes bibliographical references.
    1. Cancer—Prevention—Congresses.
2. Carcinogenesis—Congresses.   I. Magee, Peter N.
II. Takamatsu no Miya Hi Gan Kenkyū Kikin.
[DNLM: 1. Neoplasms—Prevention and control—
Congresses.   QZ200 F982 1976]
RC268. F86   616.9′94′05   76-50548
ISBN 0-8391-0965-2

© UNIVERSITY OF TOKYO PRESS, 1976
UTP No. 3047-68494-5149
Printed in Japan

Originally published by
UNIVERSITY OF TOKYO PRESS

Princess Takamatsu Cancer Research Fund

* Dr. Nakahara was deprived of his earthly life on January 21, 1976, at the age of 79.
He was Scientific Advisor of the Proceedings of the International Symposium of
The Princess Takamatsu Cancer Research Fund from 1968 to 1976.

Organizing Committee of the 6th International Symposium

Peter N. MAGEE
    Fels Research Institute, Temple University, Philadelphia, U.S.A.
Shozo TAKAYAMA
    Cancer Institute, Japanese Foundation for Cancer Research, Tokyo, Japan
Takashi SUGIMURA
    National Cancer Center Research Institute, Tokyo, Japan
Taijiro MATSUSHIMA
    Institute of Medical Science, University of Tokyo, Tokyo, Japan

Participants

Bootsma, D.
Department of Cell Biology and Genetics, Erasmus University, Rotterdam, The Netherlands

Butler, W. H.
Department of Histopathology, St. George's Hospital Medical School, Blackshaw Road, Tooting, London SW17 OQT, England

Craddock, V. M.
MRC Toxicology Unit, Medical Research Council Laboratories, Carshalton, Surrey SM5 4EF, England

Farber, E.
Department of Pathology, University of Toronto, 100 College Street, Toronto, Ontario M5G 1L5, Canada

Gelboin, H. V.
Chemistry Branch, National Cancer Institute, NIH, Bethesda, Md. 20014, U.S.A.

Goldthwait, D. A.
Department of Biochemistry, Case Western Researve University, 2109 Adelbert Road, Cleveland, Ohio 44106, U.S.A.

Hashimoto, Y.
Department of Hygienic Chemistry, Faculty of Pharmaceutical Sciences, Tohoku University, Aoba Aramaki, Sendai 980, Japan

Kondo, S.
Department of Fundamental Radiology, Faculty of Medicine, Osaka University, Kita-ku, Osaka 530, Japan

LAUFS, R.
Hygiene-Institut der Universität, D-34 Göttingen, Kreuzbergring 57, West Germany

LIEBERMAN, M. W.
Environmental Mutagenesis Branch, National Institute of Environmental Health Sciences, Research Triangle Park, N.C. 27709, U.S.A.

MAGEE, P. N.
Fels Research Institute, Temple University School of Medicine, Philadelphia, Penn. 19140, U.S.A.

MAHER, V. M.
Carcinogenesis Laboratory, Division of Biological Sciences, Michigan Cancer Foundation, 110 East Warren Avenue, Detroit, Mich. 48201, U.S.A.

MATSUSHIMA, T.
Department of Molecular Oncology, Institute of Medical Science, University of Tokyo, Minato-ku, Tokyo 108, Japan

McCALLA, D. R.
Department of Biochemistry, Faculty of Science, McMaster University, Hamilton, Ontario L8S 4J9, Canada

NEWBERNE, P. M.
Department of Nutrition and Food Science, Room E. 18-611, Massachusetts Institute of Technology, Cambridge, Mass. 02139, U.S.A.

OKADA, M.
Tokyo Biochemical Research Institute, Takada 3-41-8, Toshima-ku, Tokyo 171, Japan

RAJEWSKY, M. F.
Max-Planck Institut für Virusforschung, 74 Tübingen, Spemannstrasse 35, West Germany

SAFFIOTTI, U.
Division of Cancer Cause & Prevention, National Cancer Institute, NIH, Bethesda, Md. 20014, U.S.A.

SUGIMURA, T.
National Cancer Center Research Institute, Chuo-ku, Tokyo 104, Japan

SUTHERLAND, B. M.
Department of Molecular Biology & Biochemistry, School of Biological Sciences, University of California, Irvine, Calif. 92664, U.S.A.

TADA, M.
Department of Biochemistry, Aichi Cancer Center Research Institute, Tashiro-cho, Chikusa-ku, Nagoya 464, Japan

TAKAYAMA, S.
Cancer Institute, Japanese Foundation for Cancer Research, Toshima-ku, Tokyo 170, Japan

TAKEBE, H.
Department of Fundamental Radiology, Faculty of Medicine, Osaka University, Kita-ku, Osaka 530, Japan

TROLL, W.
Institute of Environmental Medicine, New York University Medical Center, 550 1st Avenue, New York, N.Y. 10016, U.S.A.

WATTENBERG, L. W.
Department of Laboratory Medicine and Pathology, University of Minnesota Medical School, Minneapolis, Mn. 55455, U.S.A.

WEISBURGER, J. H.
Naylor Dana Institute for Disease Prevention, American Health Foundation, Valhalla, N.Y. 10595, U.S.A.

WILLIAMS, R. E. O.
Public Health Laboratory Service, Lower Entrance, Colindale Hospital, Colindale Avenue, London NW9 5EQ, England

Observers

Toshio ANDO, Institute of Medical Science, University of Tokyo, Tokyo

Takaaki AOYAGI, Institute of Microbial Chemistry, Tokyo

Misako ARAKI, Institute of Medical Science, University of Tokyo, Tokyo

Ryuichi DOHUKU, Cancer Institute, Tokyo

Hideya ENDO, Cancer Research Institute, Faculty of Medicine, Kyushu University, Fukuoka

Janos FODOR, National Institute of Oncology, Budapest

Setsuro FUJII, Institute for Enzyme Research, School of Medicine, Tokushima University, Tokushima

Masao FUJIMORI, Saitama Cancer Center Research Institute, Saitama

Yoshisada FUJIWARA, Kobe University School of Medicine, Kobe

Hisayuki FUKUTOMI, National Cancer Center Hospital, Tokyo

Osamu HAYAISHI, Faculty of Medicine, Kyoto University, Kyoto

Yuzo HAYASHI, Hatano Research Institute, Food & Drug Safety Center, Hatano

Yorio HINUMA, School of Medicine, Kumamoto University, Kumamoto

Takeshi HIRAYAMA, National Cancer Center Research Institute, Tokyo

Iwao HIRONO, School of Medicine, Gifu University, Gifu

Thomas HOFSTAETTER, National Cancer Center Research Institute, Tokyo

Masakatsu HORIKAWA, Faculty of Pharmaceutical Sciences, Kanazawa University, Kanazawa

Motoo HOZUMI, Saitama Cancer Center Research Institute, Saitama

Yoji IKAWA, Cancer Institute, Tokyo

Yoshio IKEDA, National Institute of Hygienic Sciences, Tokyo

Mitsuo IKENAGA, Medical School, Osaka University, Osaka

Naomichi INUI, Biological Research Center, JTS, Hatano

Nobuyuki ITO, Medical School, Nagoya City University, Nagoya

Motoi ISHIDATE, JR., National Institute Hygienic Sciences, Tokyo

Takatoshi ISHIKAWA, Cancer Institute, Tokyo

Tsuneo KADA, National Institute of Genetics, Misima

Shiro KATOH, Research Institute for Microbial Diseases, Osaka University, Osaka

Tadao KAKIZOE, National Cancer Center

Research Institute, Tokyo

Takashi KAWACHI, National Cancer Center Research Institute, Tokyo

Yutaka KAWAZOE, National Cancer Center Research Institute, Tokyo

Nadao KINOSHITA, School of Health Sciences, Kyushu University, Fukuoka

Hisayo S. KITAGAWA, Tokyo Biochemical Research Institute, Tokyo

Tomoyuki KITAGAWA, Cancer Institute, Tokyo

Susumu KODAIRA, National Cancer Center Hospital, Tokyo

Katsuro KOIKE, Cancer Institute, Tokyo

Yasuo KOYAMA, National Cancer Center Hospital, Tokyo

Yukiaki KURODA, National Institute of Genetics, Misima

Akihiko MAEKAWA, National Institute of Hygienic Sciences, Tokyo

H. I. H. Prince MASAHITO

Hiromu MATSUMOTO, Institute of Medical Science, University of Tokyo, Tokyo

Mutsushi MATSUYAMA, Aichi Cancer Center Research Institute, Nagoya

Masanao MIWA, National Cancer Center Research Institute, Tokyo

Masataka MOCHIZUKI, Tokyo Biochemical Research Institute, Tokyo

Wataru MORI, Faculty of Medicine, University of Tokyo, Tokyo

Minako NAGAO, National Cancer Center Research Institute, Tokyo

Chikayoshi NAGATA, National Cancer Center Research Institute, Tokyo

Takeo NAGAYO, Aichi Cancer Center Research Insitute, Nagoya

Masahiro NAKADATE, National Institute of Hygienic Sciences, Tokyo

Tomio NARISAWA, Akita University School of Medicine, Akita

Taisei NOMURA, Institute for Cancer Research, Medical School, Osaka University, Osaka

Atsushi OIKAWA, The Research Institute for Tuberculosis, Leprosy and Cancer, Tohoku University, Sendai

Shigehumi OKADA, Faculty of Medicine, University of Tokyo, Tokyo

Kiwamu OKITA, Yamaguchi University, School of Medicine, Ube

Shigeyoshi ODASHIMA, National Institute of Hygienic Sciences, Tokyo

Tetsuo ONO, Cancer Institute, Tokyo

Tamenori ONOÉ, Sapporo Medical College, Sapporo

Melvin D. REUBER, National Institute of Hygienic Sciences, Tokyo

Yoshio SAKURAI, Cancer Institute, Tokyo

Shigeaki SATO, National Cancer Center Research Institute, Tokyo

Makoto SEIJI, Tohoku University School of Medicine, Sendai

Haruo SUGANO, Cancer Institute, Tokyo

Emako SUZUKI, Tokyo Biochemical Research Institute, Tokyo

Mariko TADA, Aichi Cancer Center Research Institute, Nagoya

Yasuyuki TAKAGI, Faculty of Medicine, Kyushu University, Fukuoka

Nozomu TAKEMURA, The Jikei University School of Medicine, Tokyo

Mieko TAKEUCHI, National Cancer Center Research Institute, Tokyo

Tomio TAKEUCHI, Institute of Microbial Chemistry, Tokyo

Hiroshi TANOOKA, National Cancer Center Research Institute, Tokyo

Koichi TATSUMI, Faculty of Medicine, Kyoto University, Kyoto

Yataro TAZIMA, National Institute of Genetics, Misima

Reiko TOKUZEN, National Cancer Center Research Institute, Tokyo

Shigeru TSUKAGOSHI, Cancer Institute, Tokyo

Hamao UMEZAWA, Institute of Microbial Chemistry, Tokyo

Tadashi UTAKOJI, Cancer Institute, Tokyo

Tadashi WATABE, Tokyo College of Pharmacy, Tokyo

Minro WATANABE, The Research Institute for Tuberculosis, Leprosy and Cancer, Tohoku University, Sendai

George WEBER, School of Medicine, Indiana University, U.S.A.

Takie YAHAGI, National Cancer Center

Research Institute, Tokyo

Tadashi YAMAMOTO, Institute of Medical Science, University of Tokyo, Tokyo

Masanosuke YOSHIKAWA, Institute of Medical Science, University of Tokyo, Tokyo

Opening Address

H.I.H. Princess KIKUKO TAKAMATSU

For the past several years it has been my privilege to witness the developments in various aspects of cancer research through the annual International Symposia held under the auspices of the Cancer Research Fund which bears my name. The first symposium took place in 1970 on "Human Tumor Virology and Immunology" which set the academic standard for other symposia which followed. It is a matter of satisfaction to me to recall the past five symposia which have been so highly successful.

This morning it is my pleasant duty to attend the opening meeting of the Sixth Symposium and to greet all the participants and observers. The subject chosen this time is "Fundamentals in Cancer Prevention." My scientific advisors are of the opinion that we are now in a position to discuss the prevention of cancer on the basis of the advancing knowledge of carcinogenic mechanism. There is an intimate relation between the hazards of all kinds in our environment and the causation of cancer in man. The fundamental knowledge of how each of the potential carcinogens acts may eventually point to the ways and means of practical cancer prevention.

I am especially pleased to take this opportunity of extending my cordial welcome to the participants from overseas whose co-operation makes the Symposium internationally meaningful. In this connection I should not fail to thank Dr. P. N. Magee of the United Kingdom who has taken up special responsibility for the Symposium by joining the Organizing Committee, so making the Organizing Committee itself international.

I now declare open the Sixth International Symposium of our series, with every confidence in its fruitful outcome.

Contents

FUNDAMENTALS IN CANCER PREVENTION, P. N. MAGEE ET AL. (EDS.),
UNIV. OF TOKYO PRESS, TOKYO / UNIV. PARK PRESS, BALTIMORE, PP. 1–13, 1976

Thoughts on the Prevention of Cancer

P. N. Magee

Courtauld Institute of Biochemistry, Middlesex Hospital Medical School, London, U.K.

Although the results of treatment of some forms of human cancer have greatly improved in recent years, for example, Hodgkin's disease, choriocarcinoma, and skin cancers, there still remain some types of tumour for which treatment is relatively unsuccessful, for example, tumours of the lung, bladder, and stomach. There is thus very good reason to attempt to improve methods for the prevention of human cancer. It should be remembered that many forms of microbial disease were controlled by the established methods of preventive medicine and hygiene before the advent of chemotherapy and antibiotics and certainly before knowledge of the mechanisms of causation of the disease were elucidated. There are, in fact, many diseases of microbial origin where the molecular mechanisms involved are still unknown but which can be controlled by preventive measures. An attempt is made in this communication to indicate some of the ways in which cancer can or might be prevented.

Known Causes of Cancer

Although a small proportion of cancers in man are inherited in Mendelian fashion and there are several hereditary preneoplastic syndromes, it appears that environmental influences are mainly responsible for the distribution of cancer in the human population (*1*). Thus hopes of preventing cancer must be largely based on attempts to influence external or internal environmental factors.

The principle known causes of cancer are radiation, chemicals, and viruses. The evidence that some forms of human cancer are induced by ionizing or ultraviolet irradiation or by certain chemicals is too well known to require repetition. With viruses however, the evidence is not conclusive, but has become much more impressive in recent years. Further consideration of the possible viral aetiology of some human tumours will be deferred until after discussion of possible mechanisms of carcinogenesis.

1

Mechanisms of Carcinogenesis

The exact mechanisms by which exposure to radiations, chemicals, or viruses causes transformation of normal into malignant cells are not known but there is substantial experimental data which gives some clarification of the processes involved.

Ionizing radiation, as the name implies, exerts its biological effects either as the direct result of an ionizing track or indirectly by the action of free radicals produced in the target tissues (*2*), this mechanism resembling that now widely accepted for chemical carcinogens. Ultraviolet radiation induces the formation of pyrimidine dimers in DNA which can be removed by enzymic repair mechanisms (*3*). The discovery by Cleaver (*4*) that this repair enzyme system is defective or absent in skin cells of human sufferers from the hereditary condition xeroderma pigmentosum, who are also highly prone to cancer of the exposed skin, is the main evidence for a central role of DNA in the induction of cancer.

The majority of chemical carcinogens are now thought to require metabolic activation by enzymes in the target organs in order to induce cancer (*5, 6*). The terms precarcinogen, proximate carcinogen, and ultimate carcinogen (*7*) have been introduced to describe the relatively inactive parent compound, metabolites with greater activity and the final product that reacts with the crucial cellular target to cause the malignant change. All known ultimate carcinogens are highly reactive electrophiles that react with nucleophilic centres in DNA, RNA, and proteins, as well as elsewhere in the cell. The nature of the crucial cellular target is not known, but, as with irradiation, there is increasing evidence in favour of DNA. Oncogenic viruses may contain either DNA or RNA. After entry into the cell, the DNA of the DNA viruses becomes stably integrated into the genome of the host cell, and this is followed by the change to a cancer cell (*8*). The RNA of RNA tumour viruses acts as a template for the RNA-dependent DNA polymerase (reverse transcriptase) that is present in the virion (*9, 10*). The DNA product is then incorporated into the cellular DNA, as with oncogenic DNA viruses and replicates with the host DNA (*11*).

Recent Evidence of the Possible Viral Causation of Some Human Tumours

Although some tumours in animals are transmitted horizontally, for example cat leukaemia (*12*), Day (*13*) has pointed out that very few human cancers exhibit behaviour that can be interpreted as horizontal transmission of tumour risk. Recently, however, a considerable body of evidence has accumulated which suggests that both RNA and DNA viruses may be responsible for some human cancers.

The possible role of RNA viruses is indicated by the various demonstrations by Spiegelman *et al.* (*14*) of the presence of RNA in human cancer cells related to the RNA of mouse leukaemia and the reports of C-type viruses associated with human leukemic cells recently discussed by Boiron (*15*) and by Weiss (*16*). There is also increasing evidence implicating the involvement of DNA viruses in human cancer, including the Epstein-Barr virus in Burkitt's lymphoma and nasopharyngeal carcinoma (*17–19*) with less strong evidence implicating herpes simplex virus type II in human cervical carcinoma (*20*). If these claims for a viral aetiology of human cancer can be substantiated, the possible importance of vaccination procedures, to be discussed below, is obvious.

Possible Ways of Preventing Cancer

From the above brief outline of suggested mechanisms of carcinogenesis it is clear that the disease could be prevented by blocking any stage in the pathway between the environmental agent and the interaction of its activated form with the critical cellular targets. Such a block could be accomplished by avoidance of exposure to the carcinogen, by interference with its transport or activation, or by competition for the active form by scavenger molecules. Even after the initial interaction with the cell, repair processes might be stimulated and finally immunological defence mechanisms might be increased, thus preventing the initial small foci of tumour cells from developing into clinically overt cancer.

Avoidance of Exposure to Carcinogens

Radiation

Cancer hazards can obviously be reduced to a minimum by proper screening of radioactive sources, monitoring of exposure to ionizing radiation, and avoidance of excessive exposure to sunlight.

Chemicals

a)   Industrial exposure.   It is now clearly established that prohibition of manufacture, or proper precautions in handling, of β-naphthylamine and certain other aromatic amines in the dye industry and of various tars and oils has greatly reduced the incidence of cancer of the bladder or scrotum respectively in exposed workers. Similar beneficial results can be expected from appropriate regulations applied to other industrial materials such as asbestos and vinyl chloride.

b)   Cigarette smoke.   The initial reports of a causal relationship between smoking and carcinoma of the lung (*21, 22*) have been extensively confirmed by subsequent work and, with few exceptions, the relationship is now generally accepted. There can be little doubt that a substantial proportion of lung cancer, in men and women, could be prevented by giving up smoking. In view of the difficulties encountered by many in trying to abandon the habit, extensive research is in progress to devise safer smoking materials.

c)   Environmental chemicals of unknown carcinogenic potential.   Apart from the large numbers of synthetic chemicals already present in the environment, many new ones are introduced every year, including drugs, food additives, pesticides, and various industrial chemicals. Conventional tests for carcinogenic activity involve the use of large numbers of experimental animals and are extremely costly and time consuming. Much work is in progress to devise simpler and more rapid screening methods including procedures dependent on suggested similarities between the mechanisms of mutagenesis and carcinogenesis (*23*).

d) Dietary fat, intestinal microbial flora, and cancer of the large bowel. There is epidemiological evidence that large bowel cancer is associated with high dietary fat intake (*24*) and the suggestion has been made that a chemical carcinogen might be present in faeces. Recently Williams, Hill, and their colleagues (*25*) have reported a correlation between high faecal bile-acid concentrations in the presence of faecal clostridia able to dehydrogenate the bile-acid nucleus in people with cancer of the large bowel and suggested a causal relationship. If this hypothesis proves correct it might prove possible to prevent some of these tumours by modification of the faecal microbial flora by dietary or other means.

e) Aflatoxins and primary cancer of the liver. The very high incidence of primary cancer of the liver in parts of Africa and Asia is well known. This marked geographical difference in liver cancer incidence is almost certainly due to environmental factors because the black population of North America resembles the white in this regard. There is increasing evidence (*26, 27*) that the largely vegetable diets consumed by the affected populations may be heavily contaminated with aflatoxins and related mycotoxins. If this relationship proves to be causal it should be possible, in principle, to reduce or even virtually eliminate this form of human primary liver cancer by exclusion of the fungi from the diets.

f) Nitrosamines and their possible role in human cancer. A large number of N-nitroso compounds are known to be carcinogenic in many animal species. Tumours have been induced in most organs by these compounds and they exhibit remarkable organ specificity or organotropism (*28–30*). There are similarities in the metabolism of dimethylnitrosamine by human and rat liver preparations *in vitro* (*31*), suggesting that human beings are susceptible to this and, therefore, other nitroso compounds. Although there is no direct evidence that any form of human cancer is caused by nitrosamines, the presence of these compounds in the environment suggests that they may constitute a human cancer hazard.

Human beings may be exposed to nitrosamines occurring in small amounts in food (*32, 33*) or they may be formed in the body, particularly in the acid environment of the stomach, from various amine precursors and nitrites (*33, 34*). Most foods investigated have been found to contain only small amounts of nitrosamines, usually in the parts per billion range and those containing relatively higher concentrations have often had nitrates and nitrites added as preservatives, for example bacon and ham. It is probable that the nitrosamine content of these foods could be reduced by reduction of the amounts of added nitrates and nitrites or their replacement by another preservative. Much current research is directed to the solution of this problem but it is proving difficult to find an entirely adequate replacement for nitrite.

There are numerous examples of the formation of carcinogenic nitrosamines in the body after simultaneous ingestion of secondary or tertiary amines or amides and nitrites. The amines may include drugs and compounds of agricultural importance. Recent work in Japan has demonstrated the formation of a mutagenic product from a food component, methylguanidine, nitrosated under weakly acid conditions in simulated gastric juice (*35*) and carcinogenic nitroso compounds have been produced by the reaction of nitrite and some types of agricultural chemicals

(*36*). Epidemiological investigations have indicated that the high incidence of gastric cancer in Chile is associated with the use of nitrate fertilizer (*37*). Further research is needed to clarify the relationship between the dietary intake of nitrate and the incidence of human cancer. If such a relationship exists, reduction in the amount of nitrate ingested might reduce the general human cancer incidence. However such a reduction would present formidable technical problems since nitrates are universally present in drinking water.

An alternative approach to the reduction of nitrosamine formation in the body is to reduce the availability of nitrite for nitrosation reactions. This has been accomplished by the simultaneous administration of ascorbic acid to animals receiving nitrites and various amines (*38*).

Prevention of Interaction between the Active Forms of Carcinogens and Crucial Cellular Targets
Radiation

Much work has been done on sulphydryl, *e.g.*, cysteamine and other compounds as possible radioprotective agents (*39*). This problem is of great current importance in relation to the possible hazards arising from the use of nuclear power in peace and war.

Chemicals

The carcinogenic activities of chemicals can be influenced by factors that affect the activating enzymes responsible for the production of the ultimate carcinogens and by factors that compete with the ultimate carcinogens and thus block their crucial interaction with cellular components. The behaviour of the microsomal hydroxylases responsible for the activation of carcinogens can be profoundly influenced by diet and by inducers and inhibitors of their activities (*40*). The altered enzyme activity may be reflected in the resulting carcinogenic potency. Examples of such modifications of tumour production are the effect of protein-deficient diets to increase the induction of renal tumours in the rat by dimethylnitrosamine (*41*) and the reduction of 7,12-dimethylbenz(a)anthracene tumourigenesis in mouse skin by treatment with 7,8-benzoflavone, an inhibitor of aryl hydrocarbon hydroxylase (*42*). Another recent example of an apparently similar mechanism is the reported protection by DDT, the ubiquitous pesticide, against mammary tumours and leukaemia induced by prolonged feeding of 7,12-dimethylbenz(a)anthracene (*43*). Most precarcinogens yield varying amounts of carcinogenically inactive metabolites and procedures that increase the production of these, at the expense of the ultimate carcinogens could reduce or prevent cancer induction.

The inhibitory action of cysteamine on mammary carcinogenesis by 7,12-dimethylbenz(a)anthracene in the rat (*44*) may represent blocking of the interaction of an ultimate carcinogen with its target site in the cell. Several other sulphur containing compounds, including disulphiram, dimethyldithiocarbamate, and benzyl thiocyanate have recently been reported to inhibit tumour induction by the same carcinogen (*45*).

Viruses

Clearly there is a better chance of preventing virally induced cancer when the disease is transmitted horizontally by virus particles than when the disease is transmitted vertically with integration of the viral genome into that of the host. Successful vaccination has now been achieved against Marek's disease, a common lymphoproliferative disease of the domestic fowl caused by a cell-associated herpesvirus (*46*), against the malignant lymphoma induced in nonhuman primates by herpesvirus saimiri (*47, 48*) and against feline leukaemia induced by an oncornavirus (*49*). These results indicate the serious possibility of effective vaccination against some human tumours (*50, 51*).

Possible Prevention of the Development of Cancer after the Initial Interaction of the Active Carcinogen with the Crucial Cellular Target

DNA repair

The probable importance of DNA repair in carcinogenesis is emphasised by the large part of the programme of the Symposium that has been allotted to it. Although it is not established with certainty that interaction between DNA and the active forms of carcinogens is causally related to cancer induction, there is considerable and increasing evidence in favour of this concept. As more and more chemicals are adequately tested, the correlation between mutagenic and carcinogenic activity becomes increasingly close (*52–54*), thus reducing the force of earlier argument against the somatic mutation hypothesis based on lack of such correlation (*55*). Perhaps the best evidence for a central role of DNA in carcinogenesis, as already briefly mentioned, comes from studies on the human disease xeroderma pigmentosum (*56*).

If cancer does result from reaction of an ultimate carcinogen with DNA, leading to a change in the genetic material which is fixed and perpetuated by cellular replication, it is theoretically possible that the malignant transformation would not follow if the DNA defect was excised and repaired by an error-free mechanism before replication had occurred. It is also possible that somatic mutation resulting in cancer might arise from error-prone mechanisms of postreplication DNA repair (*57*) which would also be prevented by prior removal of the DNA lesion. Clearly much more must be learnt about DNA repair in mammalian cells, particularly in the intact animal *in vivo*, before ways can be devised of influencing these repair processes.

It is now clear that different organs differ greatly in their capacity to remove certain alkylated bases from their DNA after treatment with alkylating carcinogens (*58–60*) and these differing capacities to repair the DNA lesions seem to play an important part in determining the sites of tumour induction.

Concepts of Preneoplasia

The concept of carcinogenesis as a sequential or multistage process has been widely discussed. Derived from the two-stage mechanism of skin carcinogenesis postulated by Berenblum (*61*) and developed by Foulds (*62*) in terms of tumour

progression, the idea has been applied by Farber and his colleagues in their extensive study on pathogenesis of chemically induced liver cancer in the rat (63). According to Farber, the development of liver cancer can be considered as a progression from multiple areas or islands of altered cells, through early to late hyperplastic nodules in which a small number of basophilic nodules appear and give rise
to one or very few hepatocellular tumours. There is thus a continual selection of
smaller and smaller numbers of cells, each with an increasingly greater probability
of developing cancer.

An alternative hypothesis is that, in some cases, the conversion to malignancy
occurs very soon after exposure to the carcinogen and that the cancer cells are somehow held in check by bodily defence mechanisms so that the tumour does not
become clinically apparent until much later. The work of Hard and Butler (64, 65)
on the induction of kidney tumours in the rat by single doses of dimethylnitrosamine
has been interpreted to favour such a process.

Whether the arrest of tumour development after the initiation stage is regarded
as prevention or treatment depends on the stage reached and is, to some extent, a
matter of semantics. There is no doubt that some of the earlier chemically induced
hyperplastic nodules of the liver are reversible in the sense that the hepatic cells
can revert to an apparently normal appearance and arrangement. There is, therefore, the theoretical possibility of causing all such nodules to revert if the factors
involved were adequately understood. The recent discovery of a preneoplastic antigen present in hyperplastic nodules as well as in primary hepatocellular carcinoma
(66) suggests the possibility of prevention of tumour development by immunological
means.

A variety of agents, including protease inhibitors (67, 68) and polyinosinic-
polycytidylic acid (69) have been shown to inhibit tumourigenesis after the stage
of the initial interaction of the carcinogen. Further work on the mechanisms of
these inhibitory actions may lead to the development of more effective agents with
potential application to cancer prevention.

Immunological prevention

The concept of immunological surveillance, largely due to Burnet (70), pos-
tulates the existence of immunological reactions in the body which respond to cells
that have undergone malignant transformation to destroy or inactivate them. If
such a mechanism exists, it might be possible to increase its activity and thus reduce
the number of cells that escape and go on to form cancers. Recently, however, the
whole concept has been challenged (71) and any practical preventive measures
based on it are obviously dependent on its validity for their success.

The possibility of vaccination against cancer has already been discussed.
There is, of course, intense research activity in the field of cancer immunotherapy
but this, as mentioned earlier, falls outside the scope of the Symposium, which is
primarily concerned with the prevention of cancer.

CONCLUSIONS

Many human cancers have been and are being successfully prevented. Many more could be prevented by more vigorous application of existing knowledge. Basic research reveals a variety of potential new ways of cancer prevention, varying from the definitely feasible to the highly speculative.

ACKNOWLEDGMENT

The author would like to acknowledge generous financial support from the Cancer Research Campaign of Great Britain.

REFERENCES

1. Fraumeni, J. F. Genetic determinants of cancer. *In;* R. Doll and I. Vodopija (eds.), Host Environment Interactions in the Etiology of Cancer in Man, pp. 49–55, International Agency for Research on Cancer, Lyon, 1973.
2. Coggle, J. E. Biological Effects of Radiation, pp. 149, Wykeham Publications, London, 1971.
3. Howard-Flanders, P. DNA repair and recombination. Brit. Med. Bull., *29*: 226–235, 1973.
4. Cleaver, J. E. Defective repair replication of DNA in Xeroderma pigmentosum. Nature, *218*: 652–656, 1968.
5. Miller, J. A. Carcinogenesis by chemicals: An overview. Cancer Res., *30*: 559–576, 1970.
6. Magee, P. N. Activation and inactivation of chemical carcinogens and mutagens in the mammal. *In;* P. N. Campbell and F. Dickens (eds.), Essays in Biochemistry, vol. 10, pp. 105–136, Academic Press, London, 1974.
7. Miller, E. C. and Miller, J. A. Mechanisms of chemical carcinogenesis: Nature of proximate carcinogens and interactions with macromolecules. Pharmacol. Rev., *18*: 805–838, 1966.
8. Westphal, H. and Dulbecco, R. Viral DNA in polyoma- and SV40-transformed cell lines. Proc. Natl. Acad. Sci. U.S., *59*: 1158–1165, 1968.
9. Temin, H. and Mizutani, S. RNA-dependent DNA polymerase in virions of RNA sarcoma virus. Nature, *226*: 1211–1213, 1970.
10. Baltimore, D. RNA-dependent DNA polymerase in virions of RNA tumour viruses. Nature, *226*: 1209–1211, 1970.
11. Temin, H. The RNA tumour viruses. Background and foreground. Proc. Natl. Acad. Sci. U.S., *69*: 1016–1020, 1972.
12. Jarrett, W. F. M., Jarrett, O., Mackey, L. J., Laird, H. M., Hardy, W., and Essex, M. Horizontal transmission of leukaemia virus and leukaemia in the cat. J. Natl. Cancer Inst., *51*: 833–841, 1973.
13. Day, N. E. Epidemiological evidence for the role of a virus in the etiology of tumours. *In;* R. Doll and I. Vodopija (eds.), Host Environmental Interactions in the Etiology of Cancer in Man, pp. 367–375, International Agency for Research on Cancer, Lyon, 1973.
14. Axel, R., Schlom, J., and Spiegelman, S. Presence in human breast cancer of RNA homologous to mouse mammary tumour virus RNA. Nature, *235*: 32–36, 1972.
15. Boiron, M. Oncorna virus et leucemies humaines. Bull. Cancer, *62*: 205–212, 1975.

16. Weiss, R.   Viruses associated with human leukaemia. Nature, *254*: 101–102, 1975.
17. Epstein, M. A. and Achong, B. G.   The EB virus. Annu. Rev. Microbiol., *27*: 413–436, 1973.
18. Klein, G.   The Epstein-Barr virus. *In;* A. S. Kaplan (ed.), The Herpesviruses, pp. 521–555, Academic Press, New York and London, 1973.
19. Henle, W. and Henle, G.   Evidence for an oncogenic potential of the Epstein-Barr virus. Cancer Res., *33*: 1419–1423, 1973.
20. Rapp, F. and Buss, E. R.   Are viruses important in carcinogenesis? Am. J. Pathol., *77*: 85–102, 1974.
21. Doll, R. and Hill, A. B.   Smoking and carcinoma of the lung.   Preliminary report. Brit. Med. J., *2*: 739–748, 1950.
22. Wynder, E. L. and Graham, E. A.   Tobacco smoking as a possible etiologic factor in bronchiogenic carcinoma. A study of six hundred and eighty-four proved cases. J. Am. Med. Assoc., *143*: 329–336, 1950.
23. Ames, B. N., Durston, W. E., Yamasaki, E., and Lee, F. D.   Carcinogens are mutagens: A simple test system combining liver homogenates for activation and bacteria for detection. Proc. Natl. Acad. Sci. U.S., *70*: 2281–2285, 1973.
24. Wynder, E. L. and Reddy, B. S.   Dietary fat and colon cancer. J. Natl. Cancer Inst., *54*: 7–10, 1975.
25. Hill, M. J., Drasar, B. S., Williams, R. E. O., Meade, T. W., Cox, A.G., Simpson, J. E. P., and Morson, B. C.   Faecal bile-acids and clostridia in patients with cancer of the large bowel. Lancet, *i*: 535–538, 1975.
26. Shank, R. C., Bhamarapravati, N., Gordon, J. E., and Wogan, G. N.   Dietary aflatoxins and human liver cancer. IV. Incidence of primary liver cancer in two municipal populations of Thailand. Food Cosmet. Toxicol., *10*: 171–179, 1972.
27. Peers, F. G. and Linsell, C. A.   Dietary aflatoxins and liver cancer—A population based study in Kenya. Brit. J. Cancer, *27*: 473–484, 1973.
28. Magee, P. N. and Barnes, J. M.   Carcinogenic nitroso compounds. Adv. Cancer Res., *10*: 163–246, 1967.
29. Druckrey, H., Preussmann, R., Ivankovic, S., and Schmahl, D.   Organotrope carcinogene Wirkungen bei 65 verschiedenen N-nitroso-Verbindungen an BD-Ratten. Z. Krebsforsch., *69*: 103–201, 1967.
30. Magee, P. N., Montesano, R., and Preussmann, R.   N-Nitroso compounds and related carcinogens. *In;* C. E. Searle (ed.), Chemical Carcinogens American Chemical Society, New York, 1976, in press.
31. Montesano, R. and Magee, P. N.   Metabolism of dimethylnitrosamine by human liver slices *in vitro*. Nature, *228*: 173–174, 1970.
32. Crosby, N. T., Foreman, J. K., Palframan, J. F., and Sawyer, R.   Estimation of steam-volatile N-nitrosamines in foods at the 1 μg/kg level. Nature, *238*: 342–343, 1972.
33. Bogovski, P. and Walker, E. A.   N-Nitroso compounds in the environment. I.A.R.C. Publications No. 9, pp. 243, International Agency for Research on Cancer, Lyon, 1974.
34. Sander, J.   Untersuchungen über die Entstehung cancerogener Nitrosoverbindungen im Magen von Versuchstieren und ihre Bedeutung für den Menschen. Arzneimittel-Forschung, *21*: 1572–1580, 1707–1713, 2034–2039, 1971.
35. Endo, H. and Takahashi, K.   Identification and property of the mutagenic principle formed from a food-component methylguanidine, after nitrosation in simulated gastric ʲuices. Biochem. Biophys. Res. Commun., *54*: 1384–1392, 1973.

36. Elespuru, R. K. and Lijinsky, W.   The formation of carcinogenic nitroso compounds from nitrite and some types of agricultural chemicals. Food Cosmet. Toxicol., *11*: 807–817, 1973.

37. Zaldivar, R. and Robinson, H.   Epidemiological investigation on stomach cancer mortality in Chileans: Association with nitrate fertilizer. Z. Krebsforsch., *80*: 289–295, 1973.

38. Mirvish, S. S., Wallcave, L., Eagen, M., and Shubik, P.   Ascorbate-nitrite reaction: Possible means of blocking the formation of carcinogenic N-nitroso compounds. Science, *177*: 65–68, 1972.

39. Bacq, Z. M.   Chemical Protection against Ionizing Radiation, p. 79, Charles C. Thomas, Springfield, 1965.

40. McLean, A. E. M.   Diet and the chemical environment as modifiers of carcinogenesis. *In;* R. Doll and I. Vodopija (eds.), Host Environment Interactions in the Etiology of Cancer in Man, pp. 223–230, International Agency for Research on Cancer, Lyon, 1973.

41. McLean, A. E. M. and Magee, P. N.   Increased renal carcinogenesis by dimethylnitrosamine in protein deficient rats. Brit. J. Exp. Pathol., *51*: 587–590, 1970.

42. Gelboin, H. V., Wiebel, F., and Diamond, L.   Dimethylbenzanthracene tumorigenesis and aryl hydrocarbon hydroxylase in mouse skin. Science, *170*: 169–171, 1970.

43. Silinskas, K. C. and Okey, A. B.   Protection by 1,1,1-trichloro-2,2-bis (*p*-chlorophenyl) ethane (DDT) against mammary tumours and leukaemia during prolonged feeding of 7,12-dimethylbenz(a)anthracene. J. Natl. Cancer Inst., *55*: 653–657, 1975.

44. Marquardt, H., Sapozink, M. D., and Zedeck, M.   Inhibition by cysteamine-HCl of oncogenesis induced by 7,12-dimethylbenz(a)anthracene without affecting toxicity. Cancer Res., *34*: 3387–3390, 1974.

45. Wattenburg, L. W.   Inhibition of carcinogenic and toxic effects of polycyclic hydrocarbons by several sulphur-containing compounds. J. Natl. Cancer Inst., *52*: 1583–1587, 1974.

46. Biggs, P. M.   Marek's disease—The disease and its prevention by vaccination. Brit. J. Cancer, *31* (Suppl. II): 152–155, 1975.

47. Laufs, R.   Immunisation of marmoset monkeys with a killed oncogenic herpesvirus. Nature, *249*: 571–572, 1974.

48. Laufs, R. and Steinke, H.   Vaccination of non-human primates against malignant lymphoma. Nature, *253*: 71–72, 1975.

49. Jarrett, W. F. H.   The relation of immune response to pathogenesis, vaccination and epidemiology of virus induced leukaemia. Brit. J. Cancer, *31* (Suppl. II): 147–151, 1975.

50. Hilleman, M. R.   Human cancer virus vaccines and the pursuit of the practical. Cancer, *34*: 1439–1445, 1974.

51. Epstein, M. A.   Towards an antiviral vaccine for a human cancer. Nature, *253*: 6, 1975.

52. Ong, T. and de Serres, F. J.   Mutagenicity of chemical carcinogens in *Neurospora crassa*. Cancer Res., *32*: 1890–1893, 1972.

53. Ames, B. N., Durston, W. E., Yamasaki, E., and Lee, F. D.   Carcinogens are mutagens: A simple test system combining liver homogenates for activation and bacteria for detection. Proc. Natl. Acad. Sci. U.S., *70*: 228–2285, 1973.

54. Rohrborn, G.   Mutagenesis and carcinogenesis. *In;* R. Montesano and L. Tomatis

(eds.), Chemical Carcinogenesis Essays, pp. 213–219, International Agency for Research on Cancer, Lyon, 1974.

55. Burdette, W. J.   The significance of mutation in relation to the origin of tumours. Cancer Res., *15*: 201–226, 1955.

56. Reed, W. B., Landing, B., Sugarman, G., Cleaver, J. E., and Melnyk, J.   *Xeroderma pigmentosum*. Clinical and laboratory investigation of its basic defect. J. Am. Med. Assoc., *207*: 2073–2079, 1969.

57. Trosko, J. E. and Chu, E. H. Y.   The role of DNA repair and somatic mutation in carcinogenesis. Adv. Cancer Res., *21*: 391–425, 1975.

58. Goth, R. and Rajewsky, M. F.   Persistence of O^6-methylguanine in rat brain DNA: Correlation with nervous system specific carcinogenesis by ethylnitrosourea. Proc. Natl. Acad. Sci. U.S., *71*: 639–643, 1974.

59. Margison, G. P. and Kleihues, P.   Chemical carcinogenesis in the nervous system. Preferential accumulation of O^6-methylguanine in rat brain deoxyribonucleic acid during repetitive administration of N-methyl-N-nitrosourea. Biochem. J., *148*: 521–525, 1975.

60. Nicoll, J. W., Swann, P. F., and Pegg, A. E.   Effect of dimethylnitrosamine on persistence of methylated guanines in rat liver and kidney DNA. Nature, *254*: 261–262, 1975.

61. Berenblum, I.   Sequential aspects of chemical carcinogenesis: Skin. *In;* F. F. Becker (ed.), Cancer, vol. 1, pp. 323–344, Plenum Press, New York, 1975.

62. Foulds, L.   Neoplastic Development, vol. 1, pp. 439, Academic Press, London, 1969.

63. Farber, E.   The biochemical pathology of experimental liver carcinogenesis. *In;* G. P. Warwick, H. M. Cameron, and C. A. Linsell (eds.), Liver Cell Cancer, 1976, in press.

64. Hard, G. C. and Butler, W. H.   Cellular analysis of renal neoplasia: Light microscopic study of the development of interstitial lesions induced in the rat kidney by a single carcinogenic dose of dimethylnitrosamine. Cancer Res., *30*: 2806–2815, 1970.

65. Hard, G. C. and Butler, W. H.   Ultrastructural study of the development of interstitial lesions leading to mesenchymal neoplasia induced in the rat renal cortex by dimethylnitrosamine. Cancer Res., *31*: 337–347, 1971.

66. Okita, K., Kligman, L. H., and Farber, E.   A new common marker for premalignant and malignant hepatocytes induced in the rat by chemical carcinogens.   J. Natl. Cancer Inst., *54*: 199–202, 1975.

67. Troll, W., Klassen, A., and Janoff, A.   Tumorigenesis in mouse skin: Inhibition by synthetic inhibitors of proteases. Science, *169*: 1211–1213, 1971.

68. Hozumi, M., Ogawa, M., Sugimura, T., Takeuchi, T., and Umezawa, H.   Inhibition of tumorigenesis in mouse skin by leupeptin, a protease inhibitor from *Actinomycetes*. Cancer Res., *32*: 1725–1728, 1972.

69. Gelboin, H. V. and Levy, H. B.   Polyinosinic-polycytidylic acid inhibits chemically induced tumorigenesis in mouse skin. Science, *167*: 205–207, 1970.

70. Burnet, F. M.   Immunological factors in the process of carcinogenesis. Brit. Med. Bull., *20*: 154–158, 1964.

71. Kripke, M. L. and Borsos, T.   Immune surveillance revisited. J. Natl. Cancer Inst., *52*: 1393–1395, 1974.

Discussion of Paper of Dr. Magee

DR. WEISBURGER: There has been much tradition in chemical carcinogenesis in Japan. In particular, data have been published on interactions between carcinogens or on the modification of carcinogenicity by giving noncarcinogens. This was usually done at the customary high dose levels. We now need to know much more about the underlying mechanisms and perhaps even more important, to concern ourselves with the quantitative relationships especially at lower dosages.

DR. MAGEE: I agree.

DR. NAKAHARA: I listened to Dr. Magee's beautiful presentation of what may be called a bird's-eye view of the subject of this Symposium. I just wish to add that the immunologic inadequacy (or failure of immunosurveillance), as Dr. Magee said, may not be of much significance in the causation of cancer. We know that tumor-bearing animals and man are deficient in immunological capacity. This immunodeficiency may be due to some substance which is produced by the growing tumor, and thus may be the result rather than the cause of tumor development. Data on this point are being accumulated in many Japanese laboratories. Dr. Kennedy, at the last Symposium of this Series, also presented evidence for this conclusion.

I seriously doubt, for instance, that a minute amount of methylcholanthrene, immunosuppressive as it may be, can account for the tumors which develop 2 to 3 months after the injection of the small amount of carcinogen needed for tumor production.

DR. TROLL: Your bird's-eye view of cancer prevention was extensive. I have two further questions. One is the hormones, which are important contributors to cancer in the U.S.A., *e.g.*, breast and prostate. They can be classified as cocarcinogens or promotors and may be amenable to prevention by protein inhibitors. My second concern is carcinogenic aromatic amines and their dye derivatives used in commerce. The dyes can be metabolically reduced to their parent amines (E. Rinde and W. J. Troll, Natl. Cancer Inst., *155*: 181, 1975; Yoshida, O and Miyakawa, M. *In;* W. Nakahara *et al.* (eds.), Analytic and Experimental Epidemiology of Cancer, pp. 31–39, Univ. of Tokyo Press, Tokyo, 1973).

DR. MAGEE: I agree about the great importance of hormonal effects in carcinogenesis. I did not say more about this aspect because of lack of time.

Also, it is possible the reduction of aromatic amine dyes may cause cancer.

DR. WEISBURGER: In relation to the immunologic situation mentioned by Prof. Nakahara, Kroes and we recently showed immunological competence was not important in primary cancer induction (Cancer Res., *35*: 2651, 1975). However, the immunologic situation may be important in metastasis, as noted, for example by H. Sato of Sendai.

DR. MAGEE: I felt that effects on metastasis should perhaps be regarded as treatment rather than prevention.

DR. IKAWA: In prevention of possible virus-induced human malignancies, you suggested a possible application of vaccines. However, there is neither epidemic form nor clustering in man, as shown in some animal cases. Thus, I think a conservative attitude on the application of vaccination for prevention of human cancer is indicated.

DR. MAGEE: I have been influenced by the view of my friend Professor A. Epstein, Bristol, England, who is a strong advocate of a trial vaccination in Burkitt's lymphoma.

DR. LAUFS: There is no doubt about clustering of Burkitt's lymphoma in Uganda, and there is a second human tumor, which is suspected to be caused by the Epstein-Barr virus, the nasopharyngeal carcinoma (NPC). NPC is the commonest tumor in the male population of Southern Chinese origin and constitutes a major health problem.

FUNDAMENTALS IN CANCER PREVENTION, P. N. MAGEE ET AL. (EDS.), UNIV. OF TOKYO PRESS, TOKYO / UNIV. PARK PRESS, BALTIMORE, PP. 15–40, 1976

Nutritional Modulation of Carcinogenesis

Paul M. NEWBERNE and Adrianne E. ROGERS

Laboratory of Nutritional Pathology, Department of Nutrition and Food Science, Massachusetts Institute of Technology, Cambridge, Massachusetts, U.S.A.

Abstract: Epidemiologic and laboratory investigations have strongly inferred that a significant share of cancer morbidity and mortality in human populations can be attributed to environmental factors. Highly important among factors associated with differences in susceptibility to cancer are diet habits and dietary nutrients. Although nutrients alone exert profound effects on the capacity of the host to respond to environmental carcinogens, the coexistence of malnutrition and dietary contaminants appears to further complicate the problem and increase the risk of developing cancer. The wide variation in incidence of cancer in selected populations or ethnic groups in different geographic areas and a change in risk of cancer in migrant populations as they assume the dietary habits and nutritive status of high- or low-risk populations attest to the importance of nutrition in the etiology of cancer.

Nutrients which have been associated with a modified risk of cancer in man and experimental animals include the quality and quantity of protein, carbohydrate, fat, lipotropes (choline, methionine, folic acid, vitamin B_{12}), vitamin A, riboflavin, and some of the trace elements.

Sites of cancer development associated with modified nutrition include the esophagus, stomach, liver, large bowel, breast, and lung. The manner in which the nutritive status of the host may modulate susceptibility to cancer is complex and no doubt multifaceted. However, recent studies indicate an influence of nutrition on microsomal enzyme systems, hormones, intestinal microflora, and the immunocompetence of the host, among others.

Dietary nutrients alone influence risk to cancer but dietary contaminants, such as mycotoxins and nitrosamines, may interact with nutritional deficiency or imbalance to further enhance a potential for the development of cancer.

Those nutrients which appear to modulate susceptibility to cancer, about which most is known, will be considered in this presentation.

Physicians, medical scientists, and laymen alike have, from earliest recorded medical history, associated diet with cancer (1), and in fact, recent epidemiologic studies and data derived from well-designed animal experiments have clearly indicated that this is the case; diet and nutrition are important factors in the etiology of a number of types of cancer. The wide variation in incidence of some types of cancer in various populations or ethnic groups living in different geographic locations (Table 1) and the change in risk of migrant populations as they relocate and assume dietary habits and nutritive status of low- or high-risk groups strongly support this concept. Other factors which may be related to differences in cancer incidence are carcinogens (or their precursors) found as contaminants in foods. These include mycotoxins, nitrosamines, pesticides, and synthetic hormones; other chemicals of less current concern include intentional food additives used to improve texture, flavor, color, or nutritive value. The association of nutritional deficiencies, or imbalances, and food contaminants, or additives, with a high incidence of some forms of cancer and the supporting experimental data indicate strongly that a relationship exists between nutrition and cancer, and this has aroused a broad segment of the scientific community to the challenges and opportunities nutrition provides in our continuing search for cause and prevention.

The effects of nutrition on carcinogenesis in experimental animals are sometimes conspicuous and easily recognized, but more often they are subtle and may be expressed only as changes in induction time or in the type or distribution of tumors. There is no reason to believe that nutritional effects on human cancer differ from those observed in animals; nutritive status relevant to human cancer is probably in the nature of a marginal deficit or imbalance rather than a severely abnormal situation which makes the job of identifying the important nutritional factors difficult indeed. Nutritional factors and conditions about which more is known in human populations, by way of epidemiological studies, along with modulation of carcinogenesis in animals will be examined in this presentation.

TABLE 1.   Age-adjusted Death Rate per 100,000 (1968–1969)

Country	Primary cancer site				
	Stomach		Colon and rectum		Breast
	Male	Female	Male	Female	Female
U.S.A.	9	4	19	16	22
Japan	66	34	9	7	4
Scotland	23	12	25	21	26
Germany F.R.	33	18	21	17	19
Netherlands	26	13	18	17	26
Chile	59	36	7	7	11

Compiled from data in Refs. 3 and 4.

Esophageal Carcinoma

There is a varied geographic distribution of esophageal cancer with a high incidence in Puerto Rico, Chile and in selected areas of Japan, France, and South and East Africa; a low incidence has been reported in Norway, and the disease is practically unknown in West Africa (2). Other reports indicate high rates of esophageal cancer in parts of the Soviet Union (3), Finland, China, Hong Kong, Iran, and the West Indies (4, 5). The high frequency in some areas appears to be a development of the past 30–40 years (6). In New York City, patients with esophageal cancer tended to be heavy smokers with high alcohol consumption and decreased consumption of milk, eggs, and green leafy vegetables (6). On the island of Curacao and in several counties of South Carolina, a high incidence of esophageal cancer has been associated with use of local plants for beverages and medicinal purposes but nutrient deficiencies have not been ruled out (7). Dietary factors have been associated with esophageal cancer in each of the areas of high incidence (8).

In Puerto Rico the diet is deficient in fresh fruits and vegetables, meat, eggs, and milk but high in carbohydrates; these deficiencies along with the consumption of hot spicy foods and beverages, and alcohol from uncontrolled fermentation have been associated with esophageal cancer (9). Similar studies in Africa have suggested that beer made from maize is a factor in esophageal cancer perhaps because of contamination of the beer by mycotoxins or nitrosamines (10).

A recent study in the United States (11) showed significant correlations between esophageal cancer, percent of the population living in urban communities, and cigarette and alcohol sales. Another study (12) identified a geographic correlation between mortality rates from esophageal cancer and per capita consumption of spirits and beer. Alcoholics may exhibit deficiencies of vitamins or of zinc and iron, all of which may contribute to tumor development (13, 14).

Dietary studies in Iran have yielded an association of low intake of vitamins A, C and riboflavin, animal protein, and fresh fruit and vegetables with an increased incidence of esophageal cancer. Further, these studies have demonstrated the occurrence of this form of cancer in wheat-eating, as opposed to rice-eating, areas but there was no association with tobacco or alcohol (15). In China the high incidence areas also are areas of wheat-eating populations rather than rice-eating peoples; a high incidence of esophageal cancer in chickens as well as in people has been reported from well-defined areas of the People's Republic of China (16, 17). In the geographical areas of very high incidence, the predominance of esophageal cancer in males decreases or disappears, and women have an equal or even slightly greater incidence. In these areas of high incidence, as in Iran, the association with tobacco and alcohol is much less strong than in areas where there is a moderate incidence of the disease. These observations may be explained by exposure to other environmental carcinogens to which women may be more susceptible than men. Contributing factors may include dietary deficiency concomitant to childbearing and poor intake of nutrients resulting from poverty, all coexistent in many of these population groups (17).

Animal studies in our laboratories have provided data which suggest that deficiencies and dietary contamination may interact in esophageal carcinogenesis. We have examined the effects of feeding N-diethylnitrosoamine (DEN) to lipotrope-deficient rats and have found a significant enhancement of esophageal carci-

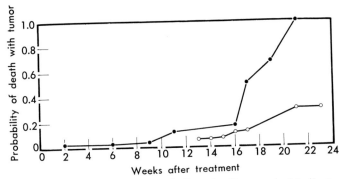

Fig. 1. Graphic representation of effect of a diet marginal in lipotropes and high in fat on development of esophageal carcinoma in rats exposed to DEN. Diet 1 (○) is control, adequately supplemented and diet 2 (●) is marginal in lipotropes, high in fat. Rats on the marginal lipotrope diet (diet 2) started developing esophageal cancer more than 10 weeks earlier than control rats (diet 2).

TABLE 2. Tumor Incidence in Rats Fed DEN

Diet	No. of rats	DEN intake (total mg/rat)	Body wt. (g)[a]	% of rats with tumor in:				
				Eso-phagus	Liver	Bladder	Lung	Any organ
Control (1)	23	179	657	35[b]	70[c]	0	4[d]	26
Marginal lipotrope (2)	34	176	702	44[b]	88[c]	3[e]	9[d]	47

[a] Average weight at end of DEN treatment. [b] Diet 1, 13% squamous carcinoma, 22% squamous polyp; diet 2, 9% squamous carcinoma, 35% squamous polyp. [c] Hepatocarcinoma in all; in 1 case in rats fed diet 1 and in 2 cases in rats fed diet 2; there was also cholangiocarcinoma. In rats fed diet 1 there was 1 case of hepatic hemangioendotheliosarcoma, which raises the percentage of liver tumors to 74%. [d] Diet 1, bronchial papilloma; diet 2, squamous carcinoma, papillary adenocarcinoma, peripheral adenoma in 1 rat each. [e] Two small transitional cell polyps were found in 1 rat.

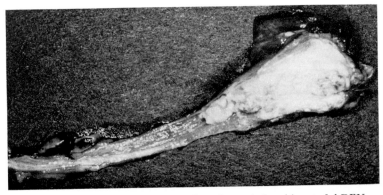

Fig. 2. Gross appearance of esophageal carcinoma induced in rats fed DEN.

nogenesis (Fig. 1 and Table 2) (*18*). The tumors induced in these investigations were invasive squamous cell carcinomas, morphologically identical to those in man (Figs. 2 and 3). In this study the diet was also high in fat resulting in more than a

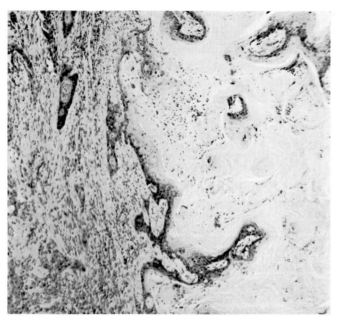

FIG. 3. Microscopic appearance of esophageal squamous cell carcinoma induced in rats by DEN. Hematoxylin and Eosin stain (H-E).   ×80.

TABLE 3. Incidence of Forestomach Papillomas Induced by Benz(a)pyrene (BP) in Hamsters

μg RA/week	No. of hamsters	% with papilloma	No. of papillomas/ papilloma-bearing hamster
100	109	50	2.9 ± 0.2[a]
1,600	111	25[b]	2.2 ± 0.3
2,400	107	26[b]	3.1 ± 0.2

RA: retinyl acetate.   [a] Mean±S.E.   [b] Compared to hamsters given 100 μg RA per week, $P<0.005$. From Ref. *19*.

simple deficiency state. High doses of vitamin A (Table 3) protected hamsters against induction of esophageal or forestomach tumors by polycyclic aromatic hydrocarbons (carcinogens present in cigarette smoke and urban air) (*19, 20*).

Both epidemiologic and experimental data point to a role for nutritional deficiencies in esophageal cancer, perhaps acting in concert with other unidentified environmental interactants; these observations require intensive followup if we are to attempt to prevent this type of cancer by rational, acceptable approaches.

Gastric Cancer

Cancer of the stomach has a remarkable variability in incidence according to geographic location. Populations in Japan, Chile, Colombia, Austria, Iceland, and Finland exhibit a high incidence while a low incidence is recorded in the United States and Canada (*2*). A number of dietary factors have been implicated in its etiology but studies about food habits in gastric cancer patients have yielded few if any significant differences in intake of specific nutrients when compared to control groups (21–23). The high incidence of gastric cancer in Iceland has been related by some to the large intake of smoked food but this hypothesis has not been substantiated (24). Talc, most of which contains asbestos, has been assigned a role in stomach cancer in Japan (25), but evidence to date has not been convincing.

There has been a marked decline in mortality from gastric cancer in the United States during the past four decades and there is a gradient of increasing frequency with decreasing socioeconomic status in which the lowest socioeconomic groups are reported to have three times the incidence of upper social groups (26). Stomach cancer in Japanese migrants to Hawaii is about equal in incidence to their native Japanese cohorts in high-risk areas even though the immigrants eat western type diets; however, their offspring have lower risks (27). Elevated risks were found for Issei and Nisei users of pickled vegetables and dried and salted fish, and low risks were associated with eating raw vegetables. In a United States study (28), it was revealed that gastric cancer patients ate raw vegetables less often than controls but there was no relation between fried foods, meats, or alcohol consumption and the disease.

There is an inverse relationship between cancer of the stomach and of the colon. Migration from a high-risk area for stomach cancer in Japan to a relatively low-risk area of California resulted in a decreasing incidence of gastric cancer and increasing incidence of colon cancer (29). On the other hand, in both cases the migrants moved more in line with the area to which they migrated (Table 4). Studies in Seventh-Day Adventist patients support migrant studies from both Japan and Colombia which have demonstrated the importance of exposure early in life to the dietary or other cultural or environmental factors which determine the incidence of gastric cancer (30, 31).

Although there is convincing evidence that environmental factors, probably nutritional, are important in the etiology of gastric carcinoma, experimental evidence is equivocal. Tatematsu et al. (32) have shown that sodium chloride increased the incidence of gastric carcinoma with either N-methyl-N-nitroso-N′-nitroguanidine (MNNG) or N-nitrosoquinoline (NQO) but the manner in which salt was

TABLE 4.   Rates of Mortality from Cancer of Gastrointestinal Sites at Ages 0 to 74 Years for Japanese in Japan and Japanese and Caucasians in California

| Number of cases | Japan | | California | | | | | |
| | Japanese | | Foreign-born Japanese | | U.S.-born Japanese | | Caucasians | |
	Men	Women	Men	Women	Men	Women	Men	Women
Stomach (151)	58.4	30.9	29.9	13.0	11.7	11.3	8.0	4.0
Colon (153)	1.9	2.1	6.1	7.0	6.3	10.4	7.9	8.3
Rectum (154)	3.3	2.8	4.0	4.0	3.1	2.0	4.2	2.8
Total (458)	63.6	35.8	40.0	24.0	21.1	23.7	20.1	15.1

From Ackerman (29).

TABLE 5. Influence of Sodium Chloride on Gastric Carcinoma

Treatment	Total malignant tumors	
	No.	%
1. 50 mg MNNG/liter drinking water, 6 g NaCl/liter drinking water, stock diet+10% NaCl	11/18	61.1
2. 50 mg MNNG/liter drinking water, 1 ml sat. NaCl 1× weekly, stock diet	12/15	80.0
3. 50 mg MNNG/liter drinking water, stock diet	12/27	44.4
4. 1 mg NQO, 1× weekly, stock diet +10% NaCl	7/18	38.9
5. 1 mg NQO saturated NaCl, 1× weekly, stock diet	9/17	52.9
6. 1 mg NQO, 1× weekly, stock diet	0/18	0.0
7. 6 g NaCl, stock diet +10% NaCl	0/10	0.0
8. 1 ml saturated NaCl, stock diet	0/10	0.0
9. Untreated—stock diet+tap water	0/10	0.0

MNNG induced adenocarcinomas of the glandular stomach; NQO induced tumors of the forestomach. From Ref. 32, abridged.

administered clearly influenced the results. Weekly doses of saturated NaCl were more effective in enhancing gastric cancer than continuous administration of salt either in water or diet (Table 5). Sodium chloride alone under these conditions was not carcinogenic, but it enhanced the effects of the two carcinogens. Moreover, these authors were unable to correlate erosion and ulceration of the gastric mucosa by salt with cancer incidence; however they suggest that salt may have

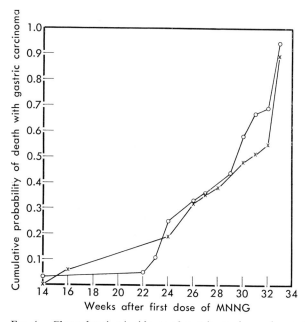

FIG. 4. Chart showing incidence of gastric carcinoma in rats fed control (diet 1) or marginal lipotrope (diet 2) and exposed to MNNG.
× diet 1+MNNG, 155 mg/kg ; ○ diet 2+MNNG, 155 mg/kg.

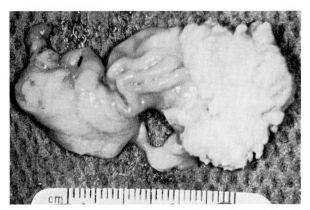

FIG. 5.   Gross appearance of gastric carcinoma induced by MNNG in rats.

modified the mucopolysaccharides and mucosal barrier rendering the stomach lining more permeable to the carcinogen.

Until the development of the model for gastric adenocarcinoma by chronic administration of MNNG, experimental studies of gastric cancer were confined to squamous tumors of the rodent forestomach, an area perhaps more closely related to esophagus than to the glandular stomach as referred to above in work from our own laboratories. We have found that increased intakes of vitamin A reduced the number of papillomas of the forestomach in hamsters given carcinogenic doses of benzo(a)pyrene intratracheally although the increased vitamin A had no influence on cancer of the respiratory tree (*19*). Other studies in our laboratory (*33*) revealed that a diet marginal in lipotropes and high in fat had no effect on the incidence of gastric squamous carcinoma (Fig. 4) induced in rats by MNNG (Fig. 5). Other investigators have shown that antioxidant food additives can reduce gastric tumor incidence in mice (*34*).

It thus appears that although there is highly suggestive evidence that nutrition is related to gastric cancer in some human populations, specific agents are still unknown and, in the case of animal experiments, the evidence is variable and sometimes conflicting.

Colon Cancer

There is a strong negative correlation between gastric and colon cancer; where one is relatively common, the other is usually rare. Cancer of the colon is associated with environmental factors and a number of studies have suggested a role for nutrition in the etiology of this type of malignancy. The mortality from colon cancer is high in Scotland, Canada, and the United States, and low in Japan and Chile (*2*).

Some epidemiological studies have implicated a high-fat diet in the etiology of colon cancer but in these same populations there is usually high protein intake since most of the dietary fat is consumed along with animal protein (*35*). In Japan where colon cancer is uncommon, fat intake is about 12% of calories and the fat is

TABLE 6. Serum Cholesterol and Relative Risk Estimates for Colon Cancer by Intakes of Processed Meats

Processed meats (times/month)	No. of men	Cholesterol (mg/100 ml)	Retrospective		Prospective	
			No. of cases	Relative risk	No. of cases	Relative risk
3	94	291	29	1.0	5	1.0
3–5	211	286	83	1.4	14	2.3
6 or more	130	271	48	2.1	6	2.0

From Bjelke (*38*), abridged.

primarily unsaturated. This compares to the 40–44% in the U.S. diet and the diet eaten by immigrants to the United States from Japan (*36, 37*). In contrast to gastric cancer, colon cancer incidence rises in the immigrants, and their children have a much higher incidence of colon cancer than those born in Japan (Table 4). The increased incidence of colon cancer is associated with adoption of a western style diet and a higher standard of living; the immigrants eat more meat and therefore take in more fat. It is interesting, however, that the incidence of colon cancer in the United States does not vary appreciably with race or ethnic group or with socioeconomic status (*3, 4*). Mortality from colon cancer in migrants from Poland and Norway to the U.S. has also shifted upward to United States levels. Bjelke (*38*) reported in Norway a negative correlation between blood-cholesterol level and mortality from colon cancer with a particularly high risk of colon cancer in people consuming an excess of processed meats (Table 6). Rose *et al.* (*39*) also found a negative correlation between blood cholesterol and colon cancer.

In most studies relative risks are higher for people ingesting meats with little or no nitrate or nitrite content, *e.g.*, beef, than for people ingesting preserved pork products which contain nitrites; there have been no associations demonstrated with dried and salted fish rich in nitrates and nitrites.

Many authors have pointed out that populations in areas with a high incidence of colon cancer consume diets high in refined foods and low in fiber. Refined foods result in small stools and long intestinal transit time while high-fiber diets are associated with large stools and rapid transit time (*40–43*). There are also differences in the bacterial flora associated with the two types of diets (*44*). Studies have indicated higher counts of anaerobic bacteria, lower counts of aerobic bacteria, higher levels of total neutral steroids and more degraded cholesterol, and bile acids in feces of individuals from areas of high risk for colon cancer. It was postulated that certain metabolites of bile salts may be carcinogenic. There is, however, some disagreement on the relative amounts of fecal bile salts in groups consuming vegetarian diets (*45*). Thus, as more recent observations illustrate (*46*), the relation of a number of dietary habits and constituents to colon cancer is a complex one, and epidemiologic studies should serve only as a point of departure for experimental studies designed to identify etiologic agents or conditions.

Cancer of the colon rarely occurs as a spontaneous disease in laboratory animals but can be induced by a number of chemical carcinogens. Bracken fern, cycasin or methylazoxymethanol (MAM) (*47, 48*), dimethylhydrazine (DMH) (*49, 50*), and aflatoxin B_1 (*51, 52*) are all inducers of or associated with colon cancer in laboratory animals. Diet can modify the incidence of the tumor, but the mechanism(s) remain to be elucidated.

Diet may modify the induction of colon cancer through its influence on the

TABLE 7.   Tumor Induction by DMH in Normal or Lipotrope-deficient Rats

Diet	Total DMH (mg/kg body wt.)	% mortality[a]	% rats dead with carcinoma of:		
			Colon[b]	Small intestine[b]	Ear duct[c]
1	300	100	86	45	75
2	300	100	100	55	44
1	150	80	56	25	56
2	150	68	85	15	15

[a] 40 weeks after initial dose of DMH.   [b] Adenocarcinoma with varying degrees of differentiation and mucus production.   [c] Squamous carcinoma. Difference between rats fed diet 1 and diet 2 is significant if two doses are combined, $P < 0.05$.

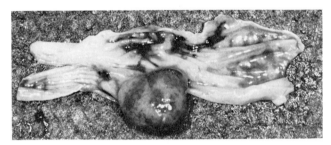

FIG. 6.   Gross appearance of colon adenocarcinoma in rats by symmetrical DMH. Most are polypoid but some are sessile with a typical napkin-ring appearance.

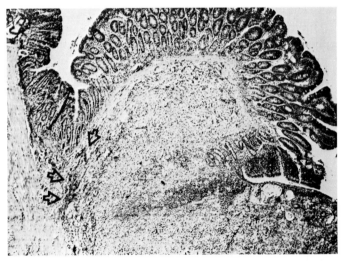

FIG. 7.   Microscopic appearance of DMH-induced colon tumor in rats. The stalk of the polypoid tumor has been infiltrated by neoplastic glandular cells (arrow).   H-E.   ×40.

intestinal microflora (53), by changing the sensitivity of the colon mucosa to carcinogens or perhaps by liberating an active metabolite or supplying promoters or accelerators to act on the colon mucosa. Rats fed a diet high in fat excreted more bile acids and steroid metabolites and were more susceptible to DMH-induced colon cancer than rats fed a diet low in fat (54).

In our own laboratories (50) we have shown that a diet high in fat and marginal in lipotropes (Table 7) increased the incidence of colon carcinoma induced by DMH (Figs. 6 and 7). We found that (Table 8) chronic dietary deficiency of vitamin A only slightly increased the incidence of DMH-induced colon tumors and slightly decreased induction time, while a high level of vitamin A in the diet did not affect tumor incidence but did decrease the number of tumors per rat (55).

Aflatoxin B_1 (AFB_1) (52), which usually causes liver cancer specifically in laboratory animals, induced a significant number of colon tumors in rats fed diets low or marginal in vitamin A (Table 9); the observation has been confirmed by more recent studies (unpublished) in which chronic vitamin A deficiency in rats fed aflatoxin resulted in a highly significant incidence of colon cancer in rats with some indication that there was a change in target organ from liver to colon (Table 10). This suggests a change in sensitivity of the colon or a change in metabolite(s) associated with vitamin A deficiency. This may be mediated through a change in gut microflora, a change in drug-metabolizing enzymes, altered quantity or quality of the secretion of colon glycopeptides which are vitamin A-dependent (56) or a combination of these.

TABLE 8.   Colon Tumors in Rats Given DMH and Vitamin A

Treatment	Amount of DMH (mg/kg body wt.)	Rats with colon carcinoma (%)
Control	420	60
10 μg/g RP	275	56
Deficient	420	100
0–1 μg/g RP	275	77
Excess	420	60
165 μg/g RP	275	60

RP : retinyl palmitate. From Ref. 55.

TABLE 9.   Liver and Colon Tumors in Rats Fed 0.1 ppm AFB_1 and Varying Amounts of Vitamin A

Treatment	No. of 2-year survivors	Liver tumors	Colon tumors	Aver. body wt. (g)
Control				
50 μg RP/day	35/50	0/50	0/50	594
50 μg RP/day+AFB_1	34/50	24/50	0/50	627
5 μg RP/day+AFB_1	23/50	11/50	6/50	397
10 μg RP/day+AFB_1	4/20	17/20	1/20	364
500 μg RP/day+AFB_1	31/50	19/50	0/50	483

Form Ref. 52.

TABLE 10.   Incidence of Liver and Colon Tumors in Rats Fed AFB$_1$ and Various Levels of Vitamin A

	Animal Nos.	Sex	Liver	Colon	Both	Liver only	Colon only
Control							
3.0 μg/g RA	1– 24	M	0/24	0/24	—	—	—
3.0 μg/g RA	25– 51	F	0/26	0/26	—	—	—
3.0 μg/g RA +AFB$_1$	52– 76	M	21/24	1/24	1/24	20/24	0/24
3.0 μg/g RA +AFB$_1$	77–101	F	19/24	2/24	2/24	17/24	0/24
Low vitamin A							
0.3 μg/g RA	102–111	M	0/10	0/10	0/10	0/10	0/10
0.3 μg/g RA	112–123	F	0/12	0/12	0/12	0/12	0/12
0.3 μg/g RA +AFB$_1$	124–190	M	59/66	19/66	17/66	41/66	2/66
0.3 μg/g RA +AFB$_1$	191–232	F	32/42	12/42	5/42	27/42	7/42
High vitamin A							
30.0 μg/g RA	233–255	M	0/23	0/23	0/23	0/23	0/23
30.0 μg/g RA	256–275	F	0/20	0/20	0/20	0/20	0/20
30.0 μg/g RA +AFB$_1$	276–301	M	24/26	2/26	2/26	22/26	2/26
30.0 μg/g RA +AFB$_1$	302–332	F	26/31	3/31	2/31	24/31	1/31

In regard to drug-metabolizing enzymes which can alter the quality or quantity of metabolites, recent studies (57, 58) have clearly shown that intestinal aryl hydrocarbon hydroxylase (AHH) can be modified by diet and this in turn can modify chemical carcinogenesis. The activity of AHH in the intestine of the rat can be changed by exogenous inducers in foods including Brussel's sprouts, turnips, cabbage, alfalfa, and other dietary components. This suggests an important role for nutrients in modulation of carcinogenesis through enzyme systems with some important implications for human cancer. We have shown a dietary effect on liver enzymes and liver cancer induction, referred to later in this paper.

Liver Cancer

In some population groups of Africa, South China, Hawaii, Thailand, Mozambique, and other areas, primary liver cancer is a major problem, particularly in males (3, 5, 59–62). Liver cancer is the most common of all forms of cancer south of the Sahara in Africa representing 10–30% of all tumors in men; in the Bantu of Mozambique it accounts for two-thirds of cancer in men. This is a rate 500 times that of the same age group in the United States; the U.S. rate is about 2.4 per 100,000.

Shank *et al.* in Thailand (60) and reports from East and South Africa clearly implicate carcinogenic dietary contaminants probably interacting with nutritional deficits or imbalances in the etiology of liver cancer (62). The tumors are mainly of the hepatocellular type. It has been suggested that the high frequency in Africa and Asia results from an increased incidence of cirrhosis which enhances susceptibility to tumor development. Cirrhosis may be induced by malnutrition or it may be the result of dietary contaminants or of a combination of these and other factors. A role for nutrition is indicated, but the complex problem is probably a result of many different interactions. In the United States, hepatocarcinoma is associated with alcoholic cirrhosis, another disease resulting from complex interactions of diet, toxins, and possibly viral liver disease.

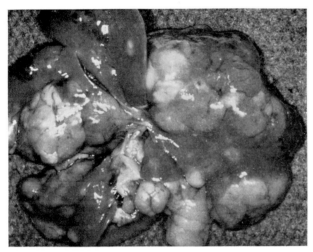

Fig. 8.   Gross appearance of hepatocellular carcinoma induced in rats by AFB₁. The nodularity is a result of hepatocarcinoma ; cirrhosis is not a component of the process unless an additional stress is imposed.

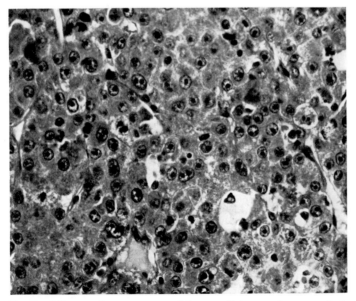

Fig. 9.   Microscopic appearance of hepatocellular carcinoma typical of those induced by AFB₁ or FAA. Trabecular or anaplastic types may be encountered with variable vascularity and glandular components.   H-E.   ×320.

Dietary effects on chemical induction of hepatocarcinoma (Figs. 8 and 9) in experimental animals have been studied extensively in our laboratory. Increased dietary lipid, particularly the unsaturated types, are associated with increased tumor incidence (63). We have found that if the diet is both high in fat and deficient in the lipotropes choline, methionine, and folic acid, induction of liver tumors by carcinogens of several chemical classes is markedly enhanced (Table 11). AFB_1, nitrosamines, and N-2-fluorenylacetamide (FAA) all induced liver tumors earlier or in higher incidence or both in deficient rats compared to rats fed adequate, balanced lipotropes (18, 33). As discussed above, the same dietary deficiency enhanced tumor induction in colon and esophagus (18, 50). The influence of vitamin A on chemical carcinogenesis is shown in Table 12. The effects of lipotropes and of vitamin A do not coincide.

The most likely mechanism by which the deficiency influences carcinogenesis is through alteration of carcinogen metabolism by the tissues. Deficient rats had decreased basal levels of hepatic microsomal oxidases (Table 13) which were

TABLE 11.   Effect of Marginal Lipotrope-High Fat Diet on Chemical Carcinogenesis in Rats

Carcinogen	Tumor induction		
	Enhanced in:	Depressed in:	Not affected in:
Males			
AFB_1	Liver	—	—
DEN	Liver, esophagus	—	—
DBN[a]	Liver	—	Esophagus, lung, bladder
DMN[b]	—	—	Liver, kidney
FAA	Liver	—	Zymbal's gland
DMH	Colon	Zymbal's gland	Small intestine
MNNG	—	—	Forestomach
FANFT[c]	—	—	Bladder
Females			
FAA (Sprague-Dawley)	—	Mammary gland	Zymbal's gland
FAA (Fischer)	Liver	—	—
DMBA	—	Mammary gland	—

[a] DBN: N, N-di-n-butylnitrosamine.   [b] DMN: N-dimethylnitrosamine.   [c] FANFT: N-[4-(5-nitro-2-furyl)-2-thiazolyl] formamide.

TABLE 12.   Effect of Vitamin A on Chemical Carcinogenesis

Carcinogen	Species	Vitamin A	Tumor induction		
			Enhanced in:	Depressed in:	Not affected in:
BP	Hamster	↑	—	Esophagus, forestomach	Respiratory tract
AFB_1	Rat	↓	Colon	Liver	—
AFB_1	Rat	↑	—	—	Liver
DMH	Rat	↓	Colon	—	Small intestine
DMH	Rat	↑	—	—	Colon, small intestine
FANFT	Rat	↑	Bladder	—	—

↑ : increase.   ↓ : decrease.   From Refs. 19 and 64.

TABLE 13. Liver Enzymes, FAA and Diet, Female Rats

Diet	PNA μg p-nitrophenol/g liver	BPOH quinine units/g liver
Control	142±16	8±4
Control+FAA	187±14	13±6
Marginal lipotrope	105±14	7±3
Marginal lipotrope+FAA	147±20	5±3

PNA: para-nitro-anisole. BPOH: benzpyrene hydroxylase.

TABLE 14. Blood Content of DEN at Intervals after Intraperitoneal Injection[a]

Time after DEN injection (min)	DEN in blood (μg/ml±S.E.)	
	Control	Deficient
4	36.1±2.0	31.2±3.1
20	19.8±2.6	19.0±1.6
40	13.9±3.0	15.0±4.4
60	11.2±3.0	12.1±1.4
120	3.1±1.5	5.5±0.9
210	None detectable[b]	0.6±0.2

[a] Rats were given 25 mg DEN/kg body wt.; 4–5 rats/diet were studied at each time period. [b] 0.05 μg/ml would have been easily detected under the experimental conditions. From Ref. *66*.

TABLE 15. Tumor Incidence in Rats Fed DEN

Diet	No. of rats	% of rats with tumor in:		
		Liver	Esophagus	Any organ[a]
1	25	24	12	28
2	25	60[b]	8	64

[a] One rat fed diet 2 bore a transitional cell carcinoma of the urinary bladder but no other tumor; one rat fed diet 1 bore an esophageal tumor but no hepatic tumor; 2 rats in each diet group bore esophageal and hepatic tumors. From Ref. *66*. [b] Difference from diet 1 significant, $P<0.05$.

induced by phenobarbital and in some cases by FAA but not by AFB$_1$ (*64–66*). Deficient rats cleared DEN from their blood slightly but significantly less rapidly than normal rats (Table 14) and this correlated with tumor incidence (Table 15).

Studies in progress on FAA metabolism, in collaboration with Poirier and Grantham at the National Cancer Institute, Bethesda, indicate that urinary excretion of N-hydroxy FAA, a compound on the pathway of activation of FAA, may be increased in deficient rats following prolonged feeding. A-Adenosylmethionine (SAM) content in the liver of deficient rats, a direct biochemical measure of lipotrope deficiency, was decreased in deficient rats. It diminished in both deficient and adequately-fed rats when FAA was fed which may indicate its participation in some aspect of FAA metabolism. Hepatic content of reduced glutathione, which reacts with many exogenous toxic chemicals to detoxify them, was normal in deficient rats and was not affected by FAA.

In collaboration with Suit and Luria at M.I.T. we are using the *in vitro* mutagenesis assay and specific bacterial strains developed by Ames (*67*) to determine whether the observed dietary effects on chemical carcinogenesis operate through alteration of hepatic activation of carcinogens. In agreement with the data on microsomal oxidases, liver preparations from deficient rats converted only about one-third to one-half as much AFB_1 to a bacterial mutagen as preparations from adequately-fed rats. Conversion of FAA also was decreased. Treatment of rats with carcinogen altered the ability of the liver preparations to convert the carcinogen to a mutagen. Preliminary studies have indicated that after FAA treatment of rats, liver preparations from lipotrope-deficient rats are as effective as preparations from normal rats in conversion of FAA to a mutagen. AFB_1 treatment either decreased the capacity of liver preparations from adequately-fed rats to convert AFB_1 to a mutagen and did not affect the conversion by preparations from deficient rats or enhanced the conversion by both groups depending on time and dose. More extensive studies, which are in progress, are required for confirmation of these results. They agree with the results of our studies of microsomal oxidases and demonstrate a diet-induced difference in hepatic carcinogen activation, insofar as it is indicated by mutagen production, but they do not fully explain the enhancement of carcinogenesis in deficient rats.

In addition to its effect on hepatic enzymes, the lipotrope-deficient diet induces and maintains increased DNA synthesis and mitosis in hepatocytes; presumably this is the result of increased cell turnover although significant necrosis is not evident histologically. Studies in collaboration with Leffert at the Salk Institute, La Jolla, have demonstrated that there is a significant drop in serum very low density lipoproteins (VLDL) in the marginally deficient animals although it is not as marked as in severely deficient ones (Table 16). Serum VLDL inhibit the initiation of hepatocyte DNA synthesis both *in vitro* and *in vivo* and may, in conjunction with several hormones, control cell division in the liver (*68*). Therefore the dietary effect on VLDL may interfere with normal regulatory growth controls and render the hepatocytes more susceptible to chemical carcinogens.

These different approaches to the problem of the mechanism by which lipotrope deficiency alters hepatocarcinogenesis all indicate that carcinogen metabolism is altered in the deficient rats and also may be altered by carcinogen treatment, in some cases in a different manner in deficient rats compared to normal control rats. The complexity of the metabolic pathways and our inability in many cases to identify the proximate carcinogen make it difficult to correlate metabolic effects with carcinogenesis. The dietary model is proving useful in separating those

TABLE 16. Effect of Lipotrope Deficiency on Hepatocyte DNA Synthesis and Serum VLDL in Weanling Rats

Diet	DNA synthesis[a]	Serum VLDL[a]
Control	0.5– 4	75
Marginal lipotrope	1– 9	50
Low lipotrope	5–20	25

[a] Expressed in arbitrary units as an index of DNA synthesis and concentration of VLDL.

aspects of carcinogen metabolism which correlate with carcinogenesis from those which do not.

Other nutrients which influence tumor induction in the liver include protein, riboflavin, and vitamin B_{12}. Protein deficiency sufficient to decrease hepatic microsomal oxidases blocked induction of hepatic tumors by DMN and enhanced induction of renal tumors, presumably because DMN was cleared from the blood less rapidly in deficient rats (69). Diets either marginally deficient or excessive in protein have variable effects on induction of liver and other tumors, most notably bladder tumors which may be increased by increased urinary levels of tryptophan metabolites (70).

Riboflavin specifically decreases hepatic tumor induction by the aminoazobenzenes since it is a cofactor for the enzymes which metabolize those compounds.

Vitamin B_{12} in high levels has been reported to be cocarcinogenic for the induction of liver tumors by dimethylaminoazobenzene (DAB) and DEN (71). No mechanism for the effect has been proposed; it may be related to an abnormality in one carbon metabolism as in lipotrope deficiency.

Both the feeding of stock diets and of antioxidants tend to decrease chemical induction of liver tumors (72). As discussed above, this may be the result of induction of microsomal oxidases by vegetable compounds or by the antioxidants.

Breast Cancer

Breast cancer incidence is correlated with socioeconomic status and therefore with ample or overnourishment. It is not common in women in developing societies nor in Japanese women but the incidence increases in these population groups when they migrate to the United States (73). Breast cancer is increasing in young women in the United States, and this has been associated by some with increased fat consumption; however, there is insufficient evidence to incriminate fat *per se* in breast cancer; increased fat intake in the United States is almost always accompanied by increased protein intake. Breast cancer patients have been reported to be obese compared to control groups but recent studies have indicated that the difference is more closely related to body mass, *i.e.*, influenced by both height and weight (74).

As to mechanisms, which are undoubtedly complex, one suggestion is that there is increased synthesis of estrogens and altered storage of hormones in people consuming a high-fat diet (75). Another possible mechanism is related to the intestinal flora; in people consuming a western, high-fat diet there is a higher proportion of strictly anaerobic microflora in the intestine. These organisms can produce estrogens from biliary steroids which also are increased in subjects consuming high-fat diets (44).

A number of other dietary factors have been associated with breast cancer in epidemiologic studies. These include iodine deficiency (76), the cadmium content of the water (77), and high rate of beer consumption (78). These suggestions are based on less than convincing evidence, however, and require more extensive epidemiologic and experimental support.

In experimental studies, diets high in corn oil enhanced mammary tumor induction in rats by 7,12-dimethylbenz(a)anthracene (DMBA). DMBA-induced mammary tumors were inhibited by the synthetic antioxidants butylated hydroxyanisole, butylated hydroxytoluene, and ethoxyquin (58) and by sulfur-containing compounds benzyl thiocyanate, disulfuram, and dimethyldithiocarbamate (79). In mice, dietary restriction (80), riboflavin deficiency (81), and phenylalanine deficiency (82) inhibited the formation of mammary gland tumors.

Experiments in our laboratory using a diet marginal in lipotropes and high in fat have yielded interesting results relative to induction of breast or liver cancer in two strains of female rats by FAA or DMBA (Fig. 10). Dietary FAA induced fewer mammary tumors in Sprague-Dawley rats fed the low-lipotrope, high-fat diet than in rats fed an adequate diet (Table 17). Tumor incidence was lower in the marginally lipotrope-deficient rats and death from mammary tumors was slowed by 4–6 weeks, compared to the controls. In Fischer rats, which are resistant to FAA induction of mammary tumors, hepatic carcinomas developed in a significantly greater incidence in the deficient rats, a result in accord with findings in male rats discussed above.

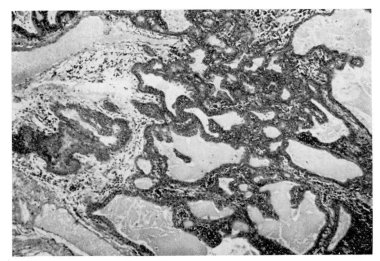

Fig. 10.   Adenocarcinoma of the mammary gland from a rat exposed to DMBA.   H-E. ×40.

TABLE 17.   Mammary Tumor Induction by FAA in Female Rats Fed Control or Marginal Lipotrope-high Fat Diets

Diet	Rat strain	No. of rats	Mammary tumors (%)		
			Carcinoma	Adenoma	Total
Control	S.D.[a]	31	65	3	68
Marginal lipotrope-high fat	S.D.	32	41	9	50
Control	Fischer	25	0	12	12
Marginal lipotrope-high fat	Fischer	25	8	0	8

[a] S.D.: Sprague-Dawley.

TABLE 18. Tumors Induced by DMBA in Sprague-Dawley Rats Fed Control or Marginal Lipotrope-high Fat Diets

Diet	No. of rats	Mammary tumors (%)		
		Carcinoma	Adenoma	Total
Control	25	40	8	48
Marginal lipotrope-high fat	27	15	0	15

In Sprague-Dawley rats fed the marginal lipotrope-high fat diet, mammary tumor incidence induced by DMBA also was reduced similar to the result with FAA (Table 18).

The alteration of mammary tumor incidence in rats fed the high-fat diet is particularly important because it is opposed to previous results in experimental animals which have shown an enhancement of mammary carcinogenesis by high-fat diets. The marginal lipotrope status of the rats may account for the observed difference in tumor induction. It should be noted, however, that the marginal deficiency of lipotropes was not of such severity as to depress growth or caloric intake and therefore this mechanism can be ruled out. There is one previous report of inhibition of DMBA induction of mammary tumors in rats fed a diet severely deficient in protein and lipotropes for 10 days before treatment. The rats lost weight and had a marked decrease in ovarian and uterine weight at the time DMBA was administered. Therefore they probably were in quite different hormonal balance compared to control rats (*83*).

DISCUSSION

The organ sites for which there is the strongest evidence in people and experimental animals for a dietary effect on tumor induction and development account for nearly one-third of the cancer incidence and deaths in the U.S. (Table 19). The definition of effective dietary factors and elucidation of their mechanisms of action offer the potential for prevention of tumors in the affected sites.

Our experimental results for the nutrients most extensively studied, lipotropes and vitamin A, are interesting in that they do not coincide. Vitamin A influences tumor induction by AFB_1 in the colon but not in the liver; lipotropes influence

TABLE 19. Morbidity and Mortality in U.S. from Cancers Possibly Related to Diet

Organ site	Estimated statistics for 1975	
	New cases	Deaths
Esophagus	7,400	6,500
Stomach	22,900	14,400
Colon	69,000	38,600
Breast	88,700	32,900
Liver (and bile ducts)	11,500	9,800
Total	199,500	102,200
All cancer	665,000	365,000

AFB$_1$ induction of tumors only in liver. Vitamin A did not significantly affect induction of colon tumors by DMH whereas lipotrope deficiency had a significant effect. Vitamin A was reported by others to block induction of bladder tumors by FANFT; lipotrope-deficiency had no effect.

It is essential to progress in cancer cause and prevention to identify nutritional factors which modify the susceptibility of an individual to environmental or endogenous carcinogens. Nutrition offers the most acceptable and direct means to attacking the cancer problem in human populations and the current surge of interest in this area of cancer studies reflects the growing recognition of the importance of nutrition in cancer prevention.

REFERENCES

1. Hoffman, F. L.   Cancer and Diet, pp. 767, Williams and Wilkins, Baltimore, 1937.
2. Levin, D. L., Devesa, S. S., Godwin, J. D., and Silverman, D. T.   Cancer Rates and Risks. D.H.E.W. Publication #75-691 (NIH), Washington D.C., 1974.
3. Doll, R.   Worldwide distribution of gastrointestinal cancer. Natl. Cancer Inst. Monogr., *25*: 173–190, 1967.
4. Bailar, J. C.   Distribution of carcinoma of esophagus, stomach, and large bowel. *In;* W. J. Burdette (ed.), Carcinoma of the Alimentary Tract, pp. 3–14, University of Utah Press, Salt Lake City, 1965.
5. Cook, P. and Burkitt, D.   Cancer in Africa. Brit. Med. Bull., *27*: 14–20, 1971.
6. Wynder, E. L. and Bross, I. J.   A study of etiological factors in cancer of the esophagus. Cancer, *14*: 389–413, 1961.
7. O'Gara, R. W., Lee, C. W., Morton, J. F., Kapadia, G. J., and Dunham, L. J. Sarcoma induced in rats by extracts of plants and by fractionated extract of *Krameria ixina*. J. Natl. Cancer Inst., *52*: 445–448, 1974.
8. Jussawalla, D. J.   Report of the International Seminar on Epidemiology of Oesophageal Cancer.   Int. J. Cancer, *10*: 436–441, 1972.
9. Martinez, I.   Factors associated with cancer of the esophagus, mouth and pharynx in Puerto Rico. J. Natl. Cancer Inst., *42*: 1069–1094, 1969.
10. Cook, P.   Cancer of the oesophagus in Africa. Brit. J. Cancer, *25*: 853–880, 1971.
11. Schoenberg, B. S., Bailar, J. C., and Fraumeni, J. F. Certain mortality patterns of esophageal cancer in the United States 1930–1967. J. Natl. Cancer Inst., *46*: 63–73, 1971.
12. Breslow, N. E. and Enstrom, J. E.   Geographic correlations between cancer mortality and alcohol-tobacco consumption in the United States. J. Natl. Cancer Inst., *53*: 631–639, 1974.
13. Leevy, C. M.   Liver disease of the alcoholic viewpoints. Digest. Dis., *3*: 1–4, 1971.
14. Halstead, J. A., Smith, J. C., Jr., and Irwin, M. I.   A conspectus of research on zinc requirements of man. J. Nutr., *104*: 345–378, 1974.
15. Hormozdiari, H., Day, N. E., Aramesh, B., and Mahbonbi, E.   Dietary factors and esophageal cancer in the Caspian littoral of Iran. Cancer Res., *35*: 3493–3498, 1975.
16. The Coordinating Group for the Research of Esophageal Carcinoma, Chinese Acad. of Medical Sciences, 1974.
17. Day, N. E.   Some aspects of the epidemiology of esophageal cancer. Cancer Res., *35*: 3304–3307, 1975.

18. Rogers, A. E., Sanchez, O., Feinsod, F. M., and Newberne, P. M. Dietary enhancement of nitrosamine carcinogenesis. Cancer Res., *34*: 96–99, 1974.

19. Smith, D. M., Rogers, A. E., and Newberne, P. M. Vitamin A and benzo(a)-pyrene carcinogenesis in the respiratory tract of hamsters fed a semisynthetic diet. Cancer Res., *35*: 1485–1488, 1975.

20. Chu, E. W. and Malmgren, R. A. An inhibitory effect of vitamin A on the induction of tumors of forestomach and cervix in the Syrian hamster by carcinogenic polycyclic hydrocarbons. Cancer Res., *25*: 884–895, 1965.

21. Graham, S., Lilienfeld, A. M., and Tidings, J. E. Dietary and purgation factors in the epidemiology of gastric cancer. Cancer, *20*: 2224–2234, 1967.

22. Acheson, E. D. and Doll, R. Dietary factors in carcinoma of the stomach: A study of 100 cases and 200 controls. Gut, *5*: 126–131, 1964.

23. Higginson, J. Etiological factors in gastrointestinal cancer in man. J. Natl. Cancer Inst., *37*: 527–545, 1966.

24. Dungal, N. and Sigurjonsson, J. Gastric cancer and diet. A pilot study on dietary habits in two districts differing markedly in respect of mortality from gastric cancer. Brit. J. Cancer, *21*: 270–276, 1967.

25. Merliss, R. R. Talc-treated rice and Japanese stomach cancer. Science, *173*: 1141–1142, 1971.

26. Lilienfeld, A. Epidemiology of gastric cancer. New Engl. J. Med., *286*: 316–317, 1972.

27. Haenszel, W., Kurihara, M., Mitsuo, S., and Lee, R. K. Stomach cancer among Japanese in Hawaii. J. Natl. Cancer Inst., *49*: 969–983, 1972.

28. Graham, S., Schotz, W., and Martino, P. Alimentary factors in the epidemiology of gastric cancer. Cancer, *30*: 927–938, 1972.

29. Ackerman, L. V. Some thoughts on food and cancer. Nutr. Today, pp. 2–9, Jan./Feb., 1972.

30. Phillips, R. L. Role of lifestyle and dietary habits in risk of cancer among seventh-day adventists. Cancer Res., *35*: 3513–3522, 1975.

31. Haenszel, W. and Correa, P. Epidemiology of stomach cancer. Cancer Res., *35*: 3452–3459, 1975.

32. Tatematsu, M., Takahashi, M., Fukushima, S., Hananouchi, M., and Shirai, T. Effects in rats of sodium chloride on experimental gastric cancers induced by N-methyl-N'-nitro-N-nitrosoguanidine or 4-nitroquinoline-1-oxide. J. Natl. Cancer Inst., *55*: 101–106, 1975.

33. Rogers, A. E. Variable effects of a lipotrope-deficient, high fat diet on chemical carcinogenesis in rats. Cancer Res., *35*: 2469–2474, 1975.

34. Wattenberg, L. W. Inhibition of carcinogenic and toxic effects of polycyclic hydrocarbons by phenolic antioxidants and ethoxyquin. J. Natl. Cancer Inst., *48*: 1425–1430, 1972.

35. Wynder, E. L. and Shigematsu, T. Environmental factors of cancer of the colon and rectum. Cancer, *20*: 1520–1561, 1967.

36. Haenszel, W. M. and Kurihara, M. Studies of Japanese migrants. I. Mortality from cancer and other diseases among Japanese in the United States. J. Natl. Cancer Inst., *40*: 43–51, 1968.

37. Haenszel, N., Berg, J. W., Segi, M., Kurihara, M., and Locke, F. B. Large bowel cancer in Hawaiian Japanese. J. Natl. Cancer Inst., *51*: 1765–1779, 1973.

38. Bjelke, E. Colon cancer and blood-cholesterol. The Lancet (June 1), 1116–1117, 1974.

39. Rose, G., Blackburn, H., Keys, A., Taylor, H., Kamel, W., Reid, P. O., and Stamler, J. Colon cancer and blood cholesterol. Lancet, *i*: 181–183, 1974.

40. Oettle, A. G. Primary neoplasms of the alimentary canal of white and Bantu of the Transvaal 1949–1953. A histopathological series. Natl. Cancer Inst. Monogr., *25*: 97–109, 1967.

41. Burkitt, D. P., Walker, A. R., and Painter, N. S. Effect of dietary fiber of stools and transit times and its role in causation of disease. Lancet, *ii*: 1408–1412, 1972.

42. Walker, A., Walker, B., and Richardon, B. D. Bowel transit times in Bantu populations. Brit. Med. J., *3*: 48–49, 1970.

43. Walker, A. R. P. Effect of high crude fiber intake on transit time and the absorption of nutrients in South African Negro school children. Am. J. Clin. Nutr., *28*: 1161–1169, 1975.

44. Hill, M. J., Drasar, B. S., Aries, V., Crowther, J. S., Hawksworth, G., and Williams, R. E. O. Bacteria and etiology of cancer of the large bowel. Lancet, *i*: 95–102, 1971.

45. Walker, A. Diet and cancer of the colon. Lancet, *i*: 593–594, 1971.

46. Wynder, E. L. and Reddy, B. S. Studies of large bowel cancer: Human leads to experimental application. J. Natl. Cancer Inst., *50*: 1099–1106, 1973.

47. Hirono, I., Fushimi, H., Mori, T., Miwa, T., and Haga, M. Comparative study of carcinogenic activity of each part of bracken. J. Natl. Cancer Inst., *50*: 1367–1371, 1973.

48. Newberne, P. M. Biologic effects of plant toxins and aflatoxin in rats J. Natl. Cancer Inst., *56*: 551–555, 1976.

49. Newberne, P. M. and Rogers, A. E. Adenocarcinoma of the colon: An animal model for human disease. Am. J. Pathol., *72*: 541–544, 1973.

50. Rogers, A. E. and Newberne, P. M. Dietary enhancement of intestinal carcinogenesis by dimethylhydrazine in rats. Nature, *246*: 491–492, 1973.

51. Newberne, P. M. and Rogers, A. E. Primary hepatocellular carcinoma: An animal model for human disease. Am. J. Pathol., *72*: 137–140, 1973.

52. Newberne, P. M. and Rogers, A. E. Rat colon carcinomas associated with aflatoxin and marginal vitamin A.. J. Natl. Cancer Inst., *50*: 439–448, 1973.

53. Reddy, B., Weisburger, J. H., Narisawa, T., and Wynder, E. L. Colon carcinogenesis in germ-free rats with 1, 2-dimethylhydrazine and N-methyl-N′-nitro-N-nitrosoguanidine. Cancer Res., *34*: 2368–2372, 1974.

54. Reddy, B., Weisburger, J. H., and Wynder, E. L. Effect of dietary fat levels and dimethylhydrazine on fecal acid and neutral sterol excretion and colon carcinogenesis in rats. J. Natl. Cancer Inst., *52*: 507–511, 1974.

55. Rogers, A. E., Herndon, B. J., and Newberne, P. M. Influence of vitamin A of dimethylhydrazine-induced colon carcinoma in rats. Cancer Res., *33*: 1003–1009, 1973.

56. Deluca, L., Schumacher, M., Wolf, G., and Newberne, P. M. Biosynthesis of a fucose-containing glycopeptide from rat small intestine in normal and vitamin A-deficient conditions. J. Biol. Chem., *245*: 4551–4558, 1970.

57. Wattenburg, L. Studies of polycyclic hydrocarbon hydroxylases of the intestine possibly related to cancer. Effect of diet on benzpyrene hydroxylase activity. Cancer, *28*: 99–110, 1971.

58. Wattenberg, L. Dietary modification of intestinal and pulmonary aryl hydrocarbon hydroxylase activity. Toxicol. Appl. Pharmacol., *23*: 741–748, 1972.

59. Higginson, J. The geographical pathology of liver disease in man. Gastroenterology, *57*: 587–598, 1969.

60. Shank, R. C., Bhamarapravati, N., Gordon, J. E., and Wogan, G. N. Dietary aflatoxins and human liver cancer. Incidence of primary liver cancer in two municipal populations of Thailand. Food Cosmet. Toxicol., *10*: 171–179, 1972.

61. Tuyns, A. J. I.A.R.C. Working Conference on the Role of Aflatoxin in Human Disease, Lyon, France, October 28–30, 1968.

62. Van Reusburg, S. J., Van Der Watt, J. J., Purchase, I. F. H., Pereira Coutenho, L., and Markham, R. Primary liver cancer rate and aflatoxin intake in a high cancer area. South African Med. J., *48*: 2508a–2508d, 1974.

63. Miller, J. A. and Miller, E. C. The carcinogenic aminoazo dyes. Adv. Cancer Res., *1*: 339–396, 1953.

64. Rogers, A. E. and Newberne, P. M. Diet and aflatoxin B_1 toxicity in rats. Toxicol. Appl. Pharmacol., *20*: 113–121, 1971.

65. Kula, N. Dietary effects on induced sleeping time and aflatoxin response in rats. Fed. Proc., *33*: 669 (Abstr.), 1974.

66. Rogers, A. E., Wishnok, J. S., and Archer, M. C. Effect of diet on DEN clearance and carcinogenesis in rats. Brit. J. Cancer, *31*: 693–695, 1975.

67. Ames, B. N. An improved bacterial test system for the detection and classification of mutagens and carcinogens. Proc. Natl. Acad. Sci. U. S., *70*: 782–786, 1973.

68. Leffert, H. L. and Weinstein, D. B. Growth control of fetal rat hepatocytes in primary monolayer culture. IX. Specific inhibition of DNA synthesis by the very low density lipoprotein fraction of rat serum and its possible significance to the problem of liver regeneration. Unpublished.

69. McLean, A. E. M. and Magee, P. N. Increased renal carcinogenesis by dimethylnitrosamine in protein-deficient rats. Brit. J. Exp. Pathol., *51*: 587–590, 1970.

70. Clayson, D. B. Nutrition and experimental carcinogenesis. Cancer Res., *35*: 3292–3300, 1975.

71. Poirier, L. A. Hepatocarcinogenesis by diethylnitrosamine in rats fed high dietary levels of lipotropes. J. Natl. Cancer Inst., *54*: 137–140, 1975.

72. Ulland, B. M., Weisburger, J. J., Yamamoto, R. S., and Weisburger, E. K. Antioxidants and carcinogenesis: Butylated hydroxytoluene, but not diphenyl-*p*-phenylene diamine, inhibits cancer induction by N-2-fluorenylacetamide in rats. Food Cosmet. Toxicol., *11*: 199–207, 1973.

73. Buell, P. Changing incidence of breast cancer in Japanese and American women. J. Natl. Cancer Inst., *51*: 1479–1483, 1973.

74. de Waard, F. Breast cancer incidence and nutritional status with particular reference to body weight and height. Cancer Res., *35*: 3351–3356, 1975.

75. Wynder, E. L. Nutrition and cancer. Symposium on Nutrition and Cancer. Fed. Proc., *35*: 1309–1315, 1975.

76. Eskin, B. A., Parker, J. A., Bassett, J. G., and George, D. L. Human breast uptake of radioactive iodine. Obstet. Gynecol., *44*: 398–402, 1974.

77. Berg, J. W. and Burbank, F. Correlations between carcinogenic trace metals in water supplies and cancer mortality. Ann. N. Y. Acad. Sci., *199*: 249–264, 1972.

78. Breslow, N. E. and Enstrom, J. E. Geographic correlation between cancer mortality rates and alcohol-tobacco consumption in the United States. J. Natl. Cancer Inst., *53*: 631–639, 1974.

79. Wattenberg, L. W. Inhibition of carcinogenic and toxic effects of polycyclic hydrocarbons by several sulfur-containing compounds. J. Natl. Cancer Inst., *52*: 1583–1587, 1974.

80. Rowlatt, L. M., Franks, M., and Sheriff, M. U.   Mammary tumor and hepatoma suppression by dietary restriction in C_3H A^{vy} Mice. Brit. J. Cancer, *28*: 83, 1973.

81. Morris, H. P.   Effects of the genesis and growth of tumors associated with vitamin intake. Ann. N.Y. Acad. Sci., *49*: 119–140, 1947.

82. Hui, Y. H., Deome, K. B., and Briggs, G. M.   The developmental noduligenic and tumorigenic potentials of transplanted mammary gland and primary ducts from C_3H mice previously fed a phenylalanine-deficient diet.   Cancer Res., *32*: 57–60, 1972.

83. Tanaka, Y. and Dao, T. L.   Effect of hepatic injury on induction of adrenal necrosis and mammary cancer by 7, 12-dimethylbenz (a) anthracene in rats. J. Natl. Cancer Inst., *35*: 631–640, 1965.

Discussion of Paper of Drs. Newberne and Rogers

DR. TAKEBE: Japanese immigrants to Hawaii have a high incidence of stomach cancer in the first generation. Is this due to an early diet exposure in childhood or due to the fact that they kept their same dietary habits? Other factors such as smoking usually start at around age of 20, but diet may affect the very sensitive stage during childhood. Also, do you have any data on people who migrated from a low-incidence to a high-incidence area, so that the age factors may be answered?

DR. NEWBERNE: The likely reason for the continued high incidence of gastric carcinoma in Japanese migrating to Hawaii is that there is an early exposure to a carcinogen which becomes expressed later in life. When born in Hawaii they do not have the same exposure in childhood and thus less chance for gastric cancer. We have no data on incidence in those going from low to high incidence areas in gastric cancer, but for colon carcinoma we know that Japanese moving from an area of low incidence in Japan to high incidence in California assume the incidence of the region to which they move.

DR. MAGEE: Could you comment on the high incidence of esophageal cancer in man and chickens in China? How good is the evidence that nitrosamines are involved in the cancer?

DR. NEWBERNE: The area northwest of Peking has a high incidence of esophageal cancer in people and chickens within the same communes. Nitrosamines have been isolated from foods consumed by both chickens and people. Further, esophageal cancer was induced in chickens by nitrosamines. The evidence has been published in a monograph but details are incomplete.

DR. LIEBERMAN: Would you please comment on the role of diethylstilbestrol in the diet and its role in breast cancer around the world?

DR. NEWBERNE: I do not have any data on diethylstilbestrol and cancer except the vaginal cancers in daughters born to mothers exposed to diethylstilbestrol. I am concerned about food exposure but even more by the "morning after" diethylstilbestrol and its potential in carcinogenesis.

DR. CRADDOCK: What might be the mechanism of the interesting effect of lipotrope-deficient diets on DNA synthesis?

DR. NEWBERNE: We have speculated that there is a defect in some phase of the cell cycle, perhaps in the S-phase of DNA synthesis. The cell turnover is about doubled and therefore cells deficient in lipotropes degrade or die sooner than normal cells. The high fat in the diet is involved in some manner; saturated fats enhance cell turnover. Furthermore, fatty acids compete with other factors for active enzyme sites, suggesting that some enzyme-activated mechanism in cell DNA synthesis and maturation is defective. In addition, hormonal factors and depressed very low density lipoprotein levels seem to "switch on" DNA synthesis in a more active fashion in lipotrope-deficient cells.

FUNDAMENTALS IN CANCER PREVENTION, P. N. MAGEE ET AL. (EDS.),
UNIV. OF TOKYO PRESS, TOKYO / UNIV. PARK PRESS, BALTIMORE, PP. 41–55, 1976

Blocking Tumor Promotion by Protease Inhibitors

Walter TROLL

Department of Environmental Medicine, New York University Medical Center, New York, New York, U.S.A.

Abstract: Cancer may be the result of exposure to a bewildering array of chemicals in our environment. Mottram and Berenblum discerned two stages in chemical carcinogenesis in mouse skin. The first stage, initiation, can result from subcarcinogenic doses of primary agents. The second stage, promotion, occurs with repeated application of specific irritants (*e.g.*, phorbol-12-myristate-13-acetate (PMA)). Initiation can result from exposure to nearly all known carcinogens and is virtually irreversible. Modification of DNA has been proposed as a general mechanism for initiation. Promotion is biologically reversible. Promotion can be modified by dietary regimens, glucocorticosteroids, and protease inhibitors. It was observed in our laboratory that PMA caused the prompt appearance of a proteolytic enzyme. A variety of protease inhibitors including Leupeptin inhibited this enzyme in mouse skin. Tumor promotion was concommittantly suppressed. Hormones can induce a variety of proteins, presumably by activation of specific regions of the genome. The comparison of hormones with PMA may be of particular interest since some hormones can be considered natural tumor promoters. We demonstrated the appearance of a protease in rat and mouse uteri given estradiol. The enzyme activates plasminogen, and hydrolyses protamine and specific histones in nuclei. It is tempting to speculate that the removal of histones by protease is responsible for the activation of specific regions of the genome. The precise role of protease in neoplastic transformation remains to be clarified, but the use of protease inhibitors to modify the development of tumors remains a promising tool in cancer therapy.

Proteases are actors who can play many parts in biological systems. Examples are: (1) blood clotting and lysis of clots; (2) activation of complement; (3) they play roles in fertilization and in embryonic development; (4) they may also play a crucial role in development and spread of tumors. The purpose of the present communication focuses on the effect of proteases in tumor promotion by specific

41

agents and hormones. Their contribution here may be the derepression of the genome. The effect of proteases may be modulated by normally occurring protease inhibitors. Tumor promotion has been successfully blocked by adding protease inhibitors and by glucocorticosteroids which may elaborate or induce protease inhibitors. Two-stage carcinogenesis employing two-stage promotion in mouse skin was the model for these studies (1). In this system, the first stage can be carried out by a variety of chemical carcinogens presumably causing DNA modification, perhaps by a somatic mutation or activation of an oncogenic virus. Support for this concept was derived from the observation that virtually all primary carcinogens tested are mutagenic in bacteria (2, 3).

Biological mechanisms of promotion are poorly understood. Initial work has concentrated on irritants and wounding (4). However, it appears that irritation is essential but insufficient for promotion (5). We have detected trypsin-like protease activity in mouse skin as early as 30 min after topical application of the purified principle of croton oil, phorbol-12-myristate-13-acetate (PMA). A number of protease inhibitors delayed tumor promotion and counteracted erythema and invasion of leukocytes. Hozumi et al. (6) confirmed the appearance of a protease caused by promotion and noted delay of tumor promotion employing the protease inhibitor Leupeptin.

Another example of two-stage carcinogenesis is the breast cancer model employing rats and mice (7). In this system, as in two-stage carcinogenesis, application of a carcinogen without the appropriate hormones does not lead to breast cancer. Levitz et al. (8) noted the appearance of a trypsin-like protease in uteri on estrogen treatment. As in the mouse skin system, the protease inhibitors Leupeptin and Antipain inhibited this activity and resulted in changes in the hormone action of estradiol.

The precise mechanism of action of protease in cancer development remains to be elucidated. Tumor promoter, as well as hormones, causes phenotypic expression of the genome allowing RNA polymerase to read a new specific portion in chromatin (9, 10). The possible action of the protease then, may be the specific removal of repressor protein from the eukaryote chromatin. We had noted that estradiol and estradiol and progesterone treatment of ovariectomized rats caused the specific removal of histones from chromatin. It is attractive to consider this mechanism of the derepression of the genome. Support for this notion has come from the successful separation of transcribable chromatin and repressed chromatin from chick embryo reticulocytes accomplished by Berkowitz and Doty (11). Here, as in the transcribable chromatin of uteri caused by protease induced by estradiol, the very lysine-rich histones (H_1) are absent (9, 10).

The judicious use of protease inhibitors in modifying phenotypic expression of damages in our genetic material may serve in delaying the appearance of tumors and delay their progression. These inhibitors offer the advantage over the use of steroid hormones which may also elaborate protease inhibitors in that they do not depend on the presence of specific receptors to exert their action.

Methods of Assay of Protease Inhibitors

Proteases are enzymes capable of hydrolyzing peptide bonds in proteins. They differ in specificity of peptide hydrolyzed, and preferences of bonds hydrolyzed. The trypsin family attacks peptides containing lysine and arginine. Members in this family are thrombin, plasmin, and plasminogen activator. These enzymes have serine as the prosthetic group. The methods described in the literature were inadequate for the convenient assay of protease and inhibitors encountered in tissue extracts. Accordingly, it was imperative to develop new, sensitive methodology in order to place our observations in quantitative perspective.

Amino acid esters and amides as substrates

N-α-tosyl-L-arginyl methyl ester (TAME), N-α-acetyl-L-lysine methyl ester (ALME), N-α-benzoyl-L-arginine anilide (BAA), and related substances are excellent substrates for trypsin, plasmin, and thrombin (*12*). By using substrates labeled with ^{3}H in the methanol or aniline moiety continuous enzyme assays can be carried out (*13, 14*). The reaction is carried out in a scintillation vial placed in a counter maintained at room temperature. The vial is filled with the usual toluene scintillant and a buffer phase containing the labeled substrate and enzyme. The unhydrolyzed substrate is concentrated in the water phase and as such is undetected by the phosphors. As hydrolysis proceeds, the liberated methanol or aniline passes into the toluene phase, giving rise to scintillation. The counts per minute are proportional to enzyme activity.

Protamine as substrate detection with Fluram

Methods used widely for the assay of proteases employ denatured proteins such as casein and urea-denatured hemoglobin as substrates (*15, 16*). The disadvantages reside in the lack of physical homogeneity of the substrate and in the requirement for separation of split peptides after precipitation with trichloroacetic acid. The basic protein, protamine, has attractive properties as substrate (*17, 18*). Arginine, a target for trypsin-like enzymes, comprises more than one-half the amino acid residues. Furthermore, arginine linkage is the preferred site for plasminogen activator. Protamine contains no lysine groups so that methods depending on the release of free amino groups for quantitation would not be complicated by high blanks. Finally, protamine (M.W. $\sim$ 5,000) exists in a single conformation, lacking tertiary structure, rendering the molecule more accessible to proteases than casein or hemoglobin. Amino groups can be assayed with speed and sensitivity by a fluorescence technique (*19*). The details of the method we have developed are published (*17*). Briefly, the enzyme to be quantitated is added to a solution of protamine chloride in borate or phosphate buffer. At the appropriate times a solution of 4-phenylspiro[Furan-2(3H), 1'-phthalan]-3,3'-dione (Fluram) in acetone is added and the fluorescence is read at 470 nm with activation at 390 nm. The protamine fluorescence blank is about 15% of that obtained after complete hydrolysis and can be rendered nil by using succinylated protamine as substrate (*18*). The protamine-Fluram method permits the linear assay of 5–500 ng trypsin in a 20-min incubation. Hydrolysis of protamine with thrombin, plasmin, and urokinase has been demonstrated. Consequently, the method is applicable to the quantitation of plasminogen activation simply by preincubating the enzyme to be tested with human plasminogen for a specified time prior to the addition of protamine. The advantages of this method over the fibrin plate method (20) are: (1) Fibrinogen is difficult to prepare free of contaminating serum factors, including proteases and their inhibitors. Protease (thrombin) must be added to produce fibrin plates. Exogenous proteases and inhibitors may perturb intracellular proteolytic systems under study. (2) The soluble substrate, protamine, provides a basis for steady-state assay conditions unhindered by biphasic interactions or by adsorption phenomena. (3) With plasminogen activator a linear assay is sensitive to subtle changes in activity and is also more accurate than a logarithmic one such as shown in the fibrin method.

Protease Activity in Tissue in the PMA-treated Mouse

Detection of protease

Groups of mice were treated with 1 μg PMA in acetone on one ear; whereas, the other ear (control) received acetone alone. At specified times mouse ears were excised, frozen in liquid nitrogen, and ground to a powder in a mortar and pestle. The powder was suspended in 0.05 M phosphate buffer, pH 7.5. The suspension was sonicated briefly, centrifuged at 10,000 rpm and aliquots of the supernatant were assayed for activity against ³H-TAME, ³H-ALME, and protamine (21).

The salient data presented in Table 1 indicate that the PMA-treated mouse ears exhibited more activities than the solvent controls. Hydrolysis of TAME was inhibited partially by N-α-tosyl-L-lysyl chloromethane (TLCK) and N-α-tosyl-L-phenylalanyl chloromethane (TPCK). On the other hand, protamine activity was inhibited completely by TLCK and not by TPCK, suggesting the presence of a mixture of enzymes. The enzyme hydrolysis of N-α-benzoyl-L-arginine ethyl ester in the mouse skin system is reported by Hozumi et al. (6), who also found that acetyl-L-leucyl-L-leucyl-L-argininal (Leupeptin) (22) is inhibitory.

TABLE 1.   Increased Esterase and Protease Activity in Mouse Skin 24 hr after Treatment with PMA

Skin homogenate treated with:	Specific activity		
	nM hydrolyzed/mg protein/hr		Fluorescence units/ mg protein/hr
	Substrate		Substrate
	TAME	ALME	Protamine
1.0 μg PMA in acetone	73	40	35
Acetone	22	21	0

Mouse ears were treated as described in text. Protein was determined with ninhydrin using crystalline bovine serum albumin as standard.

Inhibition of PMA promotion by protease inhibitors

The importance of the protease appearing in response to PMA was shown by using a variety of protease inhibitors. In the mouse ear model tumorigenesis was initiated with 7,12-dimethylbenz(a)anthracene (DMBA) and promoted with PMA. The time of first appearance of tumor was noted, but only tumors larger than 1 mm and persisting over 30 days were scored. Studies are carried out with 1 μg and 0.1 μg PMA. Applications (10 μg) of TLCK delayed the onset of tumor 50 days with 1 μg PMA and 200 days with 0.1 μg (Fig. 1).

The relative effectiveness of 1 μg TLCK, TPCK, and TAME were tested in studies where 5 μg croton oil was the promoter. Results presented in Table 2 indicate that they are all effective. TPCK virtually suppressed tumor formation for

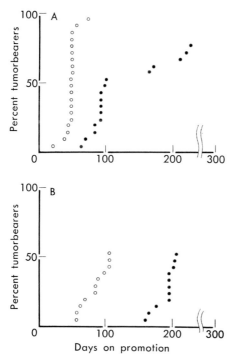

Fig. 1. Time patterns of appearance of skin tumors showing TLCK inhibition. Each point represents a single, tumor-bearing animal and is plotted according to the time of appearance of a grossly visible tumor. (A) Experiment 1. All animals were given an initiating treatment of 10 μg of DMBA in acetone. Three days after initiation, three applications per week of 1.0 μg of PMA in acetone was begun. ○ control animals ; ● animals that received 10.0 μg of TLCK together with PMA. Average time of tumor appearance in controls was 51.6 days ; in animals receiving TLCK it was increased to 122.4 days, a difference significant at $P<0.1$. The average number of tumors per animal was 2.57 for controls and 1.90 for animals receiving TLCK. This difference was significant at $P<0.05$ by a Student's t-test. (B) Experiment 2. All animals were treated as in experiment 1, except that doses of PMA and TLCK were reduced tenfold. ○ controls ; ● animals receiving TLCK. Average time of tumor appearance in controls was 83.9 days ; in animals receiving TLCK the average time was 189.6 days. Average numbers of tumors per animal were 0.71 and 0.52 for control and treated groups, respectively, not a significant difference. The difference in average time of appearance is significant at $P<0.005$.

TABLE 2. Inhibition of Tumorigenesis by Protease Inhibitors

Weeks on promotion	Inhibitor treatment							
	Control		TPCK		TLCK		TAME	
	T	S	T	S	T	S	T	S
10	8	19	0	21	0	21	0	21
12	10	19	0	21	0	21	0	21
14	11	19	0	21	1	21	3	21
16	11	19	0	21	4	21	5	21
18	11	19	0	21	4	21	5	21
20	11	19	0	21	4	21	5	21
22	11	19	0	21	5	21	5	21
24	11	19	1	21	5	21	5	21
30	11	19	1	21	5	21	5	21

Inhibition of tumorigenesis by protease inhibitors. All animals were given 10 μg of DMBA as initiator and then 5.0 μg of croton oil in acetone, applied 3 times weekly as promoter. The protease inhibitors TLCK, TPCK, and TAME were applied in DMSO 3 times weekly in 1.0 μg doses, 1 to 2 hr after applications of croton oil. All treatments were applied to ear skin of mice (the controls received DMSO alone). The average times of appearance of tumors in all 3 experimental groups are significantly different from the controls at $P<0.005$. T, number of tumor-bearing mice; S, number of survivors.

200 days and TLCK and TAME delayed and suppressed tumor formation below 50% of the control.

Inhibition of Tumor Promotion by Glucocorticoids

The mouse skin two-stage carcinogenesis is a model system for the neoplastic transformation or tumor progress. Two types of agents are involved. The primary agent initiator causes a permanent alteration which is expressed at the site where the second promoting agent is applied as a tumor. The action of the initiating agent (virtually all known carcinogens) is thought to involve the genetic material DNA. Support for this has come from the observation that virtually all carcinogens are bacterial mutagens (2, 3). On the other hand, promoting agents, *e.g.*, PMA

TABLE 3. Effect of Steroids on Tumor Incidence at 60 Days after Promotion with Croton Oil

Steroid	6 μg application		30 μg application	
	No. of papillomas/mouse	Mice with tumors (%)	No. of papillomas/mouse	Mice with tumors (%)
Control	8.4	80	8.4	80
Cortisone	8.4	75	2.8	64
Hydrocortisone	6.4	80	3.0	46
Prednisolone	5.2	60	2.0	36
Dexamethasone	0.4	18	0	0

Tumorigenesis in groups of 24 mice was initiated with 25 μg of DMBA in 0.2 ml of acetone. Thrice weekly treatments with 0.5% croton oil in 0.2 ml of acetone were begun 2 weeks later. The hormones were applied 5 times a week in 0.2 ml of acetone, starting at the same time as the croton oil.

or hormones are not mutagenic, but apparently induce proteases. The primary action of this induced enzyme in relation to tumor promotion may be to activate a portion of the genome. In addition, irritation of the type caused by the proteolytic activation of the complement system is observed. In this system a series of proteolytic enzymes are activated in a waterfall cascade after the door is opened by proteolytic activation of a trypsin-like protease (23). Both tumor promotion and irritation may be due to protease action, but involve separate actions of the enzyme. Both irritation and tumor promotion are inhibited by protease inhibitors.

The apparent relationship of inhibition of the irritation and tumor promotion led us to investigate the glucocorticosteroids with known anti-irritant properties as inhibitors of tumor promotion. We noted cortisone, hydrocortisone, prednisolone, and dexamethasone (Table 3) (24) inhibited tumor promotion in the same order as irritation.

The report of Wigler and Weinstein that dexamethasone significantly decreased the plasminogen activator concentration in HTC hepatoma cells revealed a new activity of the action of this hormone (25). We have confirmed the effect of

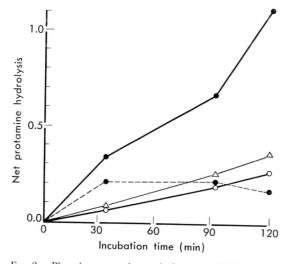

FIG. 2.   Plasminogen activator in lysates of HTC hepatoma cells treated and untreated with dexamethasone, and of a one-to-one mixture of dexamethasone and untreated lysates. ●—● dexamethasone-untreated cell lysate ;   △ buffer control ;   ●---● dexamethasone-treated cell lysate ;   ○ dexamethasone-treated and not.

TABLE 4.   Effect of Cytosol of Dexamethasone-treated or Untreated HTC Hepatoma Cells on Trypsin Hydrolysis of Protamine

	Relative protease activity with:	
	54 ng/ml trypsin	130 ng/ml trypsin
Buffer	100	187
Cytosol of treated cells	7	126
Cytosol of untreated cells	79	332

dexamethasone in the HTC-cell lysates obtained from Wigler and Weinstein using the protamine assay described above (*18*). Moreover, when we mixed cell from lysates with plasminogen activator, with those treated with 10^{-7} M dexamethasone, the plasminogen activator was decreased to the level of the dexamethasone-treated lysate (Fig. 2). This suggested the presence of a protease inhibitor in the dexamethasone-treated cells. This was confirmed by the demonstration of a trypsin inhibitor in these lysates (Table 4).

The Hormone-treated Ovariectomized Rat

While PMA is an interesting model promoter in mouse skin, it is unlikely that it has any role in human cancer. Sex hormones, on the other hand, have been considered possible promoters of uterine, breast, and prostatic cancer in man. We were able to demonstrate and partially characterize a trypsin-like protease elaborated by rat uterus in response to estradiol and estradiol plus progesterone treatment. The results of these experiments demonstrate that it is capable of activating human plasminogen.

In these studies young adult ovariectomized rats were divided into 3 groups and treated for 4 days twice daily. The first group (U) received sesame oil only. The second group (E) received estradiol and the third (EP) estradiol plus progesterone. On the fifth day the uteri were excised and subcellular fractions were prepared (*8, 26*). Protease were concentrated in nuclei and the $12,000 \times g$ granules obtained from the cytosol.

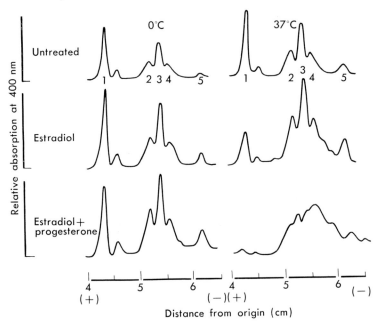

FIG. 3.   Polyacrylamide gel profiles of histones from uteri of hormone-treated, ovariectomized rats. Freshly prepared chromatin was incubated for 1 hr at 0 or 37°C, then histones were extracted and submitted to electrophoresis.

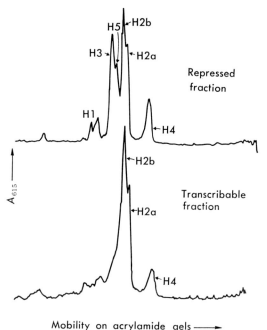

Fɪɢ. 4.   Polyacrylamide gel electrophoresis of the histones isolated from chromatin fractions. Histones extracted from 15 μg of each fraction were applied to each 10 cm gel and electrophoresed for 200 min at 2 mA/gel. From Berkowitz and Doty (*11*).

Induction of a nuclear protease

Protease activity was detected in the nucleus (associated with chromatin) using degradation of histones as the indicator. Incubation of chromatin for 1 hr at 37°C prior to extraction of histones resulted in extensive degradation of the histones from EP rat uteri, little degradation of that from E rats and no detectable breakdown of U rat histones (Fig. 3). Berkowitz and Doty (*11*) have successfully separated the transcriptionally active (TC) and repressed fraction (RC) from the 12-day-old chick embryo reticulocyte chromatin. The method involved sonication and sucrose density fractionation at 4°C. The total histone content of TC was 13% less than that of RC. The most striking difference between TC and RC was shown when histones were isolated and electrophoresed on polyacrylamide gels. The very lysine-rich histones H_1 and H_5 and one arginine-rich histone H_3 are absent from TC histones (Fig. 4). Comparison of this data with that obtained by Levitz *et al.* (*8*) (Figs. 3 and 4), reveal that the estradiol induced protease has carried out precisely the same histone deletion as observed by physical separation of the transcribable fraction by Berkowitz and Doty (*11*). This is in accord with recent experiments indicating that specific removal of histones may result in derepression of large regions of the chromatin, while much of the fine tuning of derepression is due to non-histone proteins (*27*).

Protease in the 12,000×g pellet

Extranuclear subcellular fractions were assayed for protease activity by the protamine method. Only the $12,000 \times g$ pellet was active. Activity was absent from the U rat uterine granules and was slightly higher in the E rat uterus as compared to the EP rat (Table 5). The specificity of the hormone-induced protease activity was shown in experiments in which diaphragm and thymus as well as uterus were examined. Only the uterus exhibited a significant response to sex hormone treatment.

The $12,000 \times g$ uterine pellets from U, E, and EP rats were submitted to several conditions designed to solubilize the protease(s). These included mechanical destruction, the combined application of thermal shock and detergent action, and

TABLE 5.   Protease Activity in the Extranuclear $12,000 \times g$ Pellet of Homogenates of Uteri from Hormone-treated Ovariectomized Rats

Experiment	Untreated	Hormone treatment	
		Estradiol	Estradiol+progesterone
1	3.0	33	16
2	2.5	19	13
3	5.0	30	20
4	2.5	30	19

In each experiment the $12,000 \times g$ pellets from at least 3 uteri were pooled and suspended in 0.25 M sucrose (0.4 ml per uterus). Values are in fluorescence units (per 100 μg of DNA of tissue) determined after incubation with protamine for 4 hr and reaction with Fluram. Only values greater than 4–5 can be considered significantly different from 0.

TABLE 6.   Plasminogen Activation by Extracts of Subcellular Fractions of Rat Uterus

Contents of incubation	$\varDelta$ fluorescent units/2hr
Plasminogen+protamine	1
$12,000 \times g$ supernate+protamine	3
$12,000 \times g$ supernate+plasminogen+protamine	15
Nuclear supernate+protamine	1
Nuclear supernate+plasminogen+protamine	12
Nuclear precipitate+protamine	0
Nuclear precipitate+plasminogen+protamine	6
Urokinase+protamine	0
Urokinase+plasminogen+protamine	13
Plasmin+protamine	17

Extracts are from uteri of ovariectomized rats treated with estradiol plus progesterone. The $12,000 \times g$ extranuclear pellet was incubated for 1 hr at 37°C and centrifuged. Then the supernate was tested. The nuclei were disrupted vigorously in a Polytron homogenizer, centrifuged and both the sediment and supernate were tested.   In the assay the extract was incubated with plasminogen for 1 hr, protamine was added and at specified times the protease activity was determined by the Fluram reaction.   In some controls the plasminogen was omitted, whereas in other controls, urokinase was tested in the complete system and plasmin was tested against protamine.   Note that levels of enzyme activity were selected such that in the absence of plasminogen minimal protease activity was observed.   Values presented are for 2-hr incubations with protamine.

autolysis. Autolysis gave the best results. Incubation of the $12,000 \times g$ pellet for 1 hr consistently solubilized about 50% of the protease activity. In no case was protease detected in either the soluble fraction or the pellet of the U rat.

Some of the properties of the crude solubilized protease were determined. The apparent Km toward protamine substrate is about 1.0×10^6 M. The maximum velocity is achieved by carrying out the incubations at about 45°C at pH of 8.5. The peptide aldehydes, Antipain, and Leupeptin, are effective inhibitors of the solubilized protease in the protamine-Fluram assay.

Another property of the proteases of the nucleus and $12,000 \times g$ pellet merits comment. The data in Table 6 indicate that the proteases of the $12,000 \times g$ pellet and nucleus are a plasminogen activator.

The Role of Protease in Carcinogenesis

Many roles for proteases in neoplastic transformation have been proposed. Some examples are: The removal of a cell surface glycoprotein (28); the activation of DNA polymerase by trypsin (29); the correlation of the transformed phenotype— morphology, cell locomotion, and anchorage-dependent growth in tissue culture to concentration and excretion of plasminogen activator (30, 31).

In this paper, we propose that proteases are involved in reprogramming the genome by removing repressors (10). The hopeful aspect of this concept is that reversal of genetic derepression by protease inhibitors or other means should lead to suppression of malignancy.

Indeed, the apparent reversal of a number of plant and animal tumors, including human neuroblastoma, have been ascribed to epigenetic reprogramming of the genome (32). Perhaps the best example of a correlation of suppression of tumorigenicity, together with a suppression of protease plasminogen activator, has been reported in mouse melanoma cells (33). Here, the plasminogen activator is not excreted in the presence of thymine analogue, 5-bromodeoxyuridine, together with a loss of tumorigenicity. The system is reversible in the absence of 5-bromodeoxyuridine plasminogen activator and tumorigenicity return. This presents a genetic reprogramming resulting in loss of tumorigenicity. The protease may be the reprogramming agent or a part of the genetic expression.

We are just at the beginning of understanding the mechanism of genetic expression of the eukaryote genome. The demonstration of inhibition of tumor promotion and estradiol action by specific protease inhibitors pointed to proteases as one of the agents responsible for derepression.

ACKNOWLEDGMENTS

We wish to thank Dr. Mort Levitz for his advice and assistance, Dr. Ellen Berkowitz for making her data available to us before publication, and Dr. Takashi Sugimura for his continued interest.

This work was supported by Grant NCI 16060, a grant from the National Bladder Cancer Project CA 15315, USPH ES 00606, and is part of a Center Program by the National Institute of Environmental Health Sciences Grant ES-00260.

REFERENCES

1. Boutwell, R. K. The function and mechanism of promoters of carcinogenesis. CRC Crit. Rev. Toxicol., p. 419, 1974.

2. Mukai, F. and Troll, W. The mutagenicity and initiating activity of some aromatic amine metabolites. Ann. N. Y. Acad. Sci., *163*: 828, 1969.

3. McCann, J., Choi, E., Yamasaki, E., and Ames, B. Detection of carcinogens as mutagens in the *Salmonella*/microsome test: Assay of 300 chemicals. Proc. Natl. Acad. Sci. U.S., *72*: 5135, 1975.

4. Rous, P. and Kidd, J. G. Conditional neoplasm and subthreshold neoplastic states. A study of tar tumors in rabbits. J. Exp. Med., *73*: 765, 1941.

5. Berenblum, I. A reevaluation of the concept of cocarcinogenesis. Prog. Exp. Tumor Res., *11*: 21, 1969.

6. Hozumi, M., Ogawa, M., Sugimura, T., Takeuchi, T., and Umezawa, H. Inhibition of tumorigenesis in mouse skin by Leupeptin, a protease inhibitor from *Actinomycetes*. Cancer Res., *32*: 1725, 1972.

7. Furth, J. Hormones as etiological agents in neoplasia. *In;* F. F. Becker (ed.), Cancer, a Comprehensive Treatise, pp. 75–120, Plenum Press, New York, 1975.

8. Levitz, M., Katz, J., Krone, P., Prochoroff, N. N., and Troll, W. Hormonal influences on histones and template activity in the rat uterus. Endocrinology, *94*: 633, 1974.

9. Katz, J., Troll, W., Russo, J., Filkins, K., and Levitz, M. Effect of protease inhibitors on *in vitro* breakdown of uterine histones from hormone treated rats. Endocr. Res. Commun., *1*: 331, 1974.

10. Troll, W., Rossman, T., Katz, J., Levitz, M.,and Sugimura, T. Proteinases in tumor promotion and hormone action. *In;* E. Reich, D. B. Rifkin, and E. Shaw (eds.), Proteases and Biological Control, p. 977, Cold Spring Harbor Laboratory, New York, 1975.

11. Berkowitz, E. M. and Doty, P. Chemical and physical properties of fractionated chromatin. Proc. Natl. Acad. Sci. U.S., *72*: 3328, 1975.

12. Troll, W., Sherry, S., and Wachman, J. The action of plasmin on synthetic substrates. J. Biol. Chem., *208*: 85, 1954.

13. Roffman, S., Sanocka, U., and Troll, W. Sensitive proteolytic enzyme assay using differential solubilities of radioactive substrates and products in biphasic systems. Anal. Biochem., *36*: 11, 1970.

14. Roffman, S. and Troll, W. Microassay for proteolytic enzymes using a new radioactive anilide substrate. Anal. Biochem., *61*: 1, 1974.

15. Anson, M. L. The estimation of pepsin, trypsin, papain and cathepsin with hemoglobin. J. Gen. Physiol., *22*: 79, 1938.

16. Schwabe, C. A fluorescent assay for proteolytic enzymes. Anal. Biochem., *53*: 484, 1973.

17. Brown, F., Freedman, M. L., and Troll, W. Sensitive fluorescent determination of trypsin-like proteases. Biochem. Biophys. Res. Commun., *53*: 75, 1973.

18. Kessner, A. and Troll, W. Fluorometric microassay of plasminogen activators. Hormonal effects on physiological levels. Submitted to Arch. Biochem. Biophys., 1975.

19. Udenfriend, S., Stein, S., Bohlen, P., Dairman, W., Leimgruber, W., and Weigele, M. Fluorescamine: A reagent for assay of amino acids, peptides, proteins, and primary amines in the picomole range. Science, *178*: 871, 1972.

20. Unkeless, J., Dano, K., Kellerman, G. M., and Reich, E. Fibrinolysis associated with oncogenic transformation: Partial purification and characterization of the cell factor, a plasminogen activator. J. Biol. Chem., *249*: 4295, 1974.
21. Troll, W., Klassen, A., and Janoff, A. Tumorigenesis in mouse skin: Inhibition by synthetic inhibitors of proteases. Science, *169*: 1211, 1970.
22. Maeda, K., Kamamura, K., Kondo, S., Aoyagi, T., Takeuchi, T., and Umezawa, H. The structure and activity of leupeptins and related analogs. J. Antibiol., *24*: 402, 1971.
23. Christman, J. K., Silverstein, S. C., and Acs, G. Plasminogen Activator, Chapt. 4, ASP Biological & Medical Press, Great Britain, 1976, in press.
24. Belman, S. and Troll, W. The inhibition of croton oil-promoted mouse skin tumorigenesis by steroid hormones. Cancer Res., *32*: 450, 1972.
25. Wigler, M., Ford, J. P., and Weinstein, I. B. Glucocorticoid inhibition of the fibrinolytic activity of tumor cells. *In;* E. Reich, D. B. Rifkin, and E. Shaw (eds), Proteases and Biological Control, p. 849, Cold Spring Harbor Laboratory, New York, 1975.
26. Szego, C. M., Seeler, B. J., Steadman, R. A., Hill, D. F., Kimura, A. K., and Roberts, J. A. The lysosomal membrane complex: Focal point of primary steroid hormone action. J. Biochem., *123*: 523, 1971.
27. Chiu, J. F., Wang, S., Fusitani, H., and Hnilica, L. S. DNA-binding chromosomal non-histone proteins. Isolation, characterization and tissue specificity. Biochemistry, *14*: 4552, 1975.
28. Yamada, K. M. and Weston, J. A. The synthesis, turnover, and artificial restoration of a major cell surface glycoprotein. Cell, *5*: 75, 1975.
29. Brown, R. L. and Stubbelfield, E. Enhancement of DNA synthesis in a mammalian cell-free system by trypsin treatment. Proc. Natl. Acad. Sci. U.S., *71*: 2432, 1974.
30. Ossowski, L., Quigley, J. P., Kellerman, G. M., and Reich, E. Fibrinolysis associated with oncogenic transformation. J. Exp. Med., *138*: 1056, 1973.
31. Pollack, R., Risser, R., Conlon, S., and Rifkin, D. Plasminogen activator production accompanies loss of anchorage regulation transformation of primary rat embryo cells by Simian virus 40. Proc. Natl. Acad. Sci. U.S., *71*: 4792, 1974.
32. Braun, A. C. The Biology of Cancer, Addison-Wesley Publishing Co., Reading, Massachusetts, 1974.
33. Christman, J. K., Silagi, S., Newcomb, E. W., Silverstein, S. C., and Acs, G. Correlated suppression by 5-bromodeoxyuridine of tumorigenicity and plasminogen activator in mouse melanoma cells. Proc. Natl. Acad. Sci. U.S., *72*: 47, 1975.

Discussion of Paper of Dr. Troll

DR. HOZUMI: In preventing the effect of estradiol on the uterus histone patterns, is it specific for antipain?

In your earlier work, you reported on the inhibition of the so-called initiation process of skin carcinogenesis. Is it really possible to inhibit the initiation process of carcinogenesis by protease inhibitors?

DR. TROLL: Leupeptin works too. Leupeptin plus antipain appear more effective together than either alone.

Initiation is not inhibited by nontoxic levels of protease inhibitors but the complete carcinogenicity of dibenzanthracene upon repeated application is inhibited (Proc. Am. Assoc. Cancer Res., *13*: 75, 1972).

DR. FARBER: One major complicating factor in attempting to relate tumor promotion to protease activity in the skin is the almost uniform occurrence of an infiltration of polymorphonuclear leukocytes. These cells have very active proteases. Therefore, any attempt to relate the antipromotion effect of protease inhibitors to changes in gene repression or gene activation must rule out the leukocytes as the targets. Do you have any evidence relating to this serious complication?

DR. TROLL: Protease inhibitors prevent the invasion of leukocytes and polymorphs. Thus, the induction of the initial protease-plasminogen activator must precede the invasion of leukocytes. Our measurement after 24 hr may include the leukocyte protease which needs sorting out. We have no such complication in the estradiol induction of the plasminogen activator.

DR. CRADDOCK: Is it possible that proteases used in washing powders could be carcinogenic?

DR. TROLL: I have not found papain to be a promoter in skin.

DR. RAJEWSKY: Dr. Troll, I wonder how you distinguish between the possibilities that, on the one hand, proteases activate gene transcription (*e.g.*, by removal of lysine-rich histone), and on the other, that when a certain portion of the genome is transcribed (as indicated by the absence of lysine-rich histone), protease is just a resulting protein expressed?

DR. TROLL: This is a question of which is first: the chicken or the egg. Since protease inhibitors prevent the action of the tumor promoter which induces the protease we feel that the protease is a participant causing gene depression, not merely an indicator enzyme such as ornithine decarboxylase (Cancer Res., *35*: 2426, 1975).

DR. GOLDTHWAIT: Is it possible that the lysine-rich histones are decreased in any normal, rapidly dividing cell?

DR. TROLL: This is certainly worth investigating. I am not sure what the answer is. I would expect lysine-rich histone to be absent, in any case, where protease levels are high.

DR. OKADA: You seem to rule out papain from "proteases" involved in the promotion process. Could you tell us what types of "proteases" are involved in this process?

DR. TROLL: We believe it to be a serine protease of the plasminogen activator type.

FUNDAMENTALS IN CANCER PREVENTION, P. N. MAGEE ET AL. (EDS.),
UNIV. OF TOKYO PRESS, TOKYO / UNIV. PARK PRESS, BALTIMORE, PP. 57–69, 1976

Effects of Protease-Inhibitors of Microbial Origin
on Experimental Carcinogenesis

Taijiro Matsushima,[*1] Tadao Kakizoe,[*2] Takashi Kawachi,[*2]
Kazuko Hara,[*1] Takashi Sugimura,[*2] Tomio Takeuchi,[*3] and
Hamao Umezawa[*1]

*Institute of Medical Science, University of Tokyo,[*1] National Cancer Center Research Institute,[*2] and
Institute of Microbial Chemistry,[*3] Tokyo, Japan*

Abstract: Inhibition of mouse skin tumorigenesis by protease-inhibitors was demonstrated by the pioneer work of Troll *et al.* and thus the important role played by protease in the carcinogenesis process was revealed. Tumor induction is apparently suppressed by protease-inhibitors through the inhibition of the promotion process in the two-stage skin carcinogenesis. A new approach to cancer prevention has been opened by this discovery of the inhibition of carcinogenesis by protease-inhibitors.

Several protease-inhibitors isolated from culture media of *Actinomycetes* have been characterized. These protease-inhibitors are non-toxic to small experimental animals and are suitable for use in the evaluation of the usefulness of protease-inhibitors in the prevention of cancer. The effects of leupeptin, one of protease-inhibitors of microbial origin, on chemical carcinogenesis studied in our laboratories and other laboratories in Japan are reviewed.

Leupeptin, N-acetyl (or N-propionyl)-L-leucyl-L-leucyl-L-argininal, partially suppressed tumor formation in the colon, esophagus, mammary gland of rats and in the skin of mice, and retarded leukemia induction in mice. On the other hand, leupeptin did not show any inhibitory effect on tumor formation in the liver and fore-stomach of rats and in the lung of mice, but instead enhanced tumor growth in the case of glandular stomach and bladder of rats. Leupeptin also enhanced in mice leukemia induction by X-ray.

The effects of leupeptin on carcinogenesis varied with species, organs, nature of carcinogen, and schedule of carcinogen administration. Factors which still need to be evaluated are the dosage and route of administration of the protease-inhibitors.

Prevention of cancer is an important aspect in the conquest of cancer and several approaches have been considered. Inhibition of tumorigenesis is one such approach, and many different kinds of substances have been found to inhibit tumorigenesis (1). Substances which modify the metabolic activation of carcinogens, those which enhance the detoxication of carcinogens, those which compete for target macromolecules with carcinogens, and so on, all inhibited tumor formation. A new approach to cancer prevention has been opened by the discovery of the inhibition of carcinogenesis by protease-inhibitors.

Carcinogenesis usually has a long latent period between exposure to carcinogen and tumor appearance, and several processes take place successively during this period. Protease plays an important role in the carcinogenic process, and protease-inhibitor has been shown to inhibit tumor formation. This was first demonstrated by the pioneer work of Troll et al. (2), who reported that synthetic protease inhibitors, such as N-α-tosyl-L-phenylalanyl-chloromethane and N-α-tosyl-L-lysyl-chloromethane, suppressed the two-stage mouse skin tumorigenesis. Mouse skin tumor formation was initiated by painting the carcinogen, 7, 12-dimethylbenz[a] anthracene (DMBA), and was promoted by repeated application of croton oil. Tumor induction was suppressed by the protease inhibitor through inhibition of the promotion process in the chemical carcinogenesis. This inhibition of tumorigenesis was confirmed by Hozumi et al. (3), using another type of protease-inhibitor. Leupeptin, a protease-inhibitor of microbial origin, also exhibited the suppression of mouse skin tumor formation induced by painting of DMBA, followed by croton oil. Experiments on the effects of leupeptin on chemical carcinogenesis which were carried out in our laboratories and in other laboratories in Japan are reviewed.

Protease-inhibitors of Microbial Origin

Several protease-inhibitors, isolated from culture media of *Actinomycetes*, were characterized by Umezawa and his associates (4). These protease-inhibitors have potent and highly specific inhibitory characteristics. The concentrations of in-

TABLE 1.   Specificity of Protease-inhibitors of Microbial Origin

Protease-inhibitor	Protease	ID_{50} (μg/ml)
Leupeptin	Trypsin	2
	Papain	0.5
	Plasmin	8
	Cathepsin B	0.44
Antipain	Trypsin	0.26
	Papain	0.16
	Cathepsin A	1.19
	Cathepsin B	0.60
Chymostatin	α-Chymotrypsin	0.15
	Cathepsin B	2.6
Pepstatin	Pepsin	0.0031
	Rennin	4.5
	Cathepsin D	0.011
Elastatinal	Elastase	1.8

ID_{50} is the concentration of inhibitors required for 50% inhibition of protease activity.

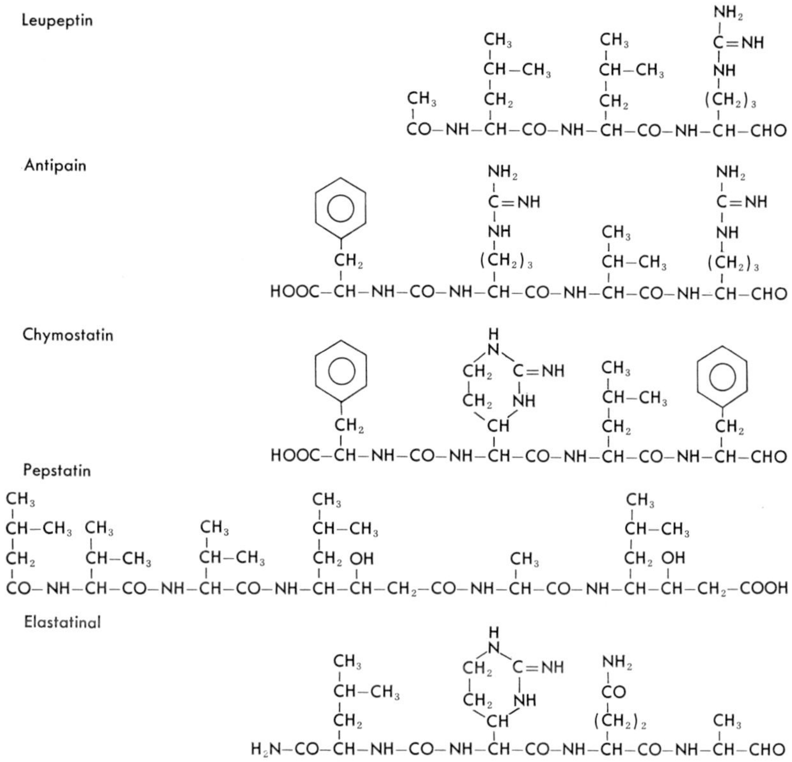

Leupeptin

```
                                         NH₂
                                          |
                 CH₃        CH₃          C=NH
                  |          |            |
                 CH−CH₃     CH−CH₃        NH
                  |          |            |
        CH₃       CH₂        CH₂         (CH₂)₃
         |        |          |            |
        CO−NH−CH−CO−NH−CH−CO−NH−CH−CHO
```

Antipain

```
                            NH₂              NH₂
                             |                |
                            C=NH             C=NH
                 ⬡           |                |
                            NH      CH₃       NH
                 |           |       |        |
                CH₂        (CH₂)₃    CH−CH₃  (CH₂)₃
                 |           |       |        |
        HOOC−CH−NH−CO−NH−CH−CO−NH−CH−CO−NH−CH−CHO
```

Chymostatin

```
                             H
                             N
                            ╱  ╲
                          CH₂   C=NH    CH₃
                           |    |        |
                          CH₂   NH      CH−CH₃       ⬡
                 ⬡          ╲   ╱        |
                 |           CH          CH₂          |
                CH₂          |           |           CH₂
                 |           |           |            |
        HOOC−CH−NH−CO−NH−CH−CO−NH−CH−CO−NH−CH−CHO
```

Pepstatin

```
CH₃                         CH₃                      CH₃
 |                           |                        |
CH−CH₃ CH₃         CH₃      CH−CH₃                    CH−CH₃
 |      |           |        |            CH₃         |
CH₂    CH−CH₃      CH−CH₃   CH₂ OH         |          CH₂ OH
 |      |           |        |            |           |
CO−NH−CH−CO−NH−CH−CO−NH−CH−CH−CH₂−CO−NH−CH−CO−NH−CH−CH−CH₂−COOH
```

Elastatinal

```
                             H
                             N
                            ╱  ╲
                          CH₂   C=NH    NH₂
                 CH₃       |    |        |
                  |       CH₂   NH       CO
                 CH−CH₃    ╲   ╱         |
                  |         CH          (CH₂)₂        CH₃
                 CH₂        |            |            |
                  |         |            |            |
        H₂N−CO−CH−NH−CO−NH−CH−CO−NH−CH−CO−NH−CH−CHO
```

Fig. 1. Chemical structures of protease-inhibitors of microbial origin.

hibitors needed to inhibit 50% of the protease activity, ID_{50}, are indicated in Table 1. Leupeptin inhibits trypsin, papain, plasmin, and cathepsin B, and antipain inhibits trypsin, papain, and cathepsin A and B. Chymostatin is an inhibitor of chymotrypsin and cathepsin B. Pepstatin is an inhibitor of acid proteases and inhibits pepsin, rennin, and cathepsin D. Elastatinal inhibits elastase. As shown in Fig. 1, these protease-inhibitors have oligopeptide-like structures with a substituted N-terminal amino-group. Leupeptin, antipain, chymostatin, and elastatinal have an aldehyde group instead of a carboxyl group at the C-terminal. This aldehyde group in these four inhibitors is essential for anti-protease activity. Pepstatin has a different structure from the other four, and has a substituted heptanoic acid, 3-hydroxy-4-amino-6-methyl-heptanoic acid at the C-terminal. These protease-inhibitors are non-toxic to rat and mouse, as shown by the LD_{50} values in Table 2. Leupeptin dissolved in buffered saline and injected intraperitoneally, at a dosage of 5 mg/100 g body weight twice a day for 3 weeks, did not show any effect on the growth of rat. Therefore, these protease-inhibitors are suitable compounds for use in the evaluation of the usefulness of protease-inhibitors in the prevention of cancer.

Leupeptin, N-acetyl (or N-propionyl)-L-leucyl-L-leucyl-L-argininal, suppressed mouse skin tumor formation induced by DMBA and croton oil (3). Therefore, the effects of leupeptin on other chemical carcinogenesis were studied. In these experiments, leupeptin was given to the animal by feeding a pellet diet containing

TABLE 2. Toxicity of Protease-inhibitors of Microbial Origin

Protease-inhibitor	Route of administration	Acute toxicity LD$_{50}$ (mg/kg)	
		Mice	Rats
Leupeptin	i.v.	118	125
	s.c.	1,450	>4,000
	p.o.	1,550	>4,000
Antipain	i.v.	187	
	s.c.	>500	
	p.o.	>500	
Chymostatin	i.p.	>500	
Pepstatin	i.p.	1,090	875
	p.o.	>2,000	>2,000
Elastatinal	i.v.	>250	

i.v. : intravenous. i.p. : intraperitoneal. s.c. : subcutaneous. p.o. : per os.

0.1% leupeptin. Leupeptin did not affect body weight gain of rats when they were fed for 30 weeks or more on a pellet diet containing 0.1% leupeptin.

Effect of Leupeptin on Carcinogenesis in Rat

Table 3 is a summary of the effects of leupeptin on chemical carcinogenesis in rat. Leupeptin suppressed tumor formation in the colon, esophagus, and mammary gland of rats, but showed no effect on tumor formation in the fore-stomach and liver of rats. On the other hand, leupeptin enhanced the growth of tumors in the glandular stomach and urinary bladder. In all experiments, leupeptin was given to the animals in a diet mixed with leupeptin at 0.1% concentration.

TABLE 3. Effects of Leupeptin on Chemical Carcinogenesis in Rat

Tumor site	Carcinogen	Effect	Reference
Colon	Azoxymethane	Inhibition	Yamamoto et al. (5)
Esophagus	Butylnitrosourethan	Inhibition	Takayama et al. (9)
Mammary gland	DMBA	Inhibition	Fukui et al. (10)
Glandular stomach	MNNG	Enhancement	Kawachi et al. (7)
Bladder	Butyl-(4-hydroxybutyl) nitrosamine	Enhancement	Kakizoe et al. (8)
Fore-stomach	Butylnitrosourethan	No effect	Takayama et al. (9)
Liver	Diethylnitrosamine	No effect	Takayama et al. (9)

1. Colon tumor

Leupeptin suppressed colon tumor formation induced by azoxymethane in the rat (5). Colon tumors were formed in male Donryu rats by subcutaneous injection of azoxymethane (0.1 mmole per kg body weight) once weekly for 10 weeks and tumor formation was observed 30 weeks after the first injection. Leupeptin was given to rat for entire experimental period. Only colon tumors developed and no small intestine tumor was observed. This is in agreement with the case of

TABLE 4. Colon Tumor Formation in Rat Treated with Azoxymethane

Group	No. of rats		Incidence (%)	Average No. of tumors per rat	Average diameter of tumors (mm)
	Total	With tumor			
Basal-diet	15	13	87	3.9±0.7	4.6±0.3
Leupeptin-diet	25	18	72	1.8±0.5	5.4±0.5

the BDIX rat, reported by Druckrey and Lange (6). Table 4 shows the results of a colon tumor experiment. The incidence of colon tumor in leupeptin-diet group was 72% which is slightly less than that of basal-diet group. However, the average number of tumors per rat was 3.9 ± 0.7 in basal-diet group and 1.8 ± 0.5 in leupeptin-diet group. This difference is significant ($P < 0.005$). Therefore, it can be safely concluded that leupeptin suppressed colon tumor formation. However, the average size of colon tumors was almost the same between the two groups. Incidences of polypoid adenoma and adenocarcinoma were also not significantly different between the two groups.

2. Glandular stomach tumor

Leupeptin did not show any inhibitory effect on tumor formation but instead enhanced tumor growth in the glandular stomach (7). Glandular stomach tumors were induced in male Wistar rats by giving drinking water containing 83 μg/ml N-methyl-N′-nitro-N-nitrosoguanidine (MNNG) for 6 months and tumor formation was examined at the 12th month. Rats were fed a pellet diet containing 0.1% leupeptin, either for the entire experimental period (12 months), or after the carcinogen administration was completed (6 months). The results are shown in Table 5. There was no significant difference in tumor incidence between basal-diet and leupeptin-diet groups, nor in the average number of tumors developed in the glandular stomach of these groups. However, the average size of tumors in the leupeptin-diet group was almost 4 times larger than that of the basal-diet group. The difference in the tumor size between these groups was significant ($P < 0.05$). In this case, leupeptin apparently enhanced tumor growth.

TABLE 5. Glandular Stomach Tumor Formation in Rats by MNNG

Group	No. of rats		Incidence (%)	Average No. of tumors per rat	Average size of tumors (mm)
	Total	With tumor			
Basal-diet	11	9	82	1.4	3.8×2.7
Leupeptin-diet (Entire period; 12 months)	13	8	62	1.4	7.1×5.2
Leupeptin-diet (After MNNG administration; 6 months)	16	11	69	1.7	7.2×5.3

3. Urinary bladder tumor

Leupeptin also enhanced the growth of urinary bladder tumors induced by N-butyl-N-(4-hydroxybutyl)nitrosamine (8). Male Wistar rats were given drink-

TABLE 6.   Bladder Tumor Formation in Rats Treated with Butyl-(4-hydroxybutyl) nitrosamine

Group	No. of rats		Incidence (%)	Average No. of tumors per rat	Average weight of bladder with tumors (g)
	Total	With tumor			
Basal-diet	15	14	93	3.1±1.7	0.26±0.22
Leupeptin-diet	14	14	100	3.4±1.8	2.14±2.10

ing water containing 0.05% of N-butyl-N-(4-hydroxybutyl)nitrosamine for 6 weeks. After ceasing the carcinogen administration, rats were fed a pellet diet with or without 0.1% leupeptin for 30 weeks. As shown in Table 6, the number of tumor-bearing animals and the average number of urinary bladder tumors per rat were not significantly different between the two groups. However, the mean weight of bladder with tumors of the leupeptin-diet group was 2.14±2.10 g which was 8 times heavier than that of the basal-diet group (0.26±0.22 g). This difference was statistically significant ($P<0.05$). There was no significant difference in the incidence of hyperplasia, papilloma, cancer, and squamous metaplasia between the two groups.

4.   Esophagus and fore-stomach tumors

Leupeptin suppressed squamous cell carcinoma formation by butylnitroso-urethan in the esophagus, but not in the fore-stomach (9). Butylnitrosourethan (0.4 mg/ml) was given to male Sprague-Dawley rats in drinking water 5 days a week for 20 weeks. Tumor formation was examined at the 30th week. The results are shown in Table 7. Tumors were induced either in the esophagus or the fore-stomach and at both sites in some cases. There was no remarkable difference in the incidence of tumors in esophagus and fore-stomach between the basal-diet group and the leupeptin-diet group. However, the frequency of squamous cell carcinoma among tumors induced in esophagus was 62% in the basal-diet group and only 32% in the leupeptin-diet group. There was no significant difference in the frequency of squamous cell carcinoma in the fore-stomach, 43% in the basal-diet group and 40% in leupeptin-diet group. Leupeptin suppressed squamous cell carcinoma formation in the esophagus, but not in the fore-stomach.

TABLE 7.   Esophagus and Fore-stomach Tumor Formation in Rats Induced with Butylnitrosourethan

Group	Total No. of rats	No. of rats with tumors in:			Incidence (%)
		Esophagus	Fore-stomach	Esophagus + fore-stomach	
Basal-diet	21	6	4	10	95
Leupeptin-diet	25	7	9	9	100

5.   Mammary tumor

Leupeptin suppressed mammary tumor formation induced by DMBA (10). DMBA was injected into female Sprague-Dawley rats from the tail vein at a dosage of 3 mg per rat on day 1 and day 4. Tumor formation was examined 120 days after the first injection. Leupeptin was fed in the diet of rats from 7 days before the first injection of DMBA to the end of experiment.

While the incidence of rat bearing mammary tumor was almost the same in both basal-diet group (100%) and leupeptin-diet group (96%), the average number of mammary tumors per rat was decreased by feeding leupeptin from 6.2 ± 3.8 in the basal-diet group to 3.3 ± 1.9 in the leupeptin-diet group. This difference was significant ($P < 0.01$). The average weight of mammary tumors was 10.4 ± 14.9 g in the basal-diet group and 4.4 ± 4.7 g in the leupeptin-diet group. The average latent period of induction of mammary tumors was also delayed by 11 days through leupeptin administration from 66 days in the basal-diet group to 77 days in the leupeptin-diet group.

6.   Liver tumor

Leupeptin showed no effect on liver tumor formation induced by diethylnitrosamine (9). Male Sprague-Dawley rats were given 100 ppm of diethylnitrosamine in drinking water for 10 weeks. Rats were fed a diet containing 0.1% leupeptin during this 10-week period of diethylnitrosamine administration. Tumor incidence was examined at the 30th week. The incidence of rats having liver tumors was 63% in the basal-diet group and 73% in the leupeptin-diet group.

Effect of Leupeptin on Experimental Carcinogenesis in Mouse

Table 8 is a summary of the effects of leupeptin on experimental carcinogenesis in mouse. Leupeptin markedly inhibited skin tumor induction by DMBA followed by croton oil and extended the induction time of leukemia formation by N-nitrosobutylurea (NBU). However, leupeptin increased the frequency of leukemia induction by X-ray irradiation. Leupeptin did not show any inhibitory effect on lung tumor formation by urethan.

TABLE 8.   Effects of Leupeptin on Carcinogenesis in Mouse

Tumor	Carcinogenic agent	Effect	Reference
Skin tumor	DMBA	Inhibition	Hozumi et al. (3)
Leukemia	NBU	Inhibition	Kakizoe et al. (unpublished)
Leukemia	X-ray	Enhancement	Kasuga et al. (11)
Lung tumor	Urethan	No effect	Matsushima et al. (unpublished)

1.   Skin tumor

Leupeptin markedly inhibited the skin tumor formation initiated by DMBA and promoted by repeated treatment of croton oil (3). Female ICR mice were given 125 μg of DMBA in 0.25 ml of acetone by a single painting on the back. After 3 weeks, 0.25 ml of 0.03% croton oil in acetone was painted 3 times a week for 30 weeks. Leupeptin solution in dimethylsulfoxide (DMSO) (0.25 ml) was painted 2 hr after croton oil painting at two-dose levels, 0.25 and 1.25 mg per mouse. The results are shown in Table 9. Leupeptin markedly inhibited not only the incidence of skin tumors, but also the fequency of the average number of

TABLE 9. Skin Tumor Formation in Mice by DMBA and Croton Oil

Treatment	Croton oil applications					
	At 10th week			At 30th week		
	No. of mice		Total No. of tumors	No. of mice		Total No. of tumors
	Total	With tumor		Total	With tumor	
DMSO	30	11	78	28	24	194
Leupeptin (0.25 mg)	30	2	3	26	9	48
Leupeptin (1.25 mg)	28	4	11	26	11	44

tumors per mouse. This inhibition of the promotion process, in the two-stage skin tumorigenesis, by protease-inhibitor of microbial origin confirmed the work of Troll *et al.* (2) who showed for the first time the inhibition of chemical carcinogenesis by protease-inhibitor. This work triggered the following studies on the effects of leupeptin on other chemical carcinogenesis in rats and mice.

2. Leukemia induction by NBU

Leupeptin extended the induction time of lymphoblastic leukemia formation in mice by NBU (Kakizoe *et al.*, unpublished). Female ICR/JCL mice were given 0.02% solution of NBU as drinking water for 10 weeks. Mice received a 0.1% leupeptin containing diet for either the entire experimental period or after the carcinogen administration was completed. Total observation period was 40 weeks. The results are shown in Table 10. Leupeptin did not show any effect on the incidence of lymphoblastic leukemia. However, leupeptin extended the induction time of leukemia. Leukemia was induced within 18 weeks in mice of the basal-diet group, but leukemia induction was retarded in mice of the leupeptin-diet group. While 80% of mice in both leupeptin-diet groups became leukemia within 18 weeks, 20% of mice became leukemia after 20 to 34 weeks. The average time of leukemia appearance was 100 days in the basal-diet group; 115 days in the leupeptin-diet group, in which leupeptin was given from the beginning of experiment through the entire period; and 112 days in the leupeptin-diet group, in which leupeptin was given after carcinogen administration was completed. Clearer effect of leupeptin might have been shown if the dose-schedule of carcinogen administration had been lower.

TABLE 10. Leukemia Induction in Mice by NBU

Group	No. of mice		Incidence (%)	Average time of appearance of leukemia (days)
	Total	With leukemia		
Basal-diet	21	20	95	100 ± 17
Leupeptin-diet (Entire period)	23	23	100	115 ± 50
Leupeptin-diet (After NBU administration)	19	19	100	112 ± 43

3.   Leukemia induction by X-ray

Leupeptin increased the frequency of lymphoblastic leukemia induction by X-ray (11). Female C57BL/6J mice were irradiated with 170R 4 times, at intervals of 7 days. Leupeptin-diet (0.1%) was fed for 35 days from 1 day before the initial irradiation until 5 days after the final irradiation. The incidence of generalized lymphoma was 18% in the basal-diet group and 20% in the leupeptin-diet group. However, the incidence of thymoma was 27% in the basal-diet group and 72% in the leupeptin-diet group. The latent period of lymphoblastic leukemia formation was shortened by leupeptin administration, from 113 days in the basal-diet group to 101 days in the leupeptin-diet group. Apparently leupeptin enhanced leukemia induction by X-ray.

Leupeptin showed an inconsistent effect on lymphoblastic leukemia induction by NBU and X-ray. The inconsistency may be due to the differences in the strain of mice and the mode of latent virus induction.

4.   Lung tumor

Leupeptin did not show any inhibitory effect on lung tumor formation by urethan (Matsushima et al., unpublished). Female A mice were given urethan at a dosage of 1 g per kg body weight in a single subcutaneous injection. Lung tumor incidence was determined after 16 weeks. Leupeptin (0.1%) feeding was started 1 week before the urethan injection and continued until the end of the experiment. There was no difference in the incidence of tumor-bearing mice, as well as in the average number of lung tumors per mouse which was 22.2 ± 9.6 in the basal-diet group and 19.6 ± 10.0 in the leupeptin-diet group.

Protease Inhibition by Leupeptin

The effects of leupeptin on carcinogenesis varied with species, sex, organs, nature of carcinogen, and route or schedule of carcinogen administration.   However, if the protease inhibition is classified according to the type of inhibition, a better relationship can be seen.

Croton oil is a promoter of skin carcinogenesis and activates skin proteases. Hozumi et al. (3) observed an increase in protease activity on mouse skin after croton oil treatment. This activated protease activity of skin was inhibited in vitro by leupeptin. Moreover, the increase in protease activity in mouse skin treated with croton oil was also abolished in vivo by leupeptin painting. Thus, leupeptin inhibited the protease(s) function in the promotion process of carcinogenesis. Troll et al. (12) also reported the activation of proteases in mouse skin by phorbol-12-myristate-13-acetate, the active principle of croton oil. They suggested that a mixture of proteases may be present, judging from the inhibition behavior by N-α-tosyl-L-lysyl-chloromethane and N-α-tosyl-L-phenylalanyl-choloromethane.

In the case of breast tumor formation, a hormone could act as the promoter and activate the proteases. Katz et al. (13) reported the activation of protease in the nuclei of uterus cells from sex hormone-treated ovariectomized rat, and the degradation of histone. Leupeptin and antipain inhibited the activated protease in the uterus. Katz *et al.* (*14*) observed the induced protease activity in the 12,000 g pellets (lysosome) obtained from the uterus of ovariectomized rat treated with estradiol or estradiol plus progesterone. The hormone-induced proteases were plasminogen activators.

Activated lysosomal proteases might have attacked chromatin and modified the template activity of the gene. This caused the promotion of the transformed cells to malignant tumor cells. The inhibition of activated lysosomal proteases resulted in a reduced number of tumor induction. One candidate for a protease in the promotion process is plasminogen activator (*12*). However, the protease working in the promotion process may not be a single species and may be different from organ to organ. This might have been one possibility for the inconsistent effect of leupeptin on carcinogenesis.

On the other hand, leupeptin could inhibit the action of proteases which are associated with the exfoliation process of epithelial cells. Such may be the case in glandular stomach and bladder tumors. In these cases, the protease-inhibitor suppressed the normal action of proteases which favor the removal of tumor cells. Thus, the tumors became larger in the leupeptin-diet group than in the basal-diet group and protease-inhibitor apparently stimulated tumor growth. This conclusion is reinforced by the observation that pepstatin also did not show any effect on glandular stomach tumor induction by MNNG, but enhanced tumor growth (*7*).

Other Possible Effects of Leupeptin

The modulation of the microflora by leupeptin could have played a role in the case of colon tumor formation. There is a possibility that co-carcinogens are produced from bile or other compounds by the microflora in the colon. The bile acids, lithocholic acid, and taurodeoxycholic acid increased the frequency of colon tumor induction by intrarectal instillation of MNNG (*15*). A high level of dietary fat also increased the excretion of fecal acid and neutral sterols and the frequency of colon tumor formation by 1, 2-dimethylhydrazine (*16*). The protease-inhibitor may have reduced the quantity of co-carcinogens produced in the colon and thus reduced the number of tumor induction per rat.

Another possible common effect of protease-inhibitor is the alteration of the carcinogen activation system. Many carcinogens (procarcinogens) need to be metabolically activated in the body to the reactive proximate or ultimate form for tumor induction (*17*). Several factors are known which alter tumor formation by chemical carcinogens. These factors exert their action by modifying the carcinogen metabolism. The reduction in the number of tumors or the size of tumors by leupeptin occurred in all cases where procarcinogens, which required metabolic activation, were used.

Prospects

Leupeptin showed effects whenever it had direct contact with organs. Therefore, it is probably necessary to maintain a higher level of leupeptin in the body in order to produce a strong systemic effect on chemical carcinogenesis. This can be done by increasing the concentration of leupeptin in the diet. Leupeptin in the pellet-diet is stable for several months of storage, but about 50% of leupeptin activity is lost during the processing of the pellet-diet. The conditions for making a pellet diet must be improved, or a powdered diet must be used to avoid the leupeptin inactivation during the process of pellet making. This 50% inactivation of leupeptin activity may be caused by racemization of the asymmetric center in argininal moiety, because only leupeptin with the L-form of argininal was active.

Injection of leupeptin solution can also increase the level in the body. Injection of leupeptin in the form of oil-water emulsion or liposome may be better in order to maintain a higher level of leupeptin and to retain its action for a longer duration.

Although it is too early to generalize on the effect of leupeptin, the animal experiments indicate that the use of protease-inhibitors in the prevention of cancer deserves further study. The studies on the effects of other protease-inhibitors of microbial origin, such as antipain, chymostatin, and pepstatin, on chemical carcinogenesis might also be considered.

ACKNOWLEDGMENT

This work was supported by grants from the Ministry of Education, Science and Culture and the Ministry of Health and Welfare, Japan.

REFERENCES

1. van Duuren, B. L. and Melchionne, S. Inhibition of tumorigenesis. *In;* F. Homburger (ed.), Progress in Experimental Tumor Research, vol. 12, pp. 55–101, S. Karger, Basel, 1969.

2. Troll, W., Klassen, A., and Janoff, A. Tumorigenesis in mouse skin: Inhibition by synthetic inhibitors of proteases. Science, *169*: 1211–1213, 1970.

3. Hozumi, M., Ogawa, M., Sugimura, T., Takeuchi, T., and Umezawa, H. Inhibition of tumorigenesis in mouse skin by leupeptin, a protease inhibitor from *Actinomycetes*. Cancer Res., *32*: 1725–1728, 1972.

4. Umezawa, H. Enzyme Inhibitors of Microbial Origin, University of Tokyo Press, Tokyo, 1972.

5. Yamamoto, R. S., Umezawa, H., Takeuchi, T., Matsushima, T., Hara, K. and Sugimura, T. Effect of leupeptin on colon carcinogenesis in rats with azoxymethane. Proc. Am. Assoc. Cancer Res., *15*: 38, 1974.

6. Druckrey, H. and Lange, A. Carcinogenicity of azoxymethane dependent on age in BD rats. Fed. Proc., *31*: 1482–1484, 1972.

7. Kawachi, T., Yamamoto, R. S., Matsushima, T., Sugimura, T., Takeuchi, T., and Umezawa, H. Effects of leupeptin and pepstatin on stomach carcinogenesis of rats induced by N-methyl-N′-nitro-N-nitrosoguanidine. Abstr. U.S.-Japan Cooperative Cancer Research Program Seminar on Action of Protease Inhibitors and Carcinogenesis, 1975.

8. Kakizoe, T., Takayasu, H., Kawachi, T., Sugimura, T., Takeuchi, T., and Umezawa, H. Effect of leupeptin, a protease inhibitor, on induction of bladder tumors

in rats by N-butyl-N-(4-hydroxybutyl) nitrosamine. J. Natl. Cancer Inst., *56*: 433–435, 1976.

9. Takayama, S., Katoh, Y., and Ishikawa, T. Effect of leupeptin in carcinogenesis of esophagus and liver in rats and leukemogenesis in mice. Abstr. U.S.-Japan Cooperative Cancer Research Program Seminar on Action of Protease Inhibitors and Carcinogenesis, 1975.

10. Fukui, Y., Takamura, C., Yamamura, M., and Yamamoto, M. Effect of leupeptin on carcinogenesis of rat mammary tumor induced by 7, 12-dimethylbenz[a]antracene. Proc. Japan. Cancer Assoc., 34th Annu. Meet., p. 20, 1975 (in Japanese).

11. Kasuga, T., Noda, Y., Furuse, T., and Terasima, T. Effect of leupeptin in the induction of radiation-induced thymic lymphoma in C57BL/6J mice. Proc. Japan. Cancer Assoc., 34th Annu. Meet., p. 40, 1975 (in Japanese).

12. Troll, W., Rossman, T., Katz, J., Levitz, M., and Sugimura, T. Proteinase in tumor promotion and hormone action. *In;* E. Reich, D. B. Rifkin, and E. Shaw (eds.), Proteases and Biological Control, pp. 977–987, Cold Spring Harbor Laboratory, Cold Spring Harbor, 1975.

13. Katz, J., Troll, W., Russo, J., Filkins, K., and Levitz, M. Effect of protease inhibitors on *in vitro* breakdown of uterine histone from hormone-treated rats. Endocr. Res. Commun., *1*: 331–337, 1974.

14. Katz, J., Troll, W., Levy, M., Filkins, K., Russo, J., and Levitz, M. Estrogen-dependent trypsin like activity in the rat uterus. Localization of activity in the 12,000 g pellet and nucleus. Arch. Biochem. Biophys., *173*: 347–354, 1976.

15. Narisawa, T., Magadia, N. E., Weisburger, J. H., and Wynder, E. L. Promoting effect of bile acids on colon carcinogenesis after intrarectal instillation of N-methyl-N'-nitro-N-nitrosoguanidine in rats. J. Natl. Cancer Inst., *53*: 1093–1097, 1974.

16. Reddy, B. S., Weisburger, J. H., and Wynder, E. L. Effects of dietary fat level and dimethylhydrazine on fecal acid and neutral sterol excretion and colon carcinogenesis in rats. J. Natl. Cancer Inst., *52*: 507–511, 1974.

17. Weisburger, J. H. and Williams, G. M. Metabolism of chemical carcinogens. *In;* F. F. Becker (ed.), Cancer, vol. 1, pp. 185–234, Plenum Press, New York, 1975.

Discussion of Paper of Drs. Matsushima et al.

DR. FARBER: Through the courtesy of Dr. Sugimura, we obtained leupeptin for studies of liver carcinogenesis with N-2-fluorenylacetamide (2-AAF). Whereas the diet containing leupeptin alone was non-toxic, the diet containing both 2-AAF and leupeptin was extremely toxic; all the animals died within 2 to 3 months. The early "pre-cancerous" changes were the same with 2-AAF and 2-AAF plus leupeptin. Dr. Matsushima, have you observed a similar effect?

DR. MATSUSHIMA: No, I have not seen such an effect of leupeptin, because the carcinogen and leupeptin were given to animals by different routes, the carcinogen by injection or in the drinking water, and leupeptin by feeding.

DR. GELBOIN: Have you or others examined the effects of leupeptin on the microsomal mixed function oxygenase system?

DR. MATSUSHIMA: Nobody seems to have studied the effect and we should do this.

DR. TROLL: The absorption of leupeptin may be the difficulty. Do you have data on absorption? Perhaps the dipeptide, acetylleucylargininal, would be better.

DR. MATSUSHIMA: About 5% of leupeptin fed to rats was excreted as the active form in feces, and less than 1% was excreted in urine. We do not know how much leupeptin is inactivated in the digestive tract and how much is absorbed. We have to determine the exact quantity absorbed by using ^{14}C-labeled leupeptin.

DR. MAGEE: In your experiment on LD_{50} determination of leupeptin, was the compound given by the oral route? Did you give leupeptin by the intraperitoneal route?

DR. MATSUSHIMA: The LD_{50} values of leupeptin, which were shown in the slide, were for the oral route. Leupeptin injected intraperitoneally into rats was not toxic at 100 mg per kg body weight, but at a higher level it was.

FUNDAMENTALS IN CANCER PREVENTION, P. N. MAGEE ET AL. (EDS.),
UNIV. OF TOKYO PRESS, TOKYO / UNIV. PARK PRESS, BALTIMORE, PP. 71–87, 1976

Precancerous Liver Cell Populations and Their Identification

Emmanuel FARBER,* Sally P. HARTMAN, Dennis SOLT, and
Ross CAMERON

Fels Research Institute, Temple University School of Medicine, Philadelphia, Pennsylvania, U.S.A.

Abstract: It is now widely appreciated that the majority of epithelial neoplasms
and perhaps even other types of cancers, seem to develop as an evolutionary process from the original cell population, with new nonmalignant cell populations as
possible intermediates. Such preneoplastic and premalignant lesions often exist in
man for many years before the appearance of unequivocal cancer and are the predominant tissue changes seen during the so-called latent period that is characteristic
of the majority of carcinogenic processes.

In the liver, at least four identifiable new hepatocyte populations are considered
as cell precursors in carcinogenesis. These are: (a) areas, islands, or foci of hepatocytes, which show decreases in several enzymes; glycogen storage, disturbance in
iron uptake or metabolism and often contain cells in S phase or in mitosis; (b) early
hyperplastic nodules, which show many of the same changes and are arranged in
two or more cell-thick plates. These can undergo maturation or differentiation to
the adult pattern of single cell plates; (c) late hyperplastic nodules, similar in many
respects to (b) but which do not differentiate or do so very slowly; and (d) hyperbasophilic foci which are seen in late hyperplastic nodules and which seem to contain the ultimate hepatocyte precursor for at least some hepatocellular carcinomas.
The possible relationship of the altered cellular organization to the abundant
biochemical evidence for "disdifferentiation," "retrodifferentiation," or "blocked
ontogeny" remains a provocative area for discussion.

Several positive markers, such as α-fetoprotein, preneoplastic antigen, selective isozymes, and other isoproteins (*e.g.*, isoferritins) and γ-glutamyl transpeptidase
seem to be associated with the carcinogenic process and/or the new cell populations
seen during carcinogenesis.

Selective resistance to cytotoxicity is considered as an attractive selection pressure for the new putative precursor cells. The possible use of this in the analysis of
liver carcinogenesis and in the development of new approaches to the rapid bioassay
of carcinogens is presented.

* Present address: Department of Pathology, University of Toronto, Toronto, Ontario, Canada.

71

It is now widely appreciated that the majority of epithelial cancers and perhaps also other types of malignant neoplasms, are preceded in time by a variety of distinctive lesions composed of altered, proliferating, or hyperplastic cells. These lesions are obviously not malignant but are possibly intermediates in a process of cellular evolution beginning with the original cell population and ending usually with a highly malignant tumor, often composed of a number of cell populations each at a different stage in this evolution or progression (*1, 2*). Even though the so-called preneoplastic or premalignant lesion has been known in some organs or tissues for quite a long time, it has not received much attention from the cancer research worker until quite recently. This relative neglect has led to a failure, especially on the part of some of the present day leaders in cancer research, to focus sufficient emphasis on the field of the precursor lesions for the control of cancer. The emphasis continues to be on the cause or causes of cancer and on the cure of the end stage. Yet, it is clear that any consideration of the prevention of cancer must encompass to an increasing degree the identification, assay, characterization, and control of the so-called preneoplastic lesions.

Firstly, as we well know from the many years of experience in dermatology and gynecology, it is easier to cure cancer by recognizing and removing preneoplastic or premalignant lesions in people than it is to treat advanced cancer. This must be a major goal for cancers in all organs or tissues. In our view, this is what should be meant when we talk about early diagnosis—the diagnosis of the early precursor lesions.

Secondly, as we identify more groups of people at high risk because of some occupational or other environmental hazard, or because of a special genetic background, we are beginning to realize that we are almost powerless to help such individuals once they already have precursor lesions, unless these are in an accessible site amenable to surgical intervention. Our ignorance does not allow us to interrupt the possible evolution of the lesions to cancer. This is perhaps most dramatically seen in the United States in the smoking asbestos worker or uranium miner.

Thirdly, although undoubtedly we will be able to identify more and more carcinogenic hazards in our environment, it may be possible to remove some of these only slowly. For example, even though the cigarette smoker is at a relatively high risk for many types of cancer and other chronic diseases, it may be many years before society will act intelligently as a response to this. Thus we are faced with the challenge to understand the carcinogenic process to a sufficient degree to interrupt the long chain reaction initiated by exposure to the cigarette hazards.

Lastly, it is becoming clear that since the properties of a malignant cell population are so many and so complex, it is doubtful if the essentials of the biochemistry and molecular biology of cancer can be dissected and understood except through an historical approach. We may have to understand the meaning and mechanism of the evolution in order to understand the end stages.

Thus, from several points of view, the study of the carcinogenic process and of the precursor cell populations that precede cancer is closely related to the overall challenge of the prevention of cancer.

Precancerous Hepatic Populations—Nodular Hyperplasia, Precursor, and Progeny

Our knowledge of epithelial precancerous lesions in man or experimental animals in most tissues and organs remains fragmentary and often speculative. Obvious exceptions to this are a few epithelial sites, especially skin, cervix, and to a lesser degree breast in man, and skin, urinary bladder, and liver in experimental animals.

New liver cell populations—nodular hyperplasia, precursors, and progeny

It is becoming increasingly evident that a major response of the liver to carcinogenic regimens is the appearance of new isolated focal hepatocyte populations. Such lesions, most frequently called hyperplastic nodules, have been seen with virtually every hepatocarcinogen since the first report with *o*-aminoazotoluene (*3*). The properties and possible biological significance of nodular hyperplasia during liver carcinogenesis has been reviewed fairly recently (*4*).

Islands of altered hepatocytes

In addition, more recent studies in several laboratories with diethylnitrosamine (DEN), nitrosomorpholine, and a few other carcinogens have suggested that an earlier precursor hepatocyte population may be identified by histochemical methods (*4–10*). These focal groups of altered liver cells are called "islands," "foci," or "areas." We shall refer to them as foci or islands. They consistently show a slight increase in cytoplasmic basophilia and a parallel decrease or loss of histochemical staining for glucose-6-phosphatase (G-6-Pase) (*11*) and nucleoside polyphosphatase (NPPase) (also called adenosine triphosphatase (ATPase)) (*12*) and a persistence of glycogen under conditions of fasting when the surrounding liver cells lose almost all of their glycogen. This property of glycogen storage has been emphasized especially by Bannasch (*13*). Such areas, induced either by 2-acetylaminofluorene (2-AAF) or by DEN, show a striking decrease in β-glucuronidase and serine dehydratase activities but not in another lysosomal enzyme, acid phosphatase (*5, 10, 14*).

Recently Dr. Williams, while at the Fels Research Institute, completed a study in which he found that these islands or foci show the same disturbance in iron metabolism as was found earlier in hyperplastic nodules (*15*).

The islands of altered hepatocytes show a considerable increase in uptake of ³H-cytidine in the nucleus and in the subsequent labeling of the cytoplasm (*12, 16*).

Recent quantitative studies indicate that the enzyme-deficient islands or foci may persist for many weeks when induced by DEN and that their number can be increased by partial hepatectomy (*7–9*). The hepatocytes in the enzyme-deficient glycogen storing foci induced by several carcinogens show some proliferation which is not constant but which is increased greatly by partial hepatectomy (*6, 17*).

In addition to altered glycogen metabolism and enzyme deficiencies, hypertrophied smooth endoplasmic reticulum (SER) has been described (*18*). The SER was closely associated with particles of glycogen, abnormal in size and shape.

The islands appear to be clones of altered hepatocytes (*19*). They are interpreted as representing a somatic mutation in liver parenchymal cells (8, 20). The basis for this hypothesis is their apparent irreversibility in that they persist long after the discontinuation of the carcinogen (DEN). Although this suggestion is reasonable, it must be recalled that many states of differentiation are equally "irreversible." The islands of altered hepatocytes could well represent inherited phenotypic alteration without necessarily being genetic mutants. Obviously this important question will require the isolation of the altered cells for more sophisticated genetic and other biological analyses.

The growth pattern of the hepatocytes in the islands of altered liver has not been clarified. Scherer *et al.* (7) have noted the compression of sinusoids and of surrounding uninvolved liver by expanding islands. However, whether the hepatocytes have the pattern of mature liver (one cell-thick plates) or of more immature liver (two or more cell-thick plates) is not known. This question is of particular importance in assessing the role, if any, of the various hyperplastic or proliferative lesions as precursors for malignant neoplasia, since both the discrete hyperplastic nodules (see later) and liver cancers have architectural arrangements of hepatocytes two or more cells thick.

Hyperplastic nodules, "ostensibly reversible" and irreversible

Hyperplastic nodules have been the subject of a recent extensive review (4). Nodules are focal collections of slowly proliferating hepatocytes with morphologic, biochemical, and biological properties that distinguish them from the surrounding original hepatocytes. Unlike the original liver cell population in the adult, the first nodule population, recognizable as such, has its hepatocytes organized in two or often more than two cell-thick plates and in various other patterns such as tubules. This has, of course, been described before in hyperplastic nodules in human cirrhosis (*e.g.*, 21, 22). These patterns, although not fetal, nevertheless resemble the liver more during fetal development than in the adult. The nodules contain bile ducts but the arrangements of the cells do not seem to be patterned after the normal liver lobule or acinus. Subsequent nodules that occur later during carcinogenesis are so far indistinguishable morphologically or biochemically from the early nodules. However, the latter ostensibly disappear on removing the carcinogen while the former do not or do so very much more slowly.

Both the early and late nodules are greyish-white in colour and readily distinguished grossly from the surrounding reddish brown liver. Under conditions of continuous feeding of carcinogens for 8 to 10 weeks or more, the nodules in general remain small, less than 0.5 cm in diameter. They appear usually by 4 to 6 weeks or sometimes later as minute greyish-white "spots" 1 mm or less in diameter and often peppering the whole surface of the liver. Some of these then grow larger and discrete but with the continuous carcinogenic regimen often remain below 5 mm in diameter and as such are very difficult to dissect cleanly.

By varying the level and the schedule of administration, very much larger nodules measuring as much as 2 cm in diameter can be obtained with several carcinogens. By increasing the amount of carcinogen administered and by allowing periodic rest periods with diets free of carcinogen, large nodules have been obtained with 2-AAF, ethionine, aflatoxin B_1 and 3'-methyl-4-dimethylaminoazo-benzene (3'-Me-DAB) (23–26). By suitable manipulation of the periods of feeding the carcinogen-containing diets and the carcinogen-free diets, large nodules that seem to regress and those that do not can be induced quite regularly.

The nodule populations show biochemical and structural differences from normal liver. Alterations or disturbances (a) in carbohydrate metabolism, such as progressive decreases in G-6-Pase and in glycogen phosphorylase, (b) in protein and nucleic acid metabolism, and (c) in SER and cell proliferation *in vivo* and *in vitro* have been found, including structural changes in DNA and in glycogen (see Farber (4) for references). The DNA content per nucleus of hepatocytes in adenomas (hyperplastic nodules?) was found to be mainly euploid in contrast to hepatomas which were frequently aneuploid (27). The nodule hepatocytes responded well to the proliferative stimulus of partial hepatectomy (28, 29). Another interesting property is the absence of stainable iron from preneoplastic (hyperplastic areas and nodules) and neoplastic lesions in animals given 2-AAF or DEN and 8-hydroxyquinoline and ferrous gluconate (15). This property may be related to the earlier findings of Reuber (23) who noted that many hyperplastic nodules and hepatocellular carcinomas, in contrast to normal liver, did not become coloured on intravenous injection of the dye, Rose Bengal. Conceivably, the observations with iron and with Rose Bengal as well as with glycogen storage could indicate some common defect in lysosome function in many putative premalignant hepatocytes as well as in malignant ones. Such an hypothesis could explain some of the diverse isolated observations on the properties of premalignant and malignant hepatocytes. Some evidence consistent with this view has been presented in studies on liver carcinogenesis induced by DAB (30–32).

Hyperplastic nodules induced by several hepatocarcinogens have been studied ultrastructurally (13, 25, 33–39). Although certain similarities were found between the nodule hepatocytes and hepatocytes in some malignant neoplasms, no identifying markers were evident. Changes in SER, nuclei, nucleoli, and annulate lamellae were regularly seen. The latter are characteristic of many fetal and adult proliferating cells. So far, no structural or biochemical properties which can be used to distinguish between the early and the late nodules have been found.

Scherer *et al.* (7) have compared the known properties of the enzyme-deficient islands with those of the nodules and have suggested that they are identical, in so far as they have been studied. This would suggest that the two types of lesions might be closely related, conceivably with the islands as the precursors for the nodules.

Apparent regression of early nodules—differentiation and maturation

The so-called regression of the early nodules is only apparent (40–42). On discontinuing the carcinogen, the early nodules undergo a process of apparent maturation, remodeling, or differentiation during which the hepatocytes in the nodule become smaller and reorganized into one cell-thick plates. The hepatocytes in the early as well as the later nodules are considerably larger than normal hepatocytes. Many show abundant pale-staining cytoplasm, often with a ground glass appearance or a vacuolization due to their abundant content of glycogen. The cytoplasmic basophilia is rarely seen as basophilic bodies but rather as a fine granularity that resembles the cytoplasm of hepatocytes during cell division. The nuclei are almost uniformly enlarged to about 1.5 to 2 times the diameter of normal liver nuclei and usually have a much looser open chromatin-staining pattern than do normal liver nuclei, usually with one or two large nucleoli. During the remodeling process, the hepatocytes come to look very much like normal liver cells with one possible exception—the frequent retention of large nucleoli.

It should be emphasized that a cellular reaction to the various nodules as well as to enzyme-deficient areas and hyperbasophilic foci is strikingly missing. The majority of these localized new cell populations evoke neither an acute polymorphonuclear leucocyte response nor a lymphocyte or plasma cell response. This is also true even when the nodules are undergoing maturation and remodeling. The absence of an observable cellular reaction to these new cell populations is in contrast to many hepatocellular carcinomas in which not infrequently one can observe a mononuclear reaction. The biological significance of the reaction and its absence may have relevance to the presence or absence of a host immunologic response but this remains to be explored.

The morphologic evidence suggesting remodeling or maturation (40, 43) is supported independently by histochemical data (10) and by studies on chromosome patterns (29). Kitagawa and Pitot (10) reported that hyperplastic areas and nodules show foci of reappearance of β-glucuronidase and serine dehydratase activities and suggested that maturation and reorganization within liver tissue may be occurring. In addition, staining for preneoplastic antigen (44) disappears in the areas of maturation in hyperplastic nodules. Becker et al. (29), in agreement with the observations of Inui et al. (27), found the hepatocyte population in hyperplastic nodules to be predominantly diploid with an obvious lack of nuclei that were tetraploid or of higher ploidy. This was considered to be evidence of some "suppression of maturation (ploidization)" in the nodule population, since normal maturation of liver is associated with a progressive increase in tetraploid and octaploid cells and cells with even higher ploidy (45, 46).

This process of maturation or remodeling can be seen on gross examination. The nodules gradually lose their greyish-white colour and acquire the reddish brown colour of normal liver. In the process, various degrees of mottling of the greyish-white appearance by brown can be seen until the nodules become indistinguishable from the surrounding nonnodular liver. We have the impression that these areas of previously altered liver cells may remain for long periods and may be induced to reappear as hyperplastic nodules by stimuli such as the induction of liver cell necrosis or partial hepatectomy. Obviously, if this impression can be scientifically established, it would indicate that a normal-appearing liver may only be apparently normal and may have islands of liver parenchyma that are still altered basically in such a manner as to remain as potential premalignant cell populations. The finding of such a liver with cancer would give the false impression that the malignant neoplasm had arisen from normal liver cells without an apparent precursor population. Some support for this concept was presented recently by Becker (*47*) who found that a single nonnecrogenic dose of dimethylnitros-amine (DMN) induced a significant number of hepatocellular carcinomas in animals previously exposed to 2-AAF for a relatively short period. The nodules induced by the latter treatment were apparently predominantly reversible and had matured.

The possible relationship of the altered patterns of cell organization and of disturbances in differentiation or maturation at the cellular and tissue level to those of "blocked ontogeny" (*48, 49*) "disdifferentiation" (*50*), "retrodifferentiation" (*51*) or "derepression of fetal enzymes" (*52*) and "anomalous gene expression" (*53*), all at the biochemical or enzymatic level, remains a fruitful and provocative area for further exploration.

Unlike the early nodules, the later ones no longer seem to become remodeled or do so only very slowly. Also, with time, one sees in some of the later nodules collections of cells that resemble more and more *bona fide* malignant hepatocytes. Increasing basophilia and nuclear-cytoplasmic ratios, more frequent mitotic figures, anisocytosis, and even atypical changes become more evident. However, no system-atic sequence of changes that could be interpreted in terms of precursor-product cells or lesions have been described. So far, the observations are consistent with the late hyperplastic nodule being considered as a precursor population for a malignant change. With time, such lesions show an increasing array of hepatocellular carci-nomas, the morphological origins of which become impossible to identify. This is partly because of the wide variation in appearance as the malignant neoplasms develop and partly because of the rapid destruction and replacement of any slowly or more slowly growing precursor lesion by neoplasms with increased growth rates.

Hyperbasophilic foci

Areas of hyperbasophilic hepatocytes were described by Opie (*54*) during the study of liver carcinogenesis induced by DAB. He suggested that these areas con-tained the ultimate or close to the ultimate precursor lesions for liver cancer. These areas have been intensively studied by Daoust *et al*. (*55–58*) in liver carcinogenesis induced predominantly by DAB and 3′-Me-DAB but also by DEN and other car-cinogens. The hyperbasophilic areas consistently show a marked decrease in RNase and DNase activities and an accelerated DNA and RNA synthesis. The majority of the hyperbasophilic hepatocytes show a much less differentiated pattern than do mature liver cells (*59*). Many of the cell organelles including the endoplasmic reticulum participate in these changes. More recently, Karasaki (*38*) found that hepatocytes in hyperbasophilic foci showed histochemical ATPase activity over the whole cell surface in contrast to normal hepatocytes or hepatocytes in hyperplastic nodules in which the staining was limited to the bile canaliculi. This and other data led Karasaki to suggest that hyperbasophilic foci might arise from hyperplastic nodules as the ultimate precursor of malignant hepatocytes or as early hepatocel-lular carcinoma. The suggestion that the relatively undifferentiated hepatocytes are precursors for liver cancer has also been made by Bruni (*39*) who described "distinctive cells similar to fetal hepatocytes" during liver carcinogenesis induced by DEN.

Resistance to Cytotoxicity as a Basis for Selection and Assay

What is the mechanism that encourages the selective growth of the putative precancerous hepatocyte populations?

An attractive hypothesis, that has experimental support, invokes selective cytotoxicity as one important selection pressure (*4*). It has been known since at least 1935 (*60*) that some carcinogens inhibit the growth of normal cells much more easily than that of neoplastic cells. Such observations formed the basis for an hypothesis suggested by Haddow in 1938 (*61*). He proposed that inhibition of cell proliferation is an early effect of carcinogens and that in response to this inhibition, an altered cell population arises which now can grow in the presence of a cytotoxic environment. Although this suggestion was derived from comparative studies with some carcinogenic polycyclic aromatic hydrocarbons using cancers in tissues other than liver, subsequent research by a variety of investigators has indicated that the liver may show the same phenomenon (*62*).

Recent evidence in our laboratory offers new support for this hypothesis. Hyperplastic nodules induced either by 2-AAF or ethionine, were found to be resistant to the necrogenic effects of CCl_4 or DMN under conditions in which the surrounding nonnodular liver showed extensive necrosis. Also, nodules showed about 50% less interaction of DMN or 2-AAF with DNA, RNA, and protein, even though the uptake of the labeled carcinogens by the nodules was the same as in the surrounding liver or in normal control liver. Thus, the nodules show about 50% less activation of these carcinogens and cytotoxic agents. These findings agree well with enzyme assays of hyperplastic nodules (*63*) and of whole liver during hepatocarcinogenesis (*64–67*). Gravela *et al.* (*63*) in particular found that hyperplastic

TABLE 1.   Levels of Cytochrome P-450 and of AHH in Hyperplastic Nodules and Surrounding Liver from Animals Fed 2-AAF and in Control Livers

Expt. No.	Rat liver	Diet[a] (0.05% 2-AAF)	Cytochrome P-450 (nmoles $\times 10^3$/mg protein)		AHH (units/mg liver)
			Homogenate	Microsome	$9,000 \times g$ supernatant
1	Nodule	21 wks. 2-AAF 1 wk. chow	7.6 (4)	236 (4)	9 (4)
	Surrounding	21 wks. 2-AAF 1 wk. chow	9.5 (4)	309 (4)	12 (4)
	Control	21 wks. basal 1 wk. chow	20.5 (4)	565 (4)	55 (4)
2	Nodule	21 wks. 2-AAF 4 wks. chow	9.8 (4)	370 (4)	2 (4)
	Surrounding	21 wks. 2-AAF 4 wks. chow	13.0 (4)	480 (4)	4 (3)
	Control	21 wks. basal 4 wks. chow	26.0 (1)	950 (1)	20 (1)

[a] Diets as described previously (*24*).   Numbers in parentheses indicate number of animals.

nodules induced by ethionine had about 50% of the cytochrome P-450, lipid peroxidation and aminopyrine demethylase activity found in the surrounding liver. The changes in primary hepatomas were even more marked. Recently we have observed a similar phenomenon in hyperplastic nodules induced by 2-AAF (Table 1). In addition, as is evident in the table, aryl hydrocarbon hydroxylase (AHH) was found to be much reduced in activity in the nodules.

If this hypothesis has any validity, it should be possible to show that cytotoxic-resistant islands of hepatocytes can be induced very early in carcinogenesis if the stimulus is a cytotoxic one. Animals are fed carcinogenic regimens containing 2-AAF for 3 weeks, at which time one observes moderate ductular proliferation and many slightly basophilic islands in which the hepatocytes show glycogen storage and lack of staining with iron. The administration of a necrogenic dose of DMN at this time fails to evoke a general regenerative response in the liver due to the general inhibition of cell proliferation. However, scattered islands of intensely basophilic proliferating cells appear. Thus, by 3 weeks with 2-AAF, a cell population is present which is not responding to the inhibitory effects of 2-AAF on cell proliferation. The relationship of these islands to the enzyme-deficient islands described previously is under study.

If this concept of cytotoxicity and its role in carcinogenesis has validity, then normal or induced variations in the level of metabolic activation in any cell or group of cells could play an important role in the early selection of hepatocytes as initial precursor cells from which a cancer could ultimately evolve. Conceivably, the induction of a mutant-like population that has a deficient carcinogen-activating system could be a key step in the initiation events for carcinogenesis. Also, given the more or less selective effect of many modulating influences on different parts of the liver lobule or acinus, one can easily see how drugs or toxic chemicals that influence liver structure or function (68) could have major effects on the carcinogenic process at the cellular level (69).

This hypothesis could be made even more specific by concentration on perhaps the most common component in the activating enzyme system for many carcinogens, the cytochrome P-450 complex. It could be postulated that an early step in the carcinogenic process is the induction of an altered cell population in which a key property is a mutation in a structural or regulatory gene related to the cytochrome P-450 system. An abnormal cytochrome or even a less active isozyme of one of the adult forms could be an important early step in the multistep process of cellular evolution to malignant neoplasia. This formulation has the appeal of relative simplicity from a biochemical viewpoint and at the same time has obvious relevance to the known biological properties of the carcinogenic process.

An attractive practical consequence of these considerations is the development of a new principle for the rapid bioassay in vivo for altered cell populations induced by carcinogens or potential carcinogens. The majority of procedures that have been or are being developed for the rapid screening of potential carcinogens have, as their endpoint, some mutation or mutation-like property that is the consequence of the interaction of an activated chemical with the DNA (or perhaps other macromolecules) of the target organism. In most instances, e.g., bacteria, yeast or other isolated eukaryocytes, it is difficult if not impossible to relate directly the properties of the endpoint observed to any carcinogenic process *in vivo*.

This new approach makes it much easier to relate, at least theoretically, the observed endpoint to carcinogenesis *in vivo*. This can be illustrated most easily with the specifics of the developing bioassay. An animal is fed a diet containing 2-AAF for one week at which time partial hepatectomy is performed. At this time, virtually no hepatocyte regeneration can be observed histologically by 3 or 4 days. Whatever regeneration takes place occurs very slowly over many days or longer. However, if one prolongs the feeding period for the 2-AAF, one begins to observe small isolated foci of highly proliferating, intensely basophilic hepatocytes. If the week of exposure of 2-AAF is preceded by a single exposure to DEN a week or two previously, and if then one performs partial hepatectomy, one now observes isolated islands or foci of proliferating hepatocytes. These isolated islands have acquired a resistence to the cytotoxic inhibitory influence of the 2-AAF feeding regimen. This histologic assay can no doubt be made quantitative by measuring DNA synthesis or one or more enzymes that are related to liver cell regeneration, such as ornithine decarboxylase, thymidine kinase, or thymidylate synthetase.

Naturally, we have to study many facets of this approach including rapidity of induction of altered resistant cells by many different carcinogens, the length such altered cells persist and their possible repair or removal, if any. However, this approach offers the possibility of measuring an endpoint of the interaction of an active carcinogen with target cells that can be related to the carcinogenic process in a single organ.

We are of the opinion that this type of approach to analysis of at least one probable step in the carcinogenic process may enable us to ask many more penetrating questions and to devise hypotheses at a biochemical or molecular level in the intact animal. This principle, in our view, is critical if we are to obtain further insight into the molecular and cellular biology of cancer development and if we are to develop novel approaches to the more rapid and more meaningful monitoring of the environment for potential carcinogenic hazards to man. It is highly probable that this cannot help but assist significantly in the development of better methods to prevent cancer in man.

ACKNOWLEDGMENTS

The authors' research included in this article was supported by research grants from the National Cancer Institute (CA-12218, CA-12227) and the National Institute of Arthritis and Metabolic Diseases (AM-14882), United States Public Health Service, American Cancer Society (BC-7) and the National Cancer Institute of Canada, and by a contract with the National Cancer Institute (U.S.A.) (NO1-CP-33262).

D. S. was a recipient of a training grant to Temple University from the National Institute of Dental Research (DE-02268) and R. C. of a Fellowship from the National Cancer Institute of Canada.

REFERENCES

1. Foulds, L. *In;* Neoplastic Development, vol. 1, pp. 41–96, Academic Press, New York, 1969.
2. Farber, E. Carcinogenesis—Cellular evolution as a unifying thread. Presidential address. Cancer Res., *33*: 2537–2550, 1973.
3. Sasaki, T. and Yoshida, T. Experimentelle Erzeugung des Lebercarcinoms durch Fütterung mit *o*-aminoazotoluol. Virchow's Arch. Pathol. Anat Physiol., *295*: 175–200, 1935.
4. Farber, E. Hyperplastic liver nodules. Methods in Cancer Res., *7*: 345–375, 1973.
5. Kitagawa, T. Histochemical analysis of hyperplastic lesions and hepatomas of the liver of rats fed 2-fluorenylacetamide. Gann, *62*: 207–216, 1971.
6. Kitagawa, T. Responsiveness of hyperplastic lesions and hepatomas to partial hepatectomy. Gann, *62*: 217–224, 1971.
7. Scherer, E., Hoffman, M., Emmelot, P., and Friedrich-Freska, H. Quantitative study on foci of altered liver cells induced in the rat by a single dose of diethylnitrosamine and partial hepatectomy. J. Natl. Cancer Inst., *49*: 93–106, 1972.
8. Schieferstein, G., Pirschel, J., Frank, W., and Friedrich-Freska, H. Quantitative Untersuchungen über den irreversiblen Verlust zweier Enzymaktivitäten in der Rattenleber nach Verfütterung von Diäthylnitrosamin. Z. Krebsforsch., *82*: 191–208, 1974.
9. Scherer, E. and Emmelot, P. Foci of altered liver cells induced by a single dose of diethylnitrosamine and partial hepatectomy: Their contribution to hepatocarcinogenesis in the rat. Eur. J. Cancer, *11*: 145–154, 1975.
10. Kitagawa, T. and Pitot, H. C. The regulation of serine dehydratase and glucose-6-phosphatase in hyperplastic nodules of rat liver during diethylnitrosamine and N-2-fluorenylacetamide feeding. Cancer Res., *35*: 1075–1084, 1975.
11. Gössner, W. and Friedrich-Freska, H. Histochemische Untersuchungen über die Glucose-6-phosphatase in der Rattenleber während der Kanzerisierung durch Nitrosamine. Z. Naturforsch. B, *19*: 862–863, 1964.
12. Schauer, A. and Kunze, E. Enzymhistochemische und autoradiographische Untersuchungen während der Diäthylnitrosamin. Z. Krebsforsch., *70*: 252–266, 1968.
13. Bannasch, P. The cytoplasm of hepatocytes during carcinogenesis; electron and light microscopical investigations of the nitrosomorpholine-intoxicated rat liver. *In;* Recent Results in Cancer Research, vol. 19, Springer-Verlag, Berlin, New York, 1968.
14. Kitagawa, T. and Sugano, H. Combined enzyme histochemical and radioautographic studies on areas of hyperplasia in the liver of rats fed N-2-fluorenylacetamide. Cancer Res., *33*: 2993–3001, 1973.
15. Williams, G. M. and Yamamoto, R. S. Absence of stainable iron from preneoplastic and neoplastic lesions in rat liver with 8-hydroxyquinoline-induced siderosis. J. Natl. Cancer Inst., *49*: 685–692, 1972.
16. Schauer, A. and Feichtner, A. Enzymhistochemische Untersuchungen über den Nucleosidphosphat und Kohlenhydratstoffwechsel während der Cancerisierung der Rattenleber mit Diäthylnitrosamine (DANA) durch dosierte orale Zufuhr des Cancerogens. Klim. Wochenschr., *46*: 1286–1288, 1972.
17. Rabes, H. M., Scholze, P., and Jantsch, B. Growth kinetics of diethyl nitrosamine-induced, enzyme-deficient "preneoplastic" liver cell populations *in vivo* and *in vitro*. Cancer Res., *32*: 2577–2586, 1972.

18. Drochmans, P. and Scherer, E. Enzyme defects in hepato-carcinogenesis. Abstr. 12th Annu. Meet. Am. Soc. Cell Biol., 63a.

19. Scherer, E. and Hoffman, M. Probable clonal genesis of diethylnitrosamine. Eur. J. Cancer, 7: 339–371, 1971.

20. Friedrich-Freska, H., Papadopulu, G., and Gössner, W. Histochemical investigations of carcinogenesis in rat liver after time limited application of diethylnitrosamine. Z. Krebsforsch., 72: 240–253, 1969.

21. Phillips, M. J. and Steiner, J. W. Electron microscopy of cirrhotic nodules. Tubularization of the parenchyma of biliary hepatocytes. Lab. Invest., 15: 801–817, 1966.

22. Rubin, E. and Popper, H. The evolution of human cirrhosis deduced from observations in experimental animals. Medicine, 46: 163–183, 1967.

23. Reuber, M. D. Development of preneoplastic and neoplastic lesions of the liver in male rats given 0.025 per cent N-2-fluorenyldiacetamide. J. Natl. Cancer Inst., 34: 697–723, 1965.

24. Epstein, S. M., Ito, N., Merkow, L., and Farber, E. Cellular analysis of liver carcinogenesis: The induction of large hyperplastic nodules in the liver with 2-fluorenylacetamide or ethionine and some aspects of their morphology and glycogen metabolism. Cancer Res., 27: 1702–1711, 1967.

25. Yasuzumi, G., Sugihara, R., Ito, N., Konishi, Y., and Hiasa, Y. Fine structure of nuclei as revealed by electron microscopy. VII. Hyperplastic liver nodules in rat induced by 3′-methyl-4-dimethylaminoazobenzene, 2-fluorenylacetamide and DL-ethionine. Exp. Cell Res., 63: 83–95, 1970.

26. Teebor, G. W. and Becker, F. F. Regression and persistence of hyperplastic nodules induced by N-2-fluorenylacetamide and their relationship to hepatocarcinogenesis. Cancer Res., 31: 1–3, 1971.

27. Inui, N., Takayama, S., and Kuwabara, N. DNA measurements on cell nucleus of normal liver, adenoma, and hepatoma in mice: Histologic features. J. Natl. Cancer Inst., 47: 47–58, 1971.

28. Becker, F. F. and Klein, K. M. The effect of L-asparaginase on mitotic activity during N-2-fluorenylacetamide hepatocarcinogenesis: Subpopulations of nodular cells. Cancer Res., 31: 169–173, 1971.

29. Becker, F. F., Fox, R. A., Klein, K. M., and Wolman, S. R. Chromosome patterns in rat hepatocytes during N-2-fluorenylacetamide carcinogenesis. J. Natl. Cancer Inst., 46: 1261–1269, 1971.

30. Deckers-Passau, L., Maisin, J., and De Duve, C. The influence of azodyes on lysosomal enzymes in rat liver. Acta Un. Int. Cancer, 13: 822–835, 1957.

31. Nodes, J. T. and Reid, E. Azo-dye carcinogenesis: Ribonucleotides and ribonucleases. Brit. J. Cancer, 17: 745–774, 1963.

32. Takano, T., Kato, N., Kunimoto-Miyata, S., Goto, S., Ohkuma, S., Mizumo, D., Kitagawa, T., and Yokoyama, T. Lysosomes of rat liver and DAB carcinogenesis. Int. J. Cancer, 7: 346–352, 1971.

33. Merkow, L. P., Epstein, S. M., Caito, B. J., and Bartus, B. The cellular analysis of liver carcinogenesis: Ultrastructural alterations within hyperplastic liver nodules induced by 2-fluorenylacetamide. Cancer Res., 27: 1712–1721, 1967.

34. Merkow, L. P., Epstein, S. M., Farber, E., Pardo, M., and Bartus, B. Cellular analysis of liver carcinogenesis. III. Comparison of the ultrastructure of hyperplastic liver nodules and hepatocellular carcinomas induced in rat liver by 2-fluorenylacetamide. J. Natl. Cancer Inst., 43: 33–63, 1969.

35. Merkow, L. P., Epstein, S. M., Slifkin, M., Farber, E., and Pardo, M. Ultrastructural alterations within hyperplastic liver nodules induced by ethionine. Cancer Res., *31*: 174–178, 1971.

36. Flaks, B. Permanent changes in the fine structure of rat hepatocytes following prolonged treatment with 2-acetylaminofluorene. Eur. J. Cancer, *4*: 297–304, 1968.

37. Sugihara, R., Hiasa, Y., and Ito, N. Ultrastructural changes in nuclei and nucleoli of rat liver cells treated with hepatocarcinogens. Gann, *63*: 419–426, 1972.

38. Karasaki, S. Subcellular localization of surface adenosine triphosphatase activity in preneoplastic liver parenchyma. Cancer Res., *32*: 1703–1712, 1971.

39. Bruni, C. Distinctive cells similar to fetal hepatocytes associated with liver carcinogenesis by diethylnitrosamine. J. Natl. Cancer Inst., *50*: 1513–1528, 1973.

40. Farber, E., Hartman, S., and Solt, D. Interruption of differentiation ("blocked ontogeny") during induction of liver cancer by hepatocarcinogens. Proc. Am. Assoc. Cancer Res., *16*: 3, 1975.

41. Goldfarb, S. and Zak, F. G. Role of injury and hyperplasia in the induction of hepatocellular carcinoma. J. Am. Med. Assoc., *178*: 729–731, 1961.

42. Goldfarb, S. A morphological and histochemical study of carcinogenesis of the liver in rats fed 3-methyl-4-dimethylaminoazobenzene. Cancer Res., *33*: 1119–1128, 1973.

43. Farber, E. Pathogenesis of liver cancer. Arch. Pathol., *98*: 145–148, 1974.

44. Okita, K., Kligman, L. H., and Farber, E. A new common marker for premalignant and malignant hepatocytes induced in the rat by chemical carcinogens. J. Natl. Cancer Inst., *54*: 199–202, 1975.

45. Carriere, R. Polyploid cell reproduction in normal adult rat liver. Exp. Cell Res., *46*: 533–540, 1967.

46. Epstein, C. J. Cell size, nuclear content and the development of polyploidy in the mammalian liver. Proc. Natl. Acad. Sci. U.S., *57*: 327–334, 1967.

47. Becker, F. F. Alteration of hepatocytes by subcarcinogenic exposure to N-2-fluorenylacetamide. Cancer Res., *35*: 1734–1736, 1975.

48. Potter, V. R. Recent trends in cancer biochemistry: The importance of studies on fetal tissue. Can. Cancer Conf., *8*: 9–30, 1969.

49. Potter, V. R., Walker, P. R., and Goodman, J. I. Survey of current studies on oncogeny as blocked ontogeny: Isozyme changes in livers of rats fed 3′-methyl-4-dimethylaminoazobenzene with collateral studies on DNA stability. GANN Monogr. Cancer Res., *13*: 121–134, 1973.

50. Sugimura, T., Matsushima, T., Kawachi, T., Kogure, K., Tanake, N., Miyake, S., Hozumi, M., Sato, S., and Sato, H. Disdifferentiation and decarcinogenesis. GANN Monogr. Cancer Res., *13*: 31–45, 1973.

51. Uriel, J. Transitory liver antigens and primary hepatoma in rat and man. Pathol. Biol., *17*: 877–884, 1969.

52. Schapira, F. Isozymes and cancer. Adv. Cancer Res., *18*: 77–153, 1973.

53. Weinhouse, S. Glycolysis, respiration, and anomalous gene expression in experimental hepatomas: G.H.A. Clowes Memorial Lecture. Cancer Res., *32*: 2007–2016, 1972.

54. Opie, E. L. Pathogenesis of tumors of liver produced by butter yellow. J. Exp. Med., *80*: 231–246, 1944.

55. Daoust, R. Cellular populations and nucleic acid metabolism in rat liver parenchyma during azo dye carcinogenesis. Can. Cancer Conf., *5*: 225–239, 1963.

56. Daoust, R. and Molnar, F. Cellular populations and mitotic activity in rat liver parenchyma during azo dye carcinogenesis. Cancer Res., *24*: 1898–1909, 1964.

57. Brière, N.   Differential staining of preneoplastic foci in rat liver parenchyma during azo dye carcinogenesis. Histochemie, *26*: 113–119, 1971.

58. Fontanière, B. and Daoust, R.   Histochemical studies on nuclease activity and neoplastic transformation in rat liver during diethylnitrosamine carcinogenesis. Cancer Res., *33*: 3108–3111, 1973.

59. Karasaki, S.   The fine structure of proliferating cells in preneoplastic rat livers during azo-dye carcinogenesis. J. Cell Biol., *40*: 322–335, 1969.

60. Haddow, A.   Influence of certain polycyclic hydrocarbons on growth of Jansen rat sarcoma. Nature, *136*: 868–869, 1935.

61. Haddow, A.   Cellular inhibition and origin of cancer. Acta Un. Contr. Cancer, *3*: 342–352, 1938.

62. Vasiliev, J. M. and Guelstein, V. I. Sensitivity of normal and neoplastic cells to the damaging action of carcinogenic substances: A review. J. Natl. Cancer Inst., *31*: 1123–1141, 1963.

63. Gravela, E., Feo, F., Canuto, R. A., Garcea, R., and Gabriel, L.   Functional and structural alterations of liver ergastoplasmic. Cancer Res., *35*: 3041–3047, 1975.

64. Barker, E. A. and Smuckler, E. A.   Altered microsome function during acute thioacetamide poisoning. Mol. Pharmacol., *8*: 318–326, 1972.

65. Meyer, D. I. and Barber, A. A.   Changes in microsomal enzyme activities during DAB carcinogenesis. Chem.-Biol. Interact., *7*: 231–240, 1973.

66. Oyanagui, Y., Sato, N., and Hagihara, B.   Spectrophotometric analysis of cytochromes in rat liver during carcinogenesis. Cancer Res., *34*: 458–462, 1974.

67. Gabriel, L., Canuto, R. A., Gravela, E., Garcea, R., and Feo, F.   Alterations of liver ergastoplasmic membranes during DL-ethionine hepatocarcinogenesis, aminopyrine dimethylase activity and ribosome-membrane interaction. Life Sci., *15*: 2119–2125, 1974.

68. Schulte-Hermann, R. Induction of liver growth by xenobiotic compounds and other stimuli. Crit. Rev. Toxicol., *3*: 97–158, 1974.

69. Farber, E.   The biochemical pathology of experimental liver carcinogenesis. *In;* G. P. Warwick, H. M. Cameron, and C. A. Linsell (eds.), Liver Cell Cancer, Elsevier, Amsterdam, in press.

Discussion of Paper of Drs. Farber et al.

Dr. Sugimura: Could you please give a little more explanation on the preneoplastic (PN) antigen? What is known on the chemical nature of PN antigen?

Dr. Farber: The PN antigen was found by Dr. Okita of the Yamaguchi Medical School while working in my laboratory in Philadelphia (Okita *et al.*, J. Natl. Cancer Inst., *54*: 199–202, 1975). It is a hyperplastic nodule microsomal protein that is antigenic in rabbits. After absorption of antiserum with normal rat liver, the serum reacts with all hyperplastic nodules and with all primary hepatomas induced by one of 5 different carcinogens. It is a protein of about 120,000 molecular weight. We are now purifying it and hope to have it pure fairly soon. We think it might be a normal component, greatly overproduced by nodules and primary hepatoma. However, we shall only know this when we obtain it in pure form and then develop a sensitive assay (radioimmunoassay?) for it.

Dr. Newberne: Would you comment on the matured nodules and what role, if any, nonspecific agents may have on reactivating these nodules, if such occurs?

What role does necrosis have in the life history of hyperplastic nodules?

Dr. Farber: We think the matured nodules can be reactivated; our evidence for this is incomplete. If we induce necrosis in a liver containing matured nodules, hyperplastic nodules reappear fairly quickly.

We believe an important stimulus for growth of hyperplastic nodules is cell damage leading to cell regeneration. This is especially clear during the carcinogen administration when the original liver cells are inhibited from proliferation by the cytotoxic action of the carcinogen (Methods Cancer Res., *1*: 345, 1973).

Dr. Ito: Do you have information on the relationship between the uptake of iron and PN antigen in hyperplastic nodules?

Do nodules induced by different carcinogens show the same change in PN antigen?

Dr. Farber: There is an inverse relationship. Nodules lacking iron contain PN antigen. Whether there is any real relationship between these two properties is not yet known.

All hyperplastic nodules induced by 2-acetylaminofluorene (2-AAF) or by ethionine, and all primary hepatomas induced by diethylnitrosamine, dimethyl-nitrosamine, 2-AAF, ethionine, or 3′-methyl-4-dimethylaminoazobenzene are positive for PN antigen. Thus it seems to be typical of all such lesions. Transplantable Morris and other hepatomas are variable. Some are positive and some negative.

DR. HOFSTAETTER: Does the open loose chromatin structure of the hyperplastic nodules reflect an increase in euchromatin, that is, in transcriptional activity? Or can it be explained by a specific removal of histones by induced protease, as found by Dr. Troll?

DR. FARBER: The loose open chromatin structure is associated with an increase in RNA synthesis, presumably by increased transcription. The possible changes— histones or other proteins associated with DNA (nonhistone chromosomal proteins) —are important areas for study.

DR. REUBER: If you transplant hyperplastic nodules to the mammary fat pad, do you find remodeling? It is difficult on a tissue section to tell whether single or double plates are forming, or *vice versa*. Thus, additional evidence is needed that remodeling is actually taking place.

Under the conditions of my experiments using 2,7-diacetylaminofluorene (di-AAF) and a well-balanced diet, the hyperplastic nodules in male rats do not contain glycogen. Could the glycogen in hyperplastic nodules in your experiment be related to the diet that you use?

DR. FARBER: We can easily determine the basic organizational pattern of the hepatocytes in sections. The differences from normal liver are striking. The transplants of normal liver or of hyperplastic nodules in mammary fat pads do not grow. They remain as they were in the liver. The possible remodeling remains to be studied carefully.

As you know, many authors in several laboratories around the world see the glycogen in hyperplastic nodules induced by one of many different carcinogens. Perhaps you don't see them because your diet is different or because the di-AAF induces additional lesions in glycogen metabolism.

DR. OKADA: Do all the nodules formed in the same liver have the same level of aryl hydrocarbon hydroxylase (AHH) activity?

DR. FARBER: Our data with 2-AAF-induced nodules and those of Dr. Okita indicate that all nodules show the low cytochrome P-450 and our data show the large decrease in the AHH activity with many different nodules. So far, it is a consistent finding.

DR. TAKAYAMA: How many hyperplastic nodules can develop into hepatic carcinoma?

DR. FARBER: I cannot give you a quantitative answer. However, it is clear that few nodules develop into hepatocellular carcinoma. As emphasized previously (see Refs. *2* and *4*) the process is statistical and probabilistic, as would be anticipated from a cellular evolutionary process (*2*).

FUNDAMENTALS IN CANCER PREVENTION, P. N. MAGEE ET AL. (EDS.),
UNIV. OF TOKYO PRESS, TOKYO / UNIV. PARK PRESS, BALTIMORE, PP. 89–102, 1976

Early Cell Changes in the Course of Chemical Carcinogenesis

W. H. BUTLER

Department of Histopathology, St. George's Hospital Medical School, London, U.K.

Abstract: The most reliable way of preventing malignant neoplasia within the population is to prevent exposure of the population to chemicals which are carcinogenic. However as this ideal will be extremely difficult to achieve, the study of the early cellular changes of neoplasia may lead to an understanding of the mechanism involved in induced carcinogenesis and lead to modification of the response.

When studying the early cellular changes which may be related to development of neoplasia it is necessary to be able to distinguish different types of phenomena occurring within a heterogeneous organ. An ideal system might be one in which a single dose of a compound induces 100% incidence of the neoplasm being studied, in the absence of any other type of toxic reaction. However, it is well recognised that chemical carcinogens are toxic to the animal under test and also to the cell type from which the neoplasm develops. Such toxicity, which may be represented by necrosis of individual cells, in itself induces a response to the damaged tissue. As a consequence of this it is always necessary to distinguish those events leading to neoplasia from those which are coincidental and reactive (*1*). A further limitation is imposed as the characterization of neoplasia requires the demonstration of autonomous growth in the primary host with the additional properties of invasion and/or metastases if the lesion is to be considered malignant. In cases of chemically induced malignant neoplasm the manifestation of these events requires time. It is possible for us to characterise cell populations based upon structural and biochemical properties, however, the all important demonstration of autonomous growth may be harder to achieve.

Neoplasia is a focal phenomenon within an organ. As I will demonstrate only a few cells within a heterogenous population become neoplastic. In order to arrive at any understanding of mechanism it is necessary to identify the cell population involved and then determine whether relevant biochemical interactions, some of which are being discussed at this symposium, occur in the affected cells.

At present we only have an association of biochemical and morphological events in a whole organ with the subsequent development of a small focal lesion.

Renal Neoplasia

We are studying this in two different systems. The first is that of renal carcinogenesis induced by dimethylnitrosamine (DMN) and the second the induction of hepatacellular carcinoma induced by aflatoxin. A single dose of DMN, as shown by Magee and Barnes (2), may induce malignant renal neoplasia following this dose. Subsequently McLean and Magee (3) demonstrated that following protein dietary depletion for 1 week prior to treatment with an LD_{50} dose of DMN, 100% of the survivors developed renal sarcoma. At the time we initiated the study of early morphological changes seen in the kidney no pathological events had been recorded for about 8 weeks following the administration of DMN. However, it seemed unreasonable to us that there should be a latent period where nothing should happen. We therefore studied the sequential development of lesions from

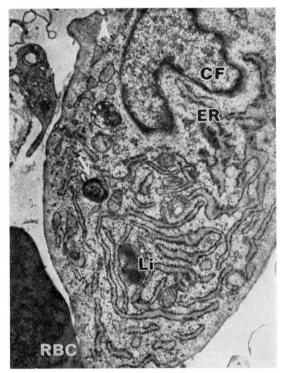

FIG. 1.   Cortical fibroblast (CF) adjacent to juxtaglomerular body 24 hr after administration of 50 mg/kg DMN. The cytoplasm contains abundant anastomosing channels of rough endoplasmic reticulum (RER) supporting characteristic clusters of ribosomes (ER). Lipid droplets (Li) and myelin figures (arrow) are early signs of intracellular damage. Arrowhead, caveola indenting the plasma membrane. An erythrocyte (RBC) is free in the interstitial space. × 13,000.

24 hr until unequivocal malignant neoplasm was recognised. This system induces both epithelial and mesenchymal neoplasia but in this paper I will only discuss the development of the mesenchymal neoplasm. This neoplasm is composed predominantly of fibroblast-like cells, smooth muscle and vascular structures (4).

The first acute toxic reaction recognised by cytoplasmic disruption, occurred by about 24 hr in some of the interstitial fibroblasts of the renal cortex, also at this time a few prominent fibroblasts were present (Fig. 1), the cytoplasm of which contained abundant anastomosing channels of rough endoplasmic reticulum (RER), lipid droplets, and myelin figures (5). At 3 days, before a significant inflammatory response occurred, mistoses were present in free interstitial cells which, ultrastructurally, were similar to the interstitial fibroblasts. This wave of proliferation, commencing at 3 days, has subsequently been confirmed by an autoradiographic study of incorporation of tritiated thymidine (6). The peak of mitotic and DNA synthetic activity of the cortical interstitial cells occurred on day 6 and returned to control levels by day 21 (Fig. 2).

As well as the acute reaction of the interstitial fibroblasts, an acute toxic response was observed in the proximal tubules of the cortex. A few tubule cells underwent necrosis by 5–6 days which initiated both a mitotic response at 5–6 days with a peak at 10 days (Fig. 3) and also an inflammatory reaction. As a result of this acute inflammatory reaction a diffuse hypercellularity of the cortex was

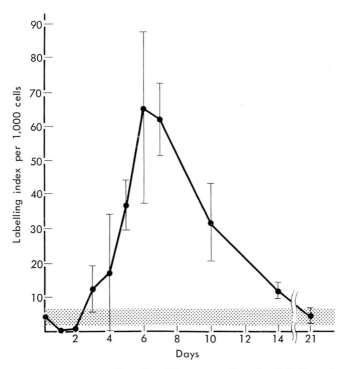

FIG. 2.   Sequential effect of DMN on mesenchymal cells in Zones 1 and 2. Labelling indices of intertubular cells 1 hr after a single pulse of ^{3}H-TdR. The stippled area represents the control range of 2 standard deviations (6).

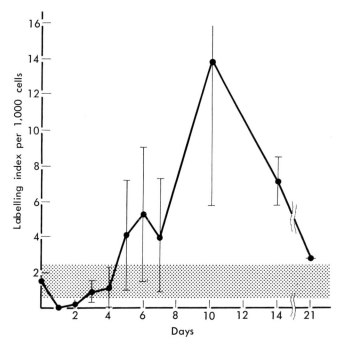

Fig. 3.   Sequential effect of DMN on epithelial cells of Zones 1 and 2. Labelling indices of cells of the nephron 1 hr after a single pulse of ^{3}H-TdR. The stippled area represents the control range of 2 standard deviations (*6*).

observed. This reaction resolved by 3–4 weeks leaving a few residual hypercellular foci within the cortex containing abnormal fibroblast-like cells (*5*). By 6–8 weeks these hypercellular foci became very prominent, the abundant cell types being plasma cells, lymphocytes, and macrophages. But also within the foci were spindle cells similar to those observed in the earlier time periods and now frequently encircling preexisting tubules (*4*). This apparent immunological response came to an abrupt end by 12 weeks following which there was rapid proliferation of mesenchymal foci so that unequivocal macroscopic invasive neoplasm was present by 22 weeks. This sequence is summarised in Fig. 4.

It is therefore clearly demonstrable that there is a continuous sequence of events from the stage of acute injury to the final demonstration of invasive malignant neoplasia. The unequivocal evidence of autonomous growth and invasion requires about 20 weeks. The best hypothesis to explain these observations is that the complete neoplasm is induced immediately following treatment with DMN. However in order to confirm this hypothesis it is necessary to demonstrate that the cell population has the properties of autonomous growth at an early stage.

In an initial series of experiments (*7*) abnormal fibroblast-like cells with many features of transformed cells were grown from the renal cortex 7 days following treatment with DMN. These cells had some of the ultrastructural characteristics of the abnormal fibroblast found both in the early-developing lesion and the invasive, metastasising sarcoma. These studies have been continued by Hard *et al.*

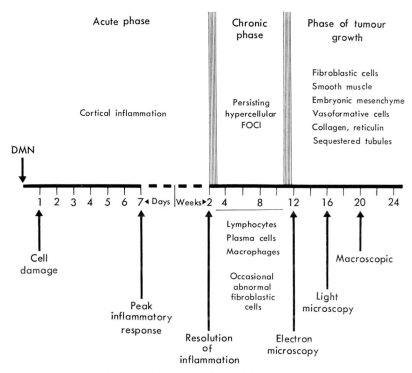

FIG. 4. Summary of sequential changes observed in the course of the development of renal mesenchymal neoplasm.

TABLE 1. Culture of Kidney Cells

Property		Normal	Tumour	DMN-treated
Life span		Limited	Unlimited	Unlimited
Contact inhibition		Yes	No	No
Transformation		No	—	Yes
Mitotic rate	{primary	High	High	Low
	{subcultures	Low	High	High
Cloning efficiency		Nil	High	High
Growth-plating efficiency		Low	High	High
Methyl cellulose gel		No	Yes	Yes
Con. A. agglutination		No	Yes	Yes

Summary of properties of renal cortical cells grown in cultures. This summary has been compiled from Borland and Hard (8) and Hard and Borland (9).

who have demonstrated the maintenance of continuous cultures obtained from animals 20 hr after *in vivo* treatment with the carcinogen. The *in vitro* behaviour of these cultures is similar to those of transformed cells and also cells derived from the final sarcoma when grown in culture (9). These characteristics are summarised in Table 1. It can be seen that the behaviour of cells derived from the renal cortex during the very early stages of the development of this lesion are similar to those of the final sarcoma and have many of the criteria for " neoplastic transformation."

Therefore these tissue culture experiments support the hypothesis that neoplasia has been induced as an acute response and only time is required for the full demonstration of autonomous growth, invasion, and metastases in the host.

If autonomous growth can be induced by very short term administration of a chemical what can be done in the way of prevention of neoplasia? Obviously as in any branch of clinical medicine prevention of the initial disease process is the ultimate aim. In the system I have described, as in most instances of induced neoplasia, there is an apparent dose response curve. However we do not know what the pattern of cell response will be when, for example, a final tumour incidence of 20% is seen. We have given some evidence that there is an early immune response to the developing neoplasm and that this is partially successful in aborting the development of focal lesions. This response comes to an abrupt end which may represent the phenomenon of "blockade." It is possible to speculate that the observed dose response reflects successful immunological defence but in order to utilise this response to combat the very early stages of malignant neoplasia in man presents a formidable challenge.

Liver Neoplasia

We have also studied the development of hepatocellular carcinoma which has been discussed by Dr. Farber at this symposium. The system we have investigated is that of feeding 5 ppm aflatoxin to inbred male Fischer rats for 6 weeks which results in a final incidence of 100% hepatic carcinoma by 40–50 weeks. There are considerable difficulties in interpreting the early events seen in the liver as we at present have no system by which a 100% incidence of malignant neoplasia may be induced by single treatment of a chemical. Feeding a toxic chemical for a num-

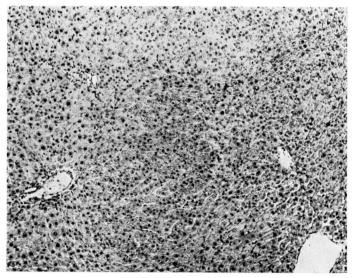

Fig. 5.   Liver of rat fed 5 ppm aflatoxin for 6 weeks showing area of small basophilic parenchymal cells. Hematoxylin and Eosin stain (H-E). × 130.

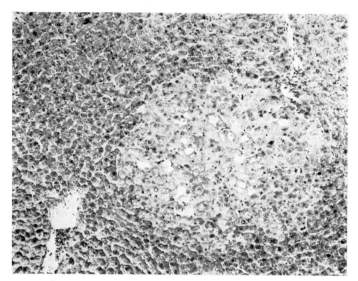

FIG. 6.   Liver of rat fed 5 ppm aflatoxin for 6 weeks showing focus of eosinophilic parenchymal cells. H-E. × 130.

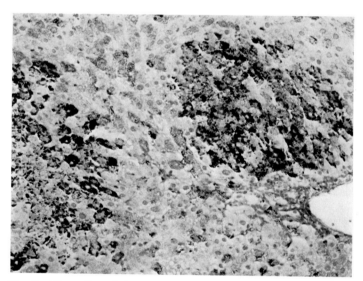

FIG. 7.   Liver of rat fed 5 ppm aflatoxin for 6 weeks and starved overnight before killing. Showing foci of basophilic parenchymal cells containing glycogen. Periodic acid-Schiff stain (P.A.S.). × 210.

ber of weeks to induce an irreversible change inevitably results in difficulties in distinguishing reactive hyperplasia from those associated with the development of neoplasia. In our experiments, at 6 weeks, when the animals are returned to a normal diet, we would suggest that the neoplasm is present in the liver but is not recognised. As with the kidney system mentioned above, and indeed other systems of induced neoplasia, time is required for the demonstration of autonomous growth in the host.

96 BUTLER

At the end of the feeding period we are able to recognise, using morphological criteria, foci of hepatic parenchymal cells which differ from the surrounding normal trabeculae. Some foci are composed of rather small basophilic parenchymal cells (Fig. 5), while other foci are composed of larger eosinophilic vacuolated cells (Fig. 6). Mitoses can be seen within both types of foci. As described by Bannasch (*10*) we have found that some of the basophilic foci contain starvation resistant glycogen

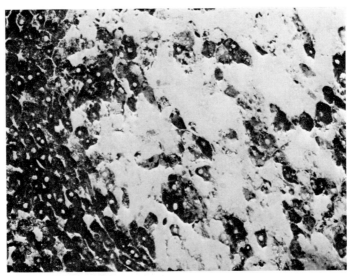

FIG. 8. Liver of rat fed 5 ppm aflatoxin for 6 weeks and fed overnight before killing. Showing foci of eosinophilic parenchymal cells showing patchy loss of glycogen. P.A.S. ×210.

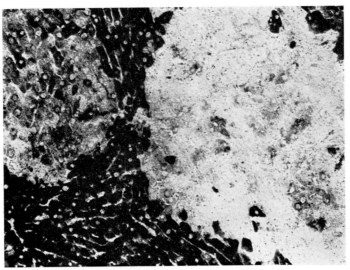

FIG. 9. Liver of rat fed 5 ppm aflatoxin for 6 weeks and fed overnight before killing. Two foci of parenchymal cells are present, the larger showing absence of glucose-6-phosphatase (G. 6-Pase) reaction and the smaller a reduction of reaction. G. 6-Pase. ×210.

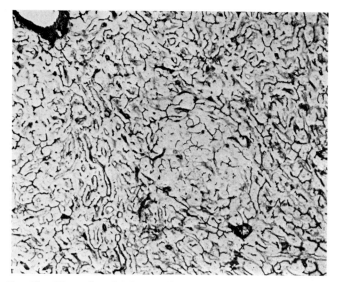

Fig. 10.   Liver of rat fed 5 ppm aflatoxin for 6 weeks and fed overnight before killing. Small focus is present with reduction of both sinusoidal and canalicular reaction. ATPase. ×210.

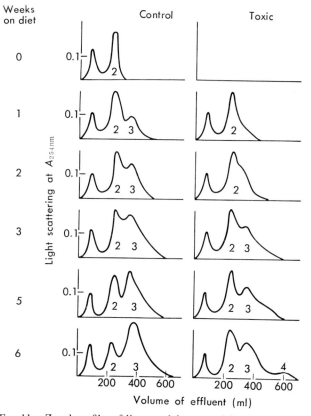

Fig. 11.   Zonal profiles of liver nuclei prepared from weanling rats fed control or toxic diet. Line light scattering at 254 nm regions of profile labelled 2 contained diploid, 3 contained tetraploid, and 4 contained octaploid nuclei (11).

(Fig. 7), while the eosinophilic vacuolated foci contain little or no glycogen (Fig. 8). When preparing tissue for a concurrent electron microscopic study, we perfuse fix the liver either *via* the portal vein or the hepatic artery. We have found that these small foci of cells perfuse very poorly *via* the portal vein but more readily *via* the hepatic artery. We are uncertain whether the modified glycogen response reflects a change within the hepatocyte or in the blood supply to the focus. We have also conducted a histochemical study of these early lesions and find that the foci contain either a reduced amount of glucose-6-phosphatase (Fig. 9) or in some instances, again associated with the eosinophilic foci, a complete absence of reaction. We also find that both foci have a reduction of succinic dehydrogenase reaction, anilene hydroxylase, and a patchy loss of membrane ATPase (Fig. 10). Although these changes are consistently seen in the proliferative foci we are uncertain of relevance to the development of hepatic carcinoma. Indeed changes are present in hepatic parenchymal cells which persist until the recognition of the final neoplasm. In collaboration with Dr. G. E. Neal, we have found that during the course of the 6-week feeding period there is a modification in the normal maturation of diploid to tetraploid parenchymal cells (Fig. 11). The tetraploid population is greatly reduced and this change in distribution persists for the life of the animal (*11*). While this change occurs through the liver which retains the normal lobular pattern and also, from preliminary densitometric studies, within the proliferative foci it is difficult to conclude this phenomenon is related to the development of neoplasia.

We would suggest that the best hypothesis to explain the observations is that at 6 weeks an irreversible change has occurred within the liver, and at that time hepatic carcinoma is present. However, the problem in interpreting the morphological findings is which, if any, of the foci seen represent neoplasia and which represent the response to toxic injury. A similar pattern of histochemical change has been described following a single dose of nitrosamine which does not lead to development of hepatic carcinoma (*12*). It is therefore necessary to be cautious in interpreting these early phenomena. If any of these foci represent developing neoplasia, many are present throughout the liver at the end of the 6-week feeding period while only relatively few carcinomas are seen. In the liver we have no evidence of an immunological response similar to that observed in the kidney to account for the decrease in number of lesions.

Again if we are interested in prevention of hepatic neoplasia in the human population the best method of achieving this is removal or reduction of recognised hepatocarcinogens from the environment. However, a proper assessment of these early lesions may make the prediction of which chemicals are hazardous more reliable. A further study of these early lesions may also give information as to how this response may be modified after induction.

REFERENCES

1. Foulds, L. *In;* "Neoplastic Development," pp. 41–90, Academic Press, London, 1969.

2. Magee, P. N. and Barnes, J. M.   Induction of kidney tumours in the rat with dimethylnitrosamine (N-nitrosodimethylamine). J. Pathol. Bacteriol., *84*: 19–31, 1962.

3. McLean, A. F. and Magee, P. N.   Increased renal carcinogenesis by dimethylnitrosamine in protein deficient rats. Brit. J. Exp. Pathol., *51*: 587–590, 1971.

4. Hard, G. C. and Butler, W. H.   Cellular analysis of renal neoplasia: Light microscopic study of the development of interstitial lesions induced in the rat kidney by a single carcinogenic dose of dimethylnitrosamine. Cancer Res., *30*: 2806–2815, 1970.

5. Hard, G. C. and Butler, W. H.   Ultrastructural study of the development of interstitial lesions leading to mesenchymal neoplasia induced in the rat renal cortex by dimethylnitrosamine. Cancer, *31*: 337–347, 1971.

6. Hard G. C. and Shaw, D. M.   Proliferative response in the rat kidney induced by a single carcinogenic dose of dimethylnitrosamine. Cell Tissue Kinet., *7*: 433–441, 1974.

7. Hard, G. C., Borland, R., and Butler, W. H.   Altered morphology and behaviour of kidney fibroblasts *in vitro*, following *in vivo* treatment of rats with a carcinogenic dose of dimethylnitrosamine. Experientia, *27*: 1208–1209, 1971.

8. Borland, R. and Hard, G. C.   Early appearance of "transformed" cells from the kidneys of rats treated with a "single" carcinogenic dose of dimethylnitrosamine (DMN) detected by tissue culture *in vivo*. Eur. J. Cancer, *10*: 177–184, 1974.

9. Hard, G. C. and Borland, R.   *In vitro* culture of cells isolated from dimethylnitrosamine—induced renal mesenchymal tumours of the rat. I. Qualitative morphology. J. Natl. Cancer Inst., *54*: 1085–1095, 1975.

10. Bannasch, P.   The cytoplasm of hepatocytes during carcinogenesis. *In;* P. Rentchnick (ed), Recent Results in Cancer Research, vol. 19, Springer-Verlag, Berlin-Heidelberg-New York, 1968.

11. Neal, G. E., Godoy, H. M., Judah, D. J., and Butler, W. H.   Some effects of acute and chronic dosing with aflatoxin B_1 on rat liver nuclei. Cancer Res., in press.

12. Scherer, E., Hoffmann, M., Emmelot, P., and Friedrich-Freska, H.   Quantitative study on foci of altered liver cells induced in the rat by a single dose of dimethylnitrosamine and partial hepatectomy. J. Natl. Cancer Inst., *49*: 93–106, 1972.

Discussion of Paper of Dr. Butler

DR. FARBER: Dr. Butler, may I ask for a point of clarification? Drs. Hard and Borland in their published papers reported that it took 5 weeks of growth in culture before growth in soft agar and other evidence for cell transformation *in vitro* was seen. Is this your interpretation, or are you saying that new evidence suggests criteria for cell transformation appear *in vitro* within 20 hr?

DR. BUTLER: In culture, the appearance of "transformed" cells only occurred after multiple subcultures. Such transformation was not seen in untreated animals. The mechanism of transformation is not understood. I do not consider that "transformation" in tissue culture can be equated directly with the induction of neoplasia, that is, autonomous growth in the primary host. What is clear is that continuous cultures are obtained from animals shortly after treatment with the carcinogen. This, in our opinion, supports the view that neoplasia is induced as an initial event in a multi-stage process.

DR. MAGEE: Have you tried the effect of immunosuppression on the lesions that you described in the kidney or in the liver?

DR. BUTLER: In collaboration with Dr. G. C. Hard (Baker Inst., Melbourne, Australia) we attempted to use anti-lymphocyte serum (ALS) for immunosuppression, but without any appreciable effect. I understand that Dr. Hard has reproduced this.

DR. WEISBURGER: With Dr. Kroes, we also studied immunosuppression by ALS on the process of primary cancer induction in liver with N-hydroxy-2-acetylaminofluorene, where we saw no remarkable effects, and on the colon by azoxymethane where again no change in incidence or rate of tumor formation was seen. In the latter case, however, liver angiosarcomas were seen in the ALS-treated groups whereas none were found in untreated controls (Cancer Res., *35*: 265, 1975).

DR. REUBER: You have done an excellent job of observing and illustrating the lesions that develop in a relatively short period of time in the kidney of rats given dimethylnitrosamine (DMN). I believe this may be related to the kidney perfusion technique that you used. You have beautifully shown that there are multiple stages in the development of carcinomas but that they only develop over a shorter period of time.

DR. BUTLER: The perfusion technique allows visualization of many changes within the kidney. Much work has been reported which demonstrates that in order to preserve the kidney in the physiological state, perfusion fixation techniques are required. Unless this is done, the degree of fixation artifact is such that any interpretation of structure change is of limited value. I interpret our observation of the development of renal sarcomas as indicating that complete neoplasia is induced within a few hours. There is then a continuous sequence of development until unequivocal malignant neoplasia can be demonstrated in the host. The development of the final lesion is modified by host reponses to the neoplasm.

DR. KITAGAWA: (1) Have you noticed an elevation of enzyme levels in "enzyme-deficient" hyperplastic areas with time? (2) The character of hyperplastic areas induced by different experimental conditions may be different, in terms of the persistency of the enzyme deficiency.

DR. BUTLER: (1) No, most foci we have studied show an enzyme depletion. (2) This is possible. Following aflatoxin we see a spectrum of changes.

DR. WATTENBERG: I have two questions. (1) Do renal fibroblasts have any unique properties? (2) Have you cultured fibroblasts from tissues in which neoplastic response does not occur?

DR. BUTLER: (1) There is evidence that pericytes and fibroblasts from the renal cortex are different from other sites in that they retain the ability of multi-potential development. In our original observation we considered that the final neoplasm exhibited most forms of mesenchymal differentiation. (2) As far as I am aware, fibroblasts from other sites will not grow in continuous culture following treatment in a host animal.

DR. OKADA: Can you quantitate these foci? I am wondering whether there is a possibility of using these foci counts as in vitro colony counts.

DR. BUTLER: We have not quantitated the foci. This could be done and is in progress in order to study the dose-response in this system.

DR. SUGANO: Mine is not a question. You mentioned a change in ploidy of the hepatic cells. Would you please explain it briefly?

DR. BUTLER: In collaboration with Dr. G. E. Neal (MRC, Carshalton, U.K.), we studied induced changes in ploidy of rat liver treated with aflatoxin. The normal maturation of the diploid population of hepatocytes to a tetraploid population is reversed in the feeding period. At the termination of treatment most hepatic parenchymal nuclei are diploid. This shift to a diploid population is present for life. Preliminary studies have shown that the small proliferative foci and the final hepatocarcinoma have a predominantly diploid population.

DR. KONDO: Does the kidney cancer induction occur only in a specific strain?

DR. BUTLER: No, many strains of rats are susceptible to the induction of renal neoplasia by nitrosamines.

DR. MAGEE: Professor Druckrey has induced similar renal tumors by single doses of DMN in his BD-IX strain of rats.

FUNDAMENTALS IN CANCER PREVENTION, P. N. MAGEE ET AL. (EDS.),
UNIV. OF TOKYO PRESS, TOKYO / UNIV. PARK PRESS, BALTIMORE, PP. 103–111, 1976

Early Cytological Changes Induced in Rat Liver Cells by Chemicals

Prince Masahito, Shozo Takayama, and Kiyomi Yamada*

*Cancer Institute, Tokyo, Japan and Clinical Research Institute, National Center Hospital, Tokyo, Japan**

Abstract: All the hepatocarcinogens administered to rats markedly increased the mitotic rate in the liver, whereas except for nitrosobutylurea, other compounds did not. Cytogenetic analyses of the ploidy rate and chromosome abnormalities showed qualitative differences between the mitotic liver cells of animals treated with hepatocarcinogens and those treated with other compounds.

This method could be used to screen for hepatocarcinogens in rats.

Previously we reported (*1*, *2*) that the mitotic rate is elevated in the liver of rats given various chemical carcinogens. It was uncertain whether this represented an initial event in carcinogenesis or liver regeneration. To elucidate this, we are now studying the histologic and cytogenetic changes in the liver during and after administration of various hepatocarcinogenic and nonhepatocarcinogenic substances to rats.

This paper reports cytogenetic studies on the mitotic rate in rat liver after administration of these substances.

Chromosome Analyses

Male Donryu rats were used. They were 8 weeks old and weighed about 150 g at the beginning of the experiments. The chemicals used were as follows: diethylnitrosamine (DEN) (Eastman Organic Chemicals, Rochester, N.Y.); 3'-methyl-4-dimethylaminoazobenzene (3'-Me-DAB) (Wako Pure Chemical Industries); 4-dimethylaminoazobenzene (DAB) (Wako Pure Chemical Industries); 2,7-acetylaminofluorene (2,7-AAF) (Tokyo Kasei Co., Ltd.); 2-acetylaminofluorene (2-AAF) (Tokyo Kasei Co., Ltd.); aflatoxin B_1 (Makor Chemicals, Jerusalem, Israel); α-benzene hexachloride (α-BHC) (Tokyo Kasei Co., Ltd.); N-nitrosobutylurea (NBU) (synthesized by Dr. Nakadate, National Institute of Hygienic Sciences, Tokyo); 2-methyl-4-dimethylaminoazobenzene (2-Me-DAB) (synthesized

TABLE 1.   Mitotic Rates (%) in Liver Cells after Administration of Various Compounds for 3 Weeks

Compound	Dose (%) and route	3 weeks		7 weeks		11 weeks		No. of rats
		Expt. 1	Expt. 2	Expt. 1	Expt. 2	Expt. 1	Expt. 2	
Hepatocarcinogen								
DEN	0.01 in drinking water	0.33	0.41	0.22	0.28	0.05	0.10	6
3'-Me-DAB	0.06 in diet	0.18	0.21	0.12	0.17	0.04	0.06	6
DAB	0.06 in diet	0.16	0.22	0.20	0.26	0.04	0.06	6
2,7-AAF	0.025 in diet	0.23	0.30	0.10	0.12	0.04	0.05	6
2-AAF	0.03 in diet	0.20	0.22	0.14	0.15	0.03	0.04	6
Aflatoxin B_1	0.01 in diet	0.17	0.22	0.16	0.51	0.06	0.09	6
α-BHC	0.06 in diet	0.09	0.13	0.08	0.11	0.02	0.02	6
Mean		0.22		0.19		0.05		
Nonhepatocarcinogen								
NBU	0.04 in drinking water	0.11	0.14	0.05	0.08	0.02	0.03	6
2-Me-DAB	0.06 in diet	0.02	0.03	0.02	0.03	0.02	0.03	6
Methionine	0.025 in diet	0.02	0.02	0.02	0.02	0.03	0.03	6
Maleic hydrazide	1.0 in diet	0.02	0.02	0.02	0.03	0.02	0.03	6
DDT	0.025 in diet	0.01	0.01	0.02	0.02	0.02	0.02	6
AF-2	0.4 in diet	0.02	0.02					2
Cigarette tar	0.02 in drinking water	0.02	0.03					2
Mean		0.03		0.02		0.03		
Control								
I (normal)		0.02	0.02	0.02	0.02	0.02		4
II (72 hr after partial hepatectomy)		0.93						1

by Dr. Hashimoto, Tohoku University, Sendai); methionine (Tokyo Kasei Co., Ltd.); maleic hydrazide (Tokyo Kasei Co., Ltd.); 1,1,1-trichloro-2,2-bis(p-chlorophenyl)ethane (DDT) (Tokyo Kasei Co., Ltd.); furylfuramide (AF-2) (provided by Dr. Nakadate, National Institute of Hygienic Sciences, Tokyo); and crude cigarette tar (produced by the Central Institute of the Japan Tobacco and Salt Public Corporation, Tokyo). Seven of these compounds (DEN, 3'-Me-DAB, DAB, 2,7-AAF, 2-AAF, aflatoxin B_1, and α-BHC) are hepatocarcinogens, and the other seven (NBU, 2-Me-DAB, methionine, maleic hydrazide, DDT, AF-2, and cigarette tar) are mostly toxic, but not hepatocarcinogenic.

These compounds were given to rats for 3 weeks at the dosages, and by the routes shown in Table 1. The dosages used were those usually adopted for induction of experimental hepatomas in rats.

Animals were killed 3, 7, and 11 weeks after the beginning of treatment, and 3 hr after i.p. injection of 0.1 mg colchicine/100 g body weight to arrest mitosis.

For comparison, some rats were partially hepatectomized, and killed 72 hr after the operation.

For examination, pieces of liver tissue were removed and suspensions of liver cells were obtained by pipetting the material up and down in 20 ml of Hanks' balanced salt solution in a test tube. The suspension was allowed to stand for a few minutes to allow relatively long pieces of tissue to precipitate and then 15 ml of the upper part of the suspension were centrifuged at 1,000 rpm for 5 min. The precipitated cells were resuspended in hypotonic solution (0.9% sodium citrate). The suspension was stood for 20 min at room temperature, and then centrifuged and the precipitated cells were fixed in methanol-acetic acid mixture (3:1, v/v). The fixative was changed 3 times at 30-min intervals and finally the cells were suspended in a small volume of the fixative. A few drops of the suspension were placed on a slide and quickly dried over a gas burner. Then the slide was stained with Giemsa, mounted, and examined under a microscope. Eighty slides were prepared to examine the effect of each compound because the mitotic rates were low and few cells were in metaphase.

The 42 chromosomes of normal male Donryu strain rats were arranged according to the numbering system proposed by the Animal Chromosome Study Group (*3*). In Donryu rats 5 pairs of autosomes (Nos. 1, 2, 11, 12, and 13) and the Y chromosome are distinguishable morphologically. In this study, chromosomes No. 11 and 12, and Y could be identified in some metaphase cells in good quality preparations, but this was usually not possible. Therefore, the normal 42 chromosomes were tentatively classified into 6 groups as follows: Nos. 1, 2, 3–12, 13, 14–18, and 19–20. Sex chromosomes were included in the Nos. 3–12 group.

The mitotic frequency was estimated by counting the number of interphase nuclei identified under the microscope before 3 mitoses had been found.

Cytogenetic Changes

The mitotic rates, ploidy rates, and chromosome abnormalities of mitotic cells in the livers of normal rats were compared with those in rats treated with hepato-carcinogens and other compounds, and those after partial hepatectomy.

Mitotic rates

The mitotic rates in the livers of rats sacrificed 3, 7, and 11 weeks after the beginning of treatment were analyzed, and the results are summarized in Table 1. The mitotic rates in the livers of rats treated with various hepatocarcinogens were 10 times higher than that in normal controls (0.02%) after 3 weeks, but decreased to 0.05% after 11 weeks (8 weeks after treatment). Of the compounds tested other than hepatocarcinogens, only NBU increased the mitotic rate in the liver and its effect was slight. 2-Me-DAB did not induce any increase in the mitotic rate, in sharp contrast to the chemically related carcinogenic compounds DAB and 3′-Me-DAB.

Ploidy rates

Ploidy rates of mitotic cells were determined by rough counts of chromosome numbers, usually made on 200 mitotic cells (Table 2). In normal controls, all the dividing cells in the liver had chromosome numbers in the diploid range and no tetraploid cells were observed. In rats sacrificed shortly after treatment with hepato-carcinogens (other than α-BHC), over 95% of the dividing cells in the livers were

TABLE 2. Ploidy Rates of Dividing Cells in the Liver Measured by Rough Counts of Chromosome Numbers

| Compound | 3 weeks | | | | 7 weeks | | | | 11 weeks | | | |
| | No. of cells analyzed | Ploidy | | | No. of cells analyzed | Ploidy | | | No. of cells analyzed | Ploidy | | |
		$2n$	$4n$	Others		$2n$	$4n$	Others		$2n$	$4n$	Others
Hepatocarcinogen												
DEN	205	99	1	0	200	79	21	0	200	99	1	0
3′-Me-DAB	203	98	2	0	95	99	1	0	112	91	9	0
DAB	202	100	0	0	200	80	20	0	136	93	7	0
2,7-AAF	202	99	1	0	122	100	0	0	200	91	9	0
2-AAF	206	97	3	0	200	100	0	0	200	95	4	1
Aflatoxin B_1	200	99	1	0	200	80	19	1	200	98	2	0
α-BHC	203	67	31	2	200	98	2	0	90	98	2	0
Nonhepatocarcinogen												
NBU	205	74	24	2	200	83	16	1	200	99	1	0
2-Me-DAB	96	97	3	0	200	79	20	1	100	81	19	0
Methionine	63	87	11	2	200	89	9	2	100	91	9	0
Maleic hydrazide	67	92	8	0	200	82	17	1	100	86	14	0
DDT	80	87	13	0	51	74	24	2	58	91	9	0
Control												
I (normal)	251	100	0	0								
II (72 hr after partial hepatectomy)	306	82	17	1								

diploid, the remainder being tetraploid. In rats treated with α-BHC, 30% of these cells were tetraploid. After 7 weeks (4 weeks after treatment), 20% of the dividing cells in rats treated with DEN, DAB, or aflatoxin B_1 were tetraploid. Administration of nonhepatocarcinogens generally increased the proportion of tetraploid cells to a value comparable to that of 17% in regenerating normal liver 72 hr after partial hepatectomy. However, in the livers of rats sacrificed after 11 weeks, the frequency of diploid cells was about 90%, irrespective of the compound that had been administered.

Chromosome abnormality

The results of chromosome analyses are shown in Table 3. The chromosome numbers were determined by exact counts in selected metaphase cells of high quality. Hyperploid cells with a chromosome count of 43 were observed in 18 of 332 cells analyzed in 12 rats treated with hepatocarcinogens. Karyotype analysis on cells with 41–43 chromosomes revealed chromosome abnormalities, characterized by monosomy, trisomy, and/or structural rearrangement of the chromosomes (Figs. 1 and 2). Chromosome abnormalities were not observed in rats given any nonhepatocarcinogens, though chromosome analysis was only possible in a few cells owing to the low mitotic rates and stickiness of the chromosomes. Chromosomal damage, probably due to the compounds tested, was analyzed in cells in which the

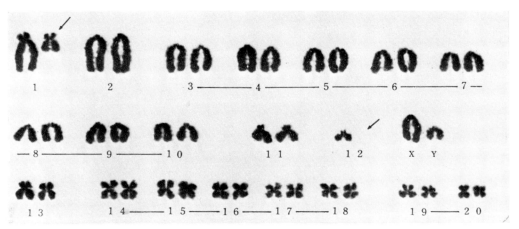

FIG. 1. Karyotype of a cell with 41 chromosomes in a rat treated with DAB. Partial deletion of the long arm in a No. 1 chromosome and monosomy No. 12 (indicated by arrows) is seen.

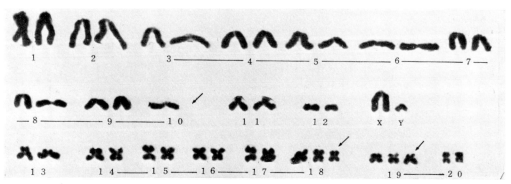

FIG. 2. Karyotype of a cell with 43 chromosomes in a rat treated with DEN. Loss of one chromosome and two extra chromosomes is seen (this abnormality was tentatively identified as monosomy No. 10 and trisomy No. 18 and No. 19, as indicated by arrows).

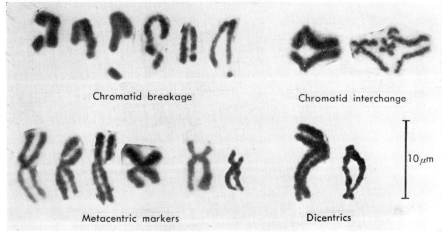

Chromatid breakage

Chromatid interchange

Metacentric markers

Dicentrics

10 μm

FIG. 3. Four types of chromosome abnormalities frequently observed in the liver cells in rats treated with hepatocarcinogens.

TABLE 3. Distribution of Chromosome Numbers and Numbers and Types of Chromosome Abnormalities in Liver Cells

Compound	No. of cells analyzed	Chromosome number							No. of cells analyzed	No. of cells with chromosome aberrations	Type of aberrations	
											Structural	
		39	40	41	42	43	44	49			Break age[a]	Rearrangement[b]
Hepatocarcinogen												
DEN	87	2	6	17	56	6			90	26	21	5
3'-Me-DAB	32		3	6	22	1			83	27	16	11
DAB	77		3	18	52	4			78	14	10	4
2,7-AAF	34		2	8	21	2		1	67	11	6	5
2-AAF	82	1	6	14	59	2			91	14	4	10
Aflatoxin B₁	13			1	9	2	1		32	8	6	2
α-BHC	7			1	5	1			37	12	7	5
Total	332	3	20	65 (20%)	224 (67%)	18 (6%)	1	1	478	112 (23%)	70	42
Nonhepatocarcinogen												
NBU	12		1	1	10				30	5	4	1
2-Me-DAB	6				6				25	5	5	0
Methionine	2				2				12	1	1	0
Maleic hydrazide	3				3				5	1	1	0
DDT	3			1	2				15	1	1	0
Total	26		1	2	23 (88%)				87	13 (15%)	12	1
Control	153	2	5	18 (12%)	128 (84%)				210	5 (3%)	5	0

[a] Including chromosomal or chromatid breaks, and fragments.   [b] Including chromatid interchanges, dicentrics, and monocentric markers.

morphology of the chromosomes was well preserved. The incidences of cells with chromosome aberrations in rats treated with the test compounds were significantly higher than the value of 3% in normal controls: the incidences in rats treated with hepatocarcinogens and with other compounds were 23% and 15%, respectively after 3 weeks and 25% and 9%, respectively after 7 weeks. The aberrations were mostly chromatid breaks and monocentric markers due to translocation between two chromosomes. Various marker chromosomes were observed in rats treated with hepatocarcinogens; large- and medium-sized metacentrics, large acrocentrics, lq-, and dicentrics (Fig. 3). In rats treated with nonhepatocarcinogens, the chromosome aberrations were mostly chromatid breaks and marker chromosomes were only observed in one cell in a rat treated with NBU.

DISCUSSION

In this study, all the hepatocarcinogens tested induced a marked increase in the mitotic rate of liver parenchymal cells, whereas, except for NBU, other compounds either had no influence on the mitotic rate of these cells or decreased it.

The cytogenetic changes produced by NBU were similar to those seen in regenerating liver after partial hepatectomy. Thus, since toxic nonhepatocarcinogens did not increase the mitotic rate the increase induced by hepatocarcinogens seems mainly due to their carcinogenic activities rather than to their toxic effects.

This conclusion is supported by the present results on the effects of these compounds on the ploidy rate and chromosome abnormalities. After treatment with hepatocarcinogens, almost all dividing liver cells were diploid and they usually had chromosome abnormalities. However, after treatment with nonhepatocarcinogens, some tetraploid cells were seen, but chromosomal abnormalities were not. Therefore this may be a good method to use in screening hepatocarcinogenic chemicals.

Carcinogens strongly inhibit the rise in the mitotic rate after partial hepatectomy (4, 5). This indicates that they reduce the regenerative potential of the liver or its ability to respond to mitotic stimuli.

The active cell proliferation and chromosome changes in cells observed in this work during carcinogen administration were probably the result of specific interactions between the carcinogens and their target tissue cells. It is uncertain whether these alterations during carcinogen treatment are prerequisites of malignant changes of liver cells, but these cytogenetic changes certainly have some relation to the initial and essential process of carcinogenesis.

ACKNOWLEDGMENT

This work was supported by a Grant-in-Aid from the Ministry of Education, Science, and Culture and the Japan Tobacco and Salt Public Corporation.

REFERENCES

1. Prince Masahito Hitachi, Yamada, K., and Takayama, S. Diethylnitrosamine-induced chromosome changes in rat liver cells. J. Natl. Cancer Inst., *53*: 507–516, 1974.
2. Prince Masahito Hitachi, Yamada, K., and Takayama, S. Cytologic changes induced in rat liver cells by short term exposure to chemical substances. J. Natl. Cancer Inst., *54*: 1245–1247, 1975.
3. Committee for a Standardized Karyotype of *Rattus norvegicus*: Standard karyotype of the Norway rat, *Rattus norvegicus*. Cytogenet. Cell Genet., *12*: 199–205, 1973.
4. Hsu, K. H. Effect of a carcinogenic substance (*o*-aminoazotoluene) on the reactivity of liver cells following partial hepatectomy. Bull. Eksped. Biol. Med., *53*: 116–118, 1962.
5. Maini, M. M. and Stich, H. F. Chromosomes of tumor cells. III. Unresponsiveness of precancerous hepatic tissue and hepatomas to a mitotic stimulus. J. Natl. Cancer Inst., *28*: 753–762, 1962.

Discussion of Paper of Drs. Takayama et al.

DR. SATO: Do you think such changes in mitotic index or chromosomal abnormalities induced by hepatocarcinogen are occurring only in hepatocytes or also in some other types of liver cells, like bile duct epithelia?

DR. TAKAYAMA: I think the possibility of small contamination of cells other than parenchymal cells cannot be completely excluded. However, this possibility was checked by examining the histologic slides of the same liver of colchicine-treated animals. Mitotic figures were observed in most cases in the hepatocytes.

DR. WEISBURGER: Dr. Takayama, in many test methods for assessing carcinogenicity, many halogenated hydrocarbons like DDT may be less active, or inactive in the rat, and yet highly active in the mouse. We have seen many reports and indeed governmental actions where these materials like Aldrin, Dieldrin, BHC were banned because of development of mouse liver tumors, without much carcinogenicity in the rat. I wonder whether your method could be broadened and extended to the mouse, to validate this question of whether these materials are really carcinogenic, in the proper sense of the word.

DR. TAKAYAMA: Thank you, Dr. Weisburger. We are now planning experiments on whether our system could be applied to mouse, hamster, and other species of animals.

DR. MAGEE: On your slide, you described DDT as a nonhepatocarcinogen in rats. Was this based on your observation or was it taken from the literature?

DR. TAKAYAMA: This was taken from the data in the IARC reports (IARC Monographs on the evaluation of carcinogenic risk of chemicals to man. Some Organic Chlorine Pesticides, vol. 5, 1974).

DR. CRADDOCK: I think you said that in control animals there was no replication in diploid cells, but in diethylnitrosamine (DEN)-treated animals diploids were found in mitosis. We have rather different results. Control animals showed some replication in tetraploid, but animals fed DEN did not show the usual increase in ploidy with age. Could you suggest any explanation for this apparent difference in response?

Dr. Takayama: We used relatively young rats (8 weeks) as controls and we did not observe tetraploid cells in the liver, and the percentage of tetraploid cells did not vary widely during 0–20 weeks of treatment with DEN.

Dr. Bootsma: Do you find evidence for the induction of specific chromosome abnormalities or for their existence at a later time in animals after drug treatment, and after partial hepatectomy?

Dr. Takayama: We did not find specific chromosomal abnormalities. We have tried but have not succeeded in obtaining good chromosome preparations in the case of partial hepatectomy with carcinogen treatment.

Dr. Kitagawa: Maini and Stich reported chromosome abnormalities in liver cells after feeding 2-methyl-4-dimethylaminoazobenzene (2-Me-DAB). Could you comment?

Dr. Takayama: Thank you, Dr. Kitagawa. Dr. Maini found mitotic irregularities in liver cells after treatment with 2-Me-DAB. I think the methods were different from ours and it is difficult to compare their results with ours.

Dr. Inui: When did you find the structural changes of chromosomes? Is it limited to just after chemical administration? How long did the changes persist?

Dr. Takayama: Chromosomal abnormalities were found as early as 3 weeks after the beginning of treatment with chemicals and these chromosomal changes persisted for 4 weeks after removal of the chemicals.

Dr. Weisburger: Our colleague in the United States, Dr. Peraino, recently published a follow-up on the observation that when he first gave limited amounts of a liver carcinogen, followed by phenobarbital he noted very much enhanced carcinogenicity. DDT did the same (Cancer Res., *35*: 2884–2890, 1975). The mechanism was not clear, but the observation is striking. I wonder whether you would comment on the possible mechanism whereby an early chromosome abnormality as you observe in 3 weeks might be potentiated into overt malignant cancer by subsequent phenobarbital or DDT feeding.

Dr. Takayama: No, I cannot now.

Prince Masahito: Tetraploid cells are present in increased numbers in the 5th week than in the 3rd week.

FUNDAMENTALS IN CANCER PREVENTION, P. N. MAGEE ET AL. (EDS.),
UNIV. OF TOKYO PRESS, TOKYO / UNIV. PARK PRESS, BALTIMORE, PP. 113–120, 1976

Anti-viral Vaccines against Herpes-associated Malignancies in Nonhuman Primates

R. Laufs

Hygiene Institut der Universität, Abteilung für Spezielle Medizinische Mikrobiologie, Göttingen, West Germany

Abstract: Antiviral vaccines against herpesvirus-induced malignancies in non-human primates were prepared by inactivation of oncogenic herpesviruses (*Herpesvirus saimiri* and *Herpesvirus ateles*) with heat and formaldehyde. The killed herpesvirus vaccines proved to be safe in 121 vaccinated monkeys of 4 different species and induced high titers of specific humoral antibodies in all vaccinated monkeys. The actively immunized monkeys (*Saguinus oedipus*) were resistant to the intramuscular challenge with 200–300 LD_{50} of cell-free oncogenic herpesviruses, while the nonvaccinated control monkeys died of malignant lymphoma 34 to 52 days after inoculation. The protected monkeys have now been under observation for two years without any sign of a clinical disease or a latent infection. The vaccination did not prevent but delayed tumor development after tumor cell transplantation. The resistance against infection *via* the oropharyngeal route remains to be determined. Killed Epstein-Barr virus (EBV) vaccines prepared in the same way proved to be safe and immunogenic in marmoset monkeys (*Callithrix jacchus* and *S. oedipus*). The fact that the killed herpesvirus vaccines were safe in different monkey species does not justify the use of such an EBV vaccine in man. The vaccines described are not free of viral DNA and the possibility that traces of viral DNA might be capable of bringing about malignant transformation cannot be excluded. The preparation of nucleic acid-free herpesvirus vaccines would solve this safety problem. Because of the anticipated long incubation period for herpesvirus cancer in man, however, it may be a long time before the protective efficacy of a killed EBV vaccine can be measured in terms of cancer prevention.

Important advances have been made in our knowledge of oncogenic herpesviruses. Herpesviruses are known to induce carcinoma, leukemia, or malignant lymphoma in different animal species. Herpesviruses are also suspected as being causal agents in human malignant neoplasia. In particular the Epstein-Barr virus (EBV) which is closely associated with Burkitt's lymphoma (BL) and nasopharyngeal carcinoma (NPC), stands first among candidate human cancer agents. According to Epstein (*1*) the reasons for this may be summarized thus: (1) cases of African BL and NPC only occur in individuals infected by the virus; (2) the viral DNA is present in all the tumor cells and determines the expression in them of virus-coded neoantigens (membrane antigen and EBV nuclear antigen) and virus production is activated in the tumor cells of BL when they are placed in tissue culture; (3) the virus causes *in vivo* a lymphoproliferative disease, the infectious mononucleosis (IM) with Paul Bunnel heterophile antibodies; (4) an impressive biologic property of EBV is its capacity to change lymphoid elements *in vitro* from resting cells into cell lines that are immortal; (5) the virus induces malignant tumors when inoculated in nonhuman primates. It seems that the first human tumor virus being identified is the EBV, a member of the herpesvirus family. The question arises whether now a vaccine against EBV can be developed.

Herpesviruses are transmitted horizontally and hence are subject to immunologic intervention, specifically by vaccines that stimulate immunity and prevent or limit proliferation of the naturally acquired virus on subsequent infection (*2*). The first example of a naturally occurring malignant tumor to be controlled in this way was the herpesvirus-induced Marek's lymphoma. Live attenuated (*3*) as well as killed (*4*) Marek's disease herpesvirus almost completely prevents this neoplastic disease of chickens. Live virus vaccines in general induce higher level and longer lasting immunity than killed vaccines and require only a small dose of virus to immunize. However, there are no reliable *in vitro* markers for the oncogenicity of live-attenuated herpesviruses that might apply to man. At present it seems impossible to administer to man a suspected oncogenic herpesvirus, however, attenuated since it may change its virulence *in vivo*. For the control of those human cancers suspected of having a herpesvirus cause, killed vaccines would be desirable.

Since experimentation in man to study the safety and efficacy of killed vaccines derived from oncogenic herpesviruses is out of the question we used a model system involving animals phylogenetically related to man. Two oncogenic simian herpesviruses, *Herpesvirus saimiri* (HVS) and *Herpesvirus ateles* (HVA) induce leukemia and/or malignant lymphoma in several New World monkey species (*5*). The oncogenic simian herpesviruses were used for the development of antiviral vaccines. The work with the primate model system offers the range of experimental possibilities necessary to study the questions in respect to safety and efficacy of killed herpesvirus vaccines.

Preparation of the Killed Vaccines

The vaccines were prepared by inactivation of HVS (strain S. 295C) and HVA (isolate No. 810) with heat (56°C for 4 hr) and formaldehyde (100 μg HCHO/ml for 6 days at 37°C and pH 6.5) as described recently (*6*). The survival curve of HVS is multicomponential after inactivation with heat as well as after treatment with formaldehyde. For vaccine production this problem could be solved by prolonged incubation periods without completely destroying the virus-specific antigenicity. As source of the viruses, cell- and serum-free supernatants of owl monkey kidney cell cultures lytically infected with HVS or HVA were used. The 100-fold concentrates of the inactivated virus suspensions were used as vaccines. The virus-specific antigenicity of the vaccines, as determined in the complement fixation (CF) test, ranged between 1 : 32 and 1 : 64. For immunization 4 to 6 intramuscular inoculations of the vaccines adsorbed onto Aluminiumhydroxydgel as adjuvant were given to each monkey within 12 weeks.

Safety of the Killed Vaccines

The killed HVS vaccine proved to be safe in 121 vaccinated monkeys of 4 different species. The three New World monkey species studied were: cotton-topped marmosets (*Saguinus oedipus*), common marmosets (*Callithrix jacchus*), and owl monkeys (*Aotus trivirgatus*). The Old World monkeys studied were African green monkeys (*Cercopithecus aethiops*). All of the vaccinated monkeys developed high titers of humoral antibodies against the oncogenic HVS: neutralizing antibodies, CF antibodies, and fluorescent antibodies. All vaccinated monkeys remained clinically well. Even 9 inoculations of the vaccine did not induce any sign of incompatibility. One of the common marmosets (*C. jacchus*) became pregnant during the vaccination procedure and delivered two healthy babies.

The vaccinated monkeys have now been under observation for more than two years. In contrast to the tumor-bearing monkeys and to the latently infected monkeys HVS could not be isolated from the vaccinated monkeys by cocultivation methods. The vaccine proved not only to be free of infectious virus particles and immunogenic but also to be nononcogenic. In spite of the fact that the killed vaccines were not free of viral DNA none of the 121 monkeys vaccinated developed a tumor. In all our *in vivo* experiments infectivity and oncogenicity of HVS were very closely correlated. One single infectious HVS particle was able to induce a tumor and all tumors examined produced complete virus particles after cocultivation *in vitro*.

Efficacy of the Killed Vaccines

The vaccinated cotton-topped marmosets (*S. oedipus*) were challenged by the intramuscular inoculation of cell-free HVS. The oncogenic virus was titrated in parallel in vaccinated monkeys and in nonvaccinated control monkeys. The vaccinated monkeys proved to be resistant against the challenge with 215 LD_{50} of the oncogenic HVS while the nonvaccinated control monkeys died of malignant lymphoma 34–52 days after inoculation. The vaccinated monkeys which had been challenged remained clinically well without signs of an infection and some of them have now been under observation for two years (7).

Under natural conditions HVS is transmitted by the oropharyngeal route of infection. The resistance of the vaccinated monkeys against this route of infection has not been examined yet. This experiment seems of great importance in respect to the prevention of the natural occurring disease.

The vaccination with the killed HVS vaccine did not prevent but delayed tumor development after tumor cell transplantation. Tumor tissue from an HVS-infected marmoset (*S. oedipus*) was transplanted in vaccinated monkeys of the same species. The tumors developed delayed in the vaccinated recipients as compared with the nonvaccinated control monkeys. The tumors which develop after transplantation are of recipient type (*8*).

The method used for the production of the killed HVS vaccine was successfully applied to the second oncogenic herpesvirus derived from monkeys, the HVA. The actively immunized cotton-topped marmosets (*S. oedipus*) were resistant to 316 LD_{50} of cell-free HVA while the nonvaccinated control monkeys died of malignant lymphoma. The challenged monkeys are clinically well and have now been under observation for one year (*9*).

Passive Immunization

The protection against malignant lymphoma achieved with the killed HVS vaccine in marmoset monkeys (*S. oedipus*) could be passively transmitted to other monkeys of the same species. Hyperimmune serum obtained from the vaccinated monkeys and used for passive immunization protected against the challenge with 32 LD_{50} of cell-free HVS and the development of malignant lymphoma was considerably delayed after challenge with doses higher than 32 LD_{50} of HVS (*10*).

Immunization with Killed EBV Vaccines

The recent demonstration of induction of lymphomas in cotton-topped marmosets (*S. oedipus*) (*11*) and an owl monkey (*12*) and the induction of a benign lymphoproliferative disease in common marmosets (*C. jacchus*) (*13*) by EBV opened the possibility to study the safety and efficacy of killed EBV vaccines in nonhuman primates. We applied the method developed for the inactivation of HVS and of HVA to EBV. For vaccine production the EBV-producing lymphoid cell line P3 HR1K (*14*) and the EBV-producing marmoset lymphoid cell line B95-8 (*15*) were used. The CF titers of the killed EBV vaccines were considerably lower than those obtained with the oncogenic simian herpesviruses and ranged between 1:4 and 1:16. The killed EBV vaccines were used for the immunization of 10 common marmosets (*C. jacchus*) and 4 cotton-topped marmosets (*S. oedipus*).

The monkeys received within 10 weeks 5 intramuscular inoculations of 1 ml vaccine adsorbed onto Aluminiumhydroxydgel as adjuvant. The vaccinated monkeys developed high titers of specific serum antibodies against EBV. The biologic property of EBV to transform human umbilical cord lymphocytes (*16*) was used to measure the neutralising antibodies. The sera obtained from the vaccinated monkeys inhibited the reaction whereas it was unaffected by the sera taken prior to vaccination. A human lymphoid cell line which did not carry the EBV genome and sera obtained from individuals in convalescence from IM and preillness sera were used as controls. All of the monkeys immunized with the killed EBV vaccine remained clinically well and have been under observation for 6 months.

DISCUSSION

These experiments clearly demonstrate that malignant tumors induced by oncogenic simian herpesviruses in nonhuman primates can be prevented by antiviral vaccines. The killed herpesvirus vaccines proved to be safe and efficient against the intramuscular challenge with cell-free oncogenic herpesviruses. Killed EBV vaccines prepared in the same way proved to be safe and immunogenic in common marmosets (*C. jacchus*), and it is likely that the vaccinated monkeys are protected against the infection with EBV. The fact that the killed herpesvirus vaccines were safe in different monkey species does not justify the use of an EBV vaccine prepared in the same way in man. The vaccines described are not free of viral nucleic acid and the possibility that traces of viral DNA in such a vaccine preparation might be capable of bringing about malignant transformation cannot be excluded. A vaccine against EBV which is free of viral DNA could be used in man. Such a vaccine could be prepared with viral subunits, soluble antigens or by purification of plasma membranes from human lymphoid cells which do have EBV-determined membrane antigens expressed on the cell surface. Antibodies to these antigens also have virus-neutralising activity (*1*). Protection of chickens against Marek's lymphoma with a vaccine free of viral nucleic acid has recently been reported (*4*).

The preparation of nucleic acid-free herpesvirus vaccines would probably solve the safety problems. But a vaccine has not only to be safe, it has to be efficient against the natural occurring infection, too. Because of the anticipated long incubation period for herpesvirus cancer in man it may be a long time before the protective efficacy of a killed EBV vaccine can be measured in terms of cancer prevention (*2*). However, trial of the vaccine in human populations could be carried out by testing its ability to protect those at risk from primary EBV infection accompanied by infectious mononucleosis (*1*). If such a field trial would prove the efficacy of the killed EBV vaccine against infectious mononucleosis the effects of vaccination on BL incidence could be tested in high incidence areas. The peak tumor incidence is at the age of 5 or 6 and it would take a decade to determine the efficacy of the vaccine. NPC is a major health problem for the population of Southern Chinese origin. However, the latent period between primary EBV infection and tumor development is even longer and the time required to obtain results could run into several decades. Nevertheless vaccination against EBV-associated tumors in man is a goal well worthy of continued study. The work with killed EBV vaccines in nonhuman primates might be expected to yield a great amount of data on safety, efficacy, and regimen that can provide important guidelines for its use in man.

ACKNOWLEDGMENT

This work was supported by the Deutsche Forschungsgemeinschaft, D 53 Bonn-Bad, Godesberg, West Germany.

REFERENCES

1. Epstein, M. A. Implications of a vaccine for the prevention of EBV infection: Ethical and logistic considerations. Cancer Res., *36*: 711–714, 1976.
2. Hilleman, M. R. Herpes simplex vaccines: Prospects and Problems. Cancer Res., *36*: 857–858, 1976.
3. Churchill, A. E., Payne, L. N., and Chubb, R. C. Immunization against Marek's disease using a live attenuated virus. Nature, *221*: 744–747, 1969.
4. Lesnik, F. and Ross, L. J. N. Immunization against Marek's disease using Marek's disease virus-specific antigens free from infectious virus. Int. J. Cancer, *16*: 153–163, 1975.
5. Deinhardt, F. *Herpesvirus saimiri. In;* A. S. Kaplan (ed.), The Herpesviruses, pp. 595–625, Academic Press, New York and London, 1973.
6. Laufs, R. and Steinke, H. Immunisation of marmoset monkeys with a killed oncogenic herpesvirus. Nature, *249*: 571–572, 1974.
7. Laufs, R. and Steinke, H. Vaccination of nonhuman primates against malignant lymphoma. Nature, *253*: 71–72, 1975.
8. Marczynska, B., Falk, L. A., Wolfe, L. G., and Deinhardt, F. Transplantation and cytogenetic studies of *Herpesvirus saimiri* induced disease in marmoset monkeys. J. Natl. Cancer Inst., *50*: 331–337, 1973.
9. Laufs, R. and Steinke, H. A killed vaccine derived from the oncogenic *Herpesvirus ateles*. J. Natl. Cancer Inst., *55*: 649–651, 1975.
10. Laufs, R. and Steinke, H. Passive immunisation of marmoset monkeys against neoplasia induced by a herpesvirus. Nature, *255*: 226–228, 1975.
11. Shope, T., Dechairo, D., and Miller, G. Malignant lymphoma in cottontop marmosets after inoculation with Epstein-Barr virus. Proc. Natl. Acad. Sci. U.S., *70*: 2487–2491, 1972.
12. Epstein, M. A., Hunt, R. D., and Rabin, H. Pilot experiments with EB virus in owl monkeys (*Aotus trivirgatus*). I. Reticuloproliferative disease in an inoculated animal. Int. J. Cancer, *12*: 309–318, 1973.
13. Deinhardt, F. Personal communication.
14. Klein, G. The Epstein-Barr virus. *In;* A. S. Kaplan (ed.), The Herpesviruses, pp. 521–555, Academic Press, New York and London, 1973.
15. Miller, G., Shope, T., Lisco, H., Stitt, D., and Lipman, M. Epstein-Barr virus: Transformation, cytopathic changes, and viral antigens in squirrel monkey and marmoset leukocytes. Proc. Natl. Acad. Sci. U.S., *69*: 383–387, 1972.
16. Miller, G. The oncogenicity of Epstein-Barr virus. J. Infect. Dis., *130*: 187–205, 1974.

Discussion of Paper of Dr. Laufs

DR. KATO: Epstein-Barr virus (EBV) persists in the human body almost throughout life even in the presence of antiviral humoral antibody. The same is true with Marek's disease (MD) virus. According to Dr. Kaaden in Germany, inactivated Turkey herpes virus (HVT) vaccine does not prevent MD lymphoma formation. Furthermore, all kinds of MD vaccine do not prevent superinfection of MD virus (MDV), and humoral antibody does not play any important role in the prevention of MD lymphoma formation. As you mentioned, your inactivated virus vaccine does prevent viral infection and humoral antibody plays a most important role in prevention of lymphoma formation of simian herpes viruses. I wonder if the situation of simian herpes virus, or EBV—monkey system is different from those of MDV—chicken system, and EBV-human system.

DR. LAUFS: The antiviral immunity induced with the killed vaccines prevents or limits the proliferation of the oncogenic herpesvirus on subsequent infection. If the virus is already established intracellularly, the humoral antibodies have little or no effect, as we know well from human infections with herpes simplex virus types 1 and 2. The antibodies have to be present prior to the virus to prevent the disease. The role of the cellular immune response in our system remains to be defined. Preliminary experiments indicate a specific cellular immunity against *Herpesvirus saimiri* in the vaccinated African green monkeys (*Cercopithecus aethiops*) and the cotton-topped marmosets (*Saguinus oedipus*). We do not know whether the vaccinated monkeys are resistant against the natural way of infection by the oropharyngeal route. The protection observed seems to be based on an *in vivo* neutralization of the cell-free virus used in the challenge experiments. Killed vaccines have been shown to be effective against the MD (Lesnik and Ross, Kaaden and Dietzschold) and our monkey system seems not to be different.

DR. WATTENBERG: Since human exposure to EBV is likely to be at a young age, possibly during the newborn period, a vaccine would presumably be given to newborns. Have you determined whether your vaccine is safe when given to newborn monkeys?

DR. LAUFS: Newborn monkeys have not been vaccinated as yet. A common marmoset monkey (*Callithrix jacchus*) received four vaccinations during pregnancy.

This monkey delivered two healthy babies which have grown up without any clinical sign of a disease.

DR. TATSUMI: Recently Dr. Nonoyama reported that EBV is present in the nucleus of the infected or transformed cells but the genome of EBV is not integrated in the genome of the host cells (episome-like virus). Does this feature of EBV have any significance for the principle of therapy using antiviral vaccines against EBV-induced malignancies?

DR. LAUFS: According to the work published by G. Klein's group in Stockholm, about 10% of the intracellular EBV-DNA is linearly integrated in the host cell DNA and 90% is present in an episomal form. The intracellular state of the EBV-DNA does not influence the principle of antiviral vaccine.

DR. SUGANO: I wonder if there is any expression of RNA tumor virus genome. You carefully excluded the existence of 70S nucleic acid. How about reverse transcriptase activity, P30 and so on?

DR. LAUFS: Attempts to demonstrate partial expression of an oncornavirus genome in the herpesvirus-induced tumors and attempts to detect an interspecies antigen related to monkey oncornaviruses were negative. The ^{3}H-DNA product of simian sarcoma virus type 1 (SSV1) did not hybridize with the polyribosomal RNA from the monkey tumor cells.

DR. RAJEWSKY: The vaccine you have so beautifully developed with neutralized virus is introduced into the animal before infection. How do you envisage the effect of the vaccination in case of a slow, clonal onset of the disease, with possibly no or very little expression of the viral genome?

DR. LAUFS: The intracellular establishment of the oncogenic herpesvirus seems to be necessary for the malignant transformation. This step is probably prevented by the antiviral antibodies. The monkey tumors are multiclonal in origin and it seems likely that the virus which enters the monkey multiplies prior to the infection of the target cell(s). The vaccination has little effect on cells already transformed by the virus, as we showed by transplantation of tumor cells into vaccinated monkeys.

FUNDAMENTALS IN CANCER PREVENTION, P. N. MAGEE ET AL. (EDS.
UNIV. OF TOKYO PRESS, TOKYO / UNIV. PARK PRESS, BALTIMORE, PP.121–142,1976

On the Etiology and Prevention of Cancer in the Gastrointestinal Tract

J. H. Weisburger, E. Fiala, T. Narisawa,* and B. S. Reddy

Naylor Dana Institute for Disease Prevention, American Health Foundation, Valhalla, New York, U.S.A.

Abstract: Current concepts on the etiology of cancers in the gastrointestinal tract are presented and the relevant mechanisms for animal models are briefly discussed.

In the Western world, cancer of the esophagus appears to be associated with population groups who smoke cigarettes and are heavy consumers of alcoholic beverages. In certain areas of the Near and Far East and Central Africa, the etiology of this cancer is as yet unclear, but is not associated with smoking and drinking. In rodents, cancer of the esophagus can be induced readily by cyclic or asymmetric dialkyl or arylalkylnitrosamines. The exact mechanism for this organotropism towards the esophagus is not yet known.

Cancer of the stomach is seen in population groups consuming diets high in carbohydrates, low in micronutrients, and also with foods or environments high in nitrate or biochemically derived nitrite. Foods treated with high levels of nitrate for preservation, or grown where the soil conditions lead to higher levels of nitrate, demonstrate appreciable amounts of nitrite when such foods are stored at room temperature, but not at constant low temperature. It is postulated that nitrite so derived reacts with an as yet unknown substrate to yield a gastric carcinogen of the alkylnitrosamide type. In animal models, these chemicals readily induce gastric cancer in the glandular stomach, comparable to that in man.

Current views are that cancer of the colon and cancer of the rectum stem possibly from distinct causes. Cancer of the colon is seen typically in populations consuming Western style diets, high in fat and meat. The contribution of the amount and type of fiber is controversial and needs further study. These diets lead to quantitative differences in the amounts of neutral sterols and bile acids in the lumen of the gut. Certain bile acids have exerted a promoting effect in animal models. The carcinogens responsible for cancer of the colon in man are unknown. In animal models, there are several effective ways to induce this cancer, including the intrarectal instillation of alkylnitrosamides, the administration of cycasin or

---

* Visiting Investigator from Akita University School of Medicine, Akita, Japan.

the derived 1,2-dimethylhydrazine, azoxymethane, or methylazoxymethanol. The metabolism of dimethylhydrazine (DMH) leading to cancer of the colon appears to occur ultimately in the colon mucosa, although the first steps of its metabolic change may take place in liver. The microbial flora of the gut may not be required for metabolism, although DMH induced fewer colon tumors in germ-free rats. However, for another type of colon carcinogen, derived from 3-methyl-4-amino-biphenyl, whose mechanism of activation is probably different but requires further elucidation, the intestinal microflora may be involved.

Promising modalities to prevent cancers in the gastrointestinal tract may involve: (1) for cancer of the esophagus, a reduction of smoking and drinking; (2) for cancer of the stomach, lowering the amount of nitrite in the food supply by utilizing lower levels of nitrate, storing food at refrigerated temperatures, and improving the quality of the diet with respect to micronutrients; (3) for cancer of the colon, lowering the dietary fat, especially hidden fat in meats.

Cancer in man has historically had an almost mythical and superstitiously fatalistic aspect. It was attributed to obscure origins and was accepted by people as much as life and death are. That cancer actually had tangible causes stems from the observations that neoplastic disease could result from occupational situations like the chimney sweeps of Pott or the aniline dye workers of Rehn (1). In this century, additional occupational group exposures to specific chemicals were found to have a cancer risk. Because of the specific nature of the exposure conditions, it was often possible to eliminate the hazard. Thus, for example, in many countries the production of 2-naphthylamine was discontinued and totally eliminated as a disease factor. In other situations, the production processes were modified to minimize exposure. In the last 60 years, after the pioneering discoveries of Yamagiwa and Ichikawa, animal models were developed in which various suspected chemicals such as tars and oils could be tested for carcinogenicity. It was the combination of the discovery that occupational situations presented a cancer risk and the fact that cancer as seen in man could be reproduced in animals which removed the mystery from cancer and established carcinogenesis and cancer research as a serious branch of medical research.

TABLE 1. Causes of Human Cancer

I.	Occupational
II.	Related to life style
	A. Tobacco-related
	B. Diet-related
III.	Cryptogenic—Virus?

Epidemiology has also assumed a key status and has provided background information on cancer incidence in various countries (2–9). Basically, the causes or mediators of human cancer can be classified into three areas (Table 1). One is cancer due to occupational or industrial exposure to carcinogens, either chemicals or radiation. There are no firm quantitative data in this field but it would seem

TABLE 2.   Cancer Related to Life Styles

A.	Tobacco—cigarettes: lung, bladder, pancreas, kidneys	
B.	Diet 1.	High carbohydrate, low micronutrients
		high nitrate, or nitrite: stomach
	2.	High fat, low fiber: colon, breast, prostate, ovary, endometrium, pancreas
C.	Combination 1.	Tobacco and alcohol: oral cavity, esophagus
	2.	Tobacco and asbestos, mining: lung

that no more than 1–5% of all cancers relate to these causes, even though there is much public interest in their occurrence (*10*). By proper medical, engineering, and industrial management these cancers are preventable.

The major types of human cancers are related to life styles in various countries (Table 2). Those cancers stem from two main environmental causes, excessive smoking of tobacco products, or intake of diets or components containing carcinogens and/or cocarcinogens, leading to the *in vivo* formation of carcinogens, or establishing metabolic patterns for such endogenous formation of carcinogens, cocarcinogens, or promoters. Much of our discussion will relate to concepts underlying the induction or development of the neoplasms in the gastrointestinal tract, formed from such events and practices (*11, 12*).

Lastly, a number of cancers in man such as leukemias, lymphomas, sarcomas, *etc.* have ill-defined origins. Despite excellent animal evidence pointing to a viral etiology, a diligent search for similar mechanisms in man has not yet been productive (*13–15*).

In the United States and in Western Europe the incidence of certain types of cancer like that in the colon, breast, and prostate is high whereas in Japan these cancers have a low incidence (*8–11*). In contrast, gastric cancer is one of the major cancers in Japan, in Eastern Europe, and in Scandinavia but at this time has a much lower incidence in the United States. This lower incidence in the United States is a recent phenomenon. While gastric cancer was quite high at the beginning of this century, a downtrend in the last 40 years has occurred. Lung cancer, on the other hand, has shown just the opposite trend—the incidence was relatively low through about 1930 but increased dramatically in the last 45 years (*9, 16*). In Japan, lung cancer exhibits the same increasing trend but with a delay of about 20 years. Similarly, lung cancer in women in the United States. has exhibited a rising pattern only in the last 20 years.

We should like to discuss current views on causative elements for the main gastrointestinal cancers. In part, this subject was covered at the Third Princess Takamatsu Symposium (*9*). Thus, in this document, we wish to give this important area a new perspective by: (1) coordinating the results of research of mechanisms in animal models to the metabolic parameters relative to the main cancers in the gastrointestinal tract of man; (2) drawing conclusions as to the key factors which mediate the development of neoplastic diseases at these target organs; and (3) presenting views on possible means of approaching modes of prevention of cancer in these organs.

Cancer of the Esophagus

Cancer at this site has a distinct incidence in different countries, and even within a country sizable variations in rates exist among different population groups. Cancer of the esophagus in Western countries, that is the American Continent including Central America, and Western Europe is generally associated with heavy smoking and drinking of alcoholic beverages (*17–19*). Individuals who smoke but do not drink alcoholic beverages rarely have cancer of the esophagus, perhaps because coronary heart disease or cancer at a more sensitive site such as the lung, also seen in heavy smokers, are competing risks. Heavy drinking alone also is not associated with cancer in the esophagus. On the other hand, in other parts of the world, especially in Eastern Iran, the southern part of the Soviet Union and in Central China, and also in select parts of Central Africa, cancer of the esophagus is a highly prevalent disease which appears to stem from causes other than smoking and drinking (*20–22*). Some aspects of the etiology of the disease in these geographic areas are under intensive investigation by groups in these regions, in cooperation with the International Agency for Cancer Research in Lyon.

Current investigations in our laboratories on the mechanism whereby smoking and drinking together may lead to cancer in the esophagus are based on two premises. One is that tobacco smoke may contain a contact carcinogen which is more effective in the esophagus in an individual who also consumes alcoholic beverages. Also, Hoffmann *et al.* (*23*) have found that tobacco tar and, indeed, also unburnt tobacco of certain types, contains sizable amounts of nitrosonornicotine which, in rats, has been demonstrated to cause cancer in the esophagus (*24*). The second point under investigation rests on the assumption that alcoholics may have a higher sensitivity in the esophagus for two reasons. The alcoholic beverages may actually alter the surface membrane structure which in turn may change the permeability and enzymology of the tissue. Furthermore, alcoholics are often malnourished, both as regards specific and essential macronutrients such as protein, and micronutrients such as minerals and vitamins, especially vitamins A and B and in particular riboflavin. Patients with Plummer-Vinson's disease originating in an iron deficiency often exhibit cancer in the esophagus (*25, 26*). This condition has been prevented by supplementation of the diet with iron. If our investigations do document that smokers are sensitive to the development of cancer in the esophagus because of nutritional abnormalities and deficiencies, it is possible to visualize that the impact of this disease can also be moderated, at least, by making efforts to fortify the diet of an alcoholic if efforts to discontinue the smoking and drinking are not successful.

Animal studies

While cancer in the esophagus was seen occasionally in rodent systems used for carcinogen testing when a variety of chemicals such as polycyclic aromatic hydrocarbons were administered, it is now easy to induce these cancers with asymmetric dialkyl- or alkylarylnitrosamines or with cyclic nitrosamines following the discoveries made by Druckrey (*27*). The mechanism whereby such compounds in-

TABLE 3. Effect of PB, NF, CH, or Limited Vitamin A on the Carcinogenicity of DNP to the Esophagus of Rats[a)]

Group	Number of rats[b)]	Number of rats with:				
		Esophagus		Pharynx	Liver	
		Papilloma	Carcinoma	Papilloma	Hyperplasia	Carcinoma
DNP	32	22(4.3)[c)]	2	4	3	1
DNP and PB[d)]	19	12(2.7)	2	2	0	0
DNP and NF[d)]	22	15(4.5)	0	0	0	0
DNP and CH[d)]	23	13(4.8)	3	2	0	0
DNP and VIT A[e)]	18	9(3.9)	2	2	1	0

[a)] Male Fischer CDF rats, 4 weeks old, were conditioned on a semipurified diet for 1 week, then diets with chemicals fed for 4 weeks, when 250 mg/liter DNP was added in the drinking water 5 days/week. The treatment continued for 8 months, then carcinogen was omitted but the test diets continued for 1 month more. All rats were killed and carefully autopsied and the tissues studied microscopically. [b)] Effective number of rats alive after 5 months. [c)] Multiplicity of tumors (papilloma and carcinoma) in the esophagus. [d)] PB, NF, and CH were fed in the diet at 500, 181, and 152 mg/kg diet, respectively. [e)] The semipurified diet contained 137 IU vitamin A/kg diet, equivalent to a daily dose of 2 IU vitamin A/rat. All the other groups received a diet with 2,670 IU vitamin A/kg a or daily intake of 40 IU/rat.

duce cancer at that location is not yet known nor is there much information about the enzymology in the esophagus especially with respect to the metabolism, particularly the biochemical activation and detoxification of these agents (*28*, *29*).

We have approached this question indirectly by administering enzyme modifiers phenobarbital (PB), chrysene (CH), or β-naphthoflavone (NF), based on the observations of Wattenberg (*73*) that some of these chemicals alter one enzyme, benzo(a)pyrene hydroxylase in the gastrointestinal tract (Table 3). At the same time, rats in various groups received 1,4-dinitrosopiperazine (DNP). One group of rats received the carcinogen alone on a normal diet, another on a diet containing only low levels of vitamin A. The group of rats given carcinogen alone had papillomas and carcinomas in the esophagus and a total of 75% of the rats were affected. A small number of the animals also had hyperplastic nodules in the liver and one had a hepatocellular carcinoma. Feeding the low-vitamin A diet or diets containing the enzyme inducers had virtually no effect in the induction of cancer in the esophagus. The animals fed the enzyme modifiers and the carcinogen, however, had normal livers. It would appear, therefore, that conditions which modify the induction of cancer in the liver do not measurably alter the process of cancer induction in the esophagus.

Prevention of esophageal cancer

Prevention of cancer of the esophagus may assume several approaches. One depends on inducing individuals to stop smoking, which would serve to diminish also the risk for the development of lung cancer and of coronary heart disease. Concomitantly, reduction of the consumption of alcoholic beverages would lower the risk for cancer of the esophagus. If ongoing research can document that one aspect of the consumption of alcoholic beverages is a specific or general type of malnutrition, then correcting this imbalance might also serve to lower the risk. It is clear that both medical advice and education of the public, as well as further research to understand mechanisms will serve overall to control the development of cancer in the esophagus.

Cancer of the Stomach

Forty years ago gastric cancer was the main visceral cancer in the United States, in Europe, in Central and Latin America, and in the Far East, especially in Japan (7, 11, 30, 31). It is now well known that this neoplasm has shown a precipitious drop in the United States in the intervening years and it is beginning at this time to also decline in Western Europe and even in Japan. Because of the past importance of this cancer there have been numerous attempts to explain its causes, the underlying mechanisms and, indeed, to develop reliable and proper animal models so this disease could be studied. The latter aim was crowned with success when Sugimura and Kawachi (32) found that the powerful mutagen N-methyl-N'-nitro-N-nitrosoguanidine (MNNG) when given in the drinking water to rats induced cancer in the glandular stomach, similar to that seen in man. This initial observation was further documented in many other laboratories and it was shown that related alkylnitrosamides also could lead to cancer in the glandular stomach. There appear to be certain species and strain-related differences in the effect (33). However, even the dog is sensitive and serves as a large animal model to study pathogenesis and better modes of diagnosis.

We have been impressed by the high degree of specificity of this type of agent in inducing gastric cancer. The high specificity, together with the discovery by Sander et al. (34) that nitrosamines and nitrosamides could be formed in the stomach from nitrite and suitable substrates, suggests that the as yet unknown chemicals responsible for gastric cancer in man might be chemicals of this general class. This concept is consistent with the specific properties of these chemicals in leading to cancer in animals even after limited administration. In man migrating from a high-risk region, like Japan, to a low-risk region, like the United States, the risk is maintained even if the individual has lived in the high-risk region for a limited period of time. Thus, our investigations were concerned with two questions: one, to establish the source of nitrite, and two, to identify the substrate which, when nitrosated at the pH of the stomach, would yield a gastric carcinogen. As to the first question, it would seem that considerable nitrate is present in many foodstuffs grown in soil containing elevated levels of nitrate due either to existing geologic conditions or because it is sometimes added during agricultural practices (35–38). Countries such as Chile, Columbia, and in Central America have higher nitrate in the soil (39). This is also true for certain other select regions of the world and in these regions, in fact, a high risk for gastric cancer is evident. Furthermore, in the past, saltpeter has been used to preserve meats and other foods, and thus these nutrients were heavily loaded with nitrates. We have demonstrated that such nitrate is reduced to nitrite during storage of these foods at room temperature, but not when refrigerated (Fig. 1) (40). Some of these foods contain several thousand ppm nitrate which

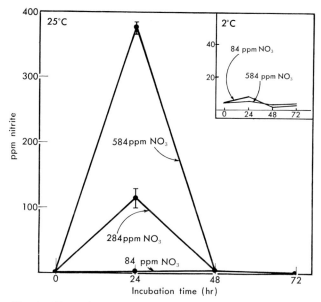

FIG. 1. Formation of nitrite on homogenized boiled potato incubated at 25° and 2°C. Five-gram samples of potato containing 84, 284, and 584 ppm of nitrate were incubated in triplicate for 24, 48 and 72 hr. The nitrite formed was extracted and the concentration was determined. The data are presented as ppm nitrite ± standard error (S.E.) (46).

even during incomplete conversion to nitrite still yields this reactive chemical in foods at levels of the order of several hundreds, if not thousands, ppm. In recent times, because of the availability of mechanical refrigeration, industrial processes for the preservation of foods, particularly of meats, have eliminated the use of nitrate. In order to inhibit the multiplication of *Clostridium botulinicum* and for other purposes, it is current practice to add 125 to 156 ppm nitrite to meats. This amount decreases relatively rapidly so that the meat products as eaten by the consumer have levels of 5 to 50 ppm nitrite (36). Mirvish (41), who has performed many kinetic studies on the nitrosation of many types of substrates, has noted that the nitrosation is quite slow with amounts of nitrite of this order of magnitude. We do not believe that the practice of adding limited amounts of nitrite to meats is responsible for gastric cancer and, in fact, it is not consistent with the decline in the gastric cancer incidence in the United States.

The problem now requiring elucidation is the nature of the substrate nitrosated. Endo (42) has demonstrated that a mutagenic and carcinogenic product is obtained when methylguanidine, present in fish and certain other foods, is nitrosated. However, inasmuch as methylguanidine nitrosates relatively slowly, additional research on other possible substrates is necessary.

The process of induction of gastric cancer involves, of course, additional parameters modifying the carcinogenic response in animal models and in man (11, 43). Populations at high risk for gastric cancer typically eat a diet high in carbohydrates, and concomitantly, low in fat, fresh fruit and vegetables. Such a diet is, therefore, limited in protein and probably in micronutrients, especially vit-

TABLE 4. Effect of Ascorbic Acid on Nitrite Levels and on the Formation of Methylnitrosourea in Potato Incubated at pH 1.5[a]

100 ppm methylurea (1 μCi [^{14}C]-methylurea)	100 ppm nitrite	Ascorbate/ nitrite	ppm	% control	Methylnitrosourea formed[b] (ppm)	% inhibition
+	—				0.0±0.0	
+	+	0	73.8±1.8[c]	100	19.2±1.1	0
+	+	1	65.4±0.7	87	12.1±0.8	37
+	+	2	47.2±0.6	64	5.0±0.4	74
+	+	4	42.0±1.2	57	1.4±0.2	93

[a] Five-gram samples of homogenized boiled potato (adjusted to pH 1.5) were incubated in triplicate at 37°C for 10 min (46). [b] Recovery of methylnitrosourea was 35.1%. [c] Mean ppm±S.E.

amins A, C, and the B type. In addition, diets are often high in salt (43). Certain of these parameters have already been studied in animal models and have been shown to enhance the carcinogenic response (44). Additional efforts are desirable in order to understand the specific mechanisms whereby this modifying effect operates. Based on the finding of Mirvish (45), we have shown that ascorbate appreciably lowers the formation of methylnitrosourea from nitrite and methylurea (46) (Table 4).

Prevention of gastric cancer

It is obvious that the data on changes in incidence of gastric cancer in the United States suggest that the factor of prevention is already operating, more so in the higher socioeconomic groups. Indeed, the lower socioeconomic groups have a higher risk of this disease, even in the United States. Several associated changes in environment have occurred in the United States during the last 50 years. The amount of nitrate used as food conditioners and preservatives has decreased very appreciably and, in fact, currently is not used, except in certain meat products. Foods tend to be stored more and more during processing as well as in homes at a constant low temperature by mechanical refrigeration. Under these conditions nitrate present in foods is not converted to nitrite. Also, people are more aware of the need of eating balanced diets, with somewhat higher levels of proteins and the addition of more fresh fruits, salads, and vegetables, all sources of essential micronutrients. Inasmuch as these overall changes in diet have served to decrease the risk for gastric cancer in the United States, it would seem eminently reasonable to recommend that in countries where the risk for gastric cancer is still high that every effort be made to institute such modified health and diet practices, namely: (1) lower or eliminate nitrate in diet; (2) avoid conversion to nitrite by low temperature storage, especially of cooked foods; (3) recommend eating of balanced diets, especially in regard to micronutrients, vitamins, *etc.* as found, for example, in vegetables and fruits. Also, since as noted above, gastric cancer can result from limited exposure for the first few years of life, it is important to implement recommendations for such alterations as soon as practical so that even the current generation in a high-risk country can benefit.

Large Bowel Cancer

Large bowel cancer has often been classified as colo-rectal cancer because of the similarity in the gross and microscopic aspects, and other parameters (*11, 47, 48*). However, in more recent years an analysis of colo-rectal cancer by subsite for ascending to descending colon cancer, and rectal cancer as separate entities made it quite apparent that the older combined treatment of the data was not warranted. Large bowel cancer has a much higher incidence in the Western world especially in the Anglo-Saxon countries, than in Central and Western South America, or in Japan. It would seem, however, that in the low-risk countries, the disease is present more in the cecum and also the ascending colon, whereas in the high-risk countries the disease is located more in the descending part with a concentration around the sigmoid colon. On the other hand, the incidence of rectal cancer is not too different in Japan than, for example, in the United States. Also, whereas colon cancer has male to female ratio of approximately unity, deviating somewhat in the older age groups, rectal cancer has a male to female ratio of 1.4. This suggests that efforts must be made to understand these distinctions in relation to causative elements. Except for the recent report that rectal cancer is more frequent in heavy beer drinkers (*49*) which is currently being investigated further through the International Agency for Cancer Research, there are no hypotheses or, indeed, specific animal models for this neoplasm.

In this report we will focus on colon cancer. On the basis of a number of lines of evidence, including consideration of data obtained from migrant studies, one key dietary element which is high in a high-risk country and much lower in a low-risk country is the amount of dietary fat and meat (*47, 48, 50*). In the Western world approximately 45% of calories stem from fat, both direct and indirect (as for example in meats), whereas in a low-risk country like Japan fat accounts for only 15 to 20% of the calories in the diet. While current evidence supports fat in the diet as a major element, the use of diets with less fiber and refined carbohydrates has been also proposed as a contributing factor (*51*). It may well be that both of these require consideration, although the evidence for fiber is not as striking.

In the last few years, considerable efforts have been made in various countries to acquire background information on causative factors of colon cancer. The United States National Cancer Institute has two major programs, the Colon Cancer Segment of the Division of Cancer Cause and Prevention, and the National Large Bowel Cancer Project, operated for the National Cancer Institute by the M.D. Anderson Hospital and Tumor Institute in Houston. This growing effort testifies to the importance of this disease which has the second highest incidence in the United States, in men after cancer in the respiratory system, and in women after cancer in the breast.

The question that needs resolution is the mechanism whereby high dietary fat leads to colon cancer. In our laboratories, we are approaching this problem through the technique of metabolic epidemiology. This area was, in part, covered by Wynder (*7*) at a preceding Princess Takamatsu Symposium. Newer results indicate that individuals on a high-fat diet excrete in their stools high amounts of total neutral

TABLE 5. Promoting Effect of Bile Acids of Colorectal Tumor Induction with Intrarectal (i.r.) MNNG in Germ-free and Conventional Fischer Rats

Treatment	Animals with tumors		Tumor classification		
	%	No.	Total	Adenocarcinoma	Adenoma
Conventional[a]					
LC (32)	0	0	0	0	0
TDC (32)	0	0	0	0	0
MNNG (32)	25	8	10	5	5
MNNG and LC (29)	52	15	30	8	22
MNNG and TDC (29)	62	18	28	4	24
Germ-free[b]					
DC (10)	0	0	0	0	0
MNNG (26)	89	14	38	7	31
MNNG and DC (22)	82	18	75	28	47

[a] MNNG group was given single dose of 4 mg i.r. MNNG; lithocholic acid (LC) or taurodeoxycholic acid (TDC) groups received 1 mg bile acid i.r. 5 times/week for 13 months; the MNNG and LC or MNNG and TDC groups were given i.r. MNNG and bile acid, as above (52). [b] MNNG group was given MNNG i.r. at a dose level of 2 mg each twice/week for 4 weeks; deoxycholate (DC) group received DC i.r., 20 mg /rat, 3 times/week for 50 weeks; MNNG and DC groups received MNNG and bile acid as above (53).

sterols and total bile acids (50). In turn, the neutral sterols are higher because the bacterially produced metabolites of cholesterol such as coprostanol and coprostanone are elevated compared to those found in a low-risk population such as vegetarians, or Japanese. Identical findings were made with respect to bile acids where the bacterial metabolites of bile acids are higher in the high-risk populations. The concentration of bile acids and cholesterol metabolites in colon cancer patients is higher than in controls, as was fecal 7α-dehydroxylation of primary bile acids (50). While other factors may stem from the high-fat diet and the resulting alteration in sterol metabolism and bacterial flora (see also the presentation by Professor Williams at this Symposium) we have demonstrated that several bile acids have a promoting effect in colon carcinogenesis in conventional animals as well as in germ-free rats (52, 53) (Table 5). The laboratory of Dr. Nigro has also produced such evidence through other approaches such as surgical transplantation of the bile duct to increase bile concentration in the large bowel or the administration of cholystyramine (54, 55).

Animal models

Sizable progress has been made in the last few years to induce colon cancer at will in different species (33) (Table 6). While this condition was seen occasionally with a number of different carcinogens, the reliable induction of colon cancer in good yield was obtained in rats through the administration of 3-methyl-4-aminobiphenyl derivatives or the analogous 3-methyl-2-naphthylamine, which induced colon cancer in male rats, but less so in female rats because of the precocious development of a competing neoplasm, breast cancer. Also, a more fundamental sex-linked biochemical difference may operate here. A second mode of inducing colon cancer stemmed from the discovery that the plant product cycasin readily induced

TABLE 6.   Effective Procedures for Cancer Induction in the Intestinal Tract

Chemical	Route[a]	Species	Organ
Cycasin	p.o.	Rat	Large bowel
1, 2-DMH	p.o., s.c., i.p., i.r.	Rat, mouse, hamster	Small and large bowel
AOM	p.o., s.c., i.r.	Rat, mouse	Small and large bowel
MAM	p.o., s.c., i.p., i.r.	Rat	Small and large bowel
N-Methylnitrosourea	i.r.	Rat, mouse, guinea pig	Distal large bowel
N-Methyl-N′-nitro-N-nitroso-guanidine	i.r.	Rat, mouse, guinea pig	Distal large bowel
3-Methyl-4-aminobiphenyl and analogs	p.o., s.c.	Rat	Small and large bowel
3-Methyl-2-aminonaphthalene	p.o., s.c.	Rat	Small and large bowel
3-Methylcholanthrene	p.o.	Hamster	Large bowel

[a] p.o., oral; s.c., subcutaneous; i.p., intraperitoneal; i.r., intrarectal.

colon cancer in rats, which eventually led to the development of a family of related chemicals 1,2-dimethylhydrazine (1,2-DMH), azoxymethane (AOM), methyl-azoxymethanol (MAM), and its acetate ester (27, 56–58). These chemicals are active as colon carcinogens in a number of different species such as the rat, mouse, and hamster, but so far not in the guinea pig (59). A third excellent and reliable way to induce colon cancer was discovered by Narisawa et al., namely the intrarectal administration of alkylnitrosamides which has been found effective in all species so far tested, including the guinea pig (60, 61). Last, Homburger (62) found that one of his inbred strains of hamster, line 15.16, developed colon cancer upon oral intake of large amounts of 3-methylcholanthrene. Here also, males were susceptible and females were not.

We are currently exploring the mode of action and metabolism of several of these carcinogens. Of key importance in this effort is the study of the modification and control of the biological and carcinogenic effect by environmental conditions, especially by diet, other chemicals, and changes in the intestinal microflora. We found that rats fed high-fat diets were more sensitive to cancer induction by dimethylhydrazine (DMH) than rats on a low-fat diet (63–65). Germ-free Fischer rats injected with DMH developed fewer colon cancers, suggesting a role for the intestinal microflora, but germ-free rats given AOM or MNNG were as, or more, sensitive than conventional rats (66, 67). The relevant mechanism may become clear as we study the metabolism of DMH under these conditions.

We have developed procedures for the separation of DMH and analogous chemicals as well as metabolites by thin-layer chromatography and by column and high-pressure liquid chromatography (Figs. 2 and 3) (68, 69). After a single dose of DMH relatively small amounts of metabolites appear in the bile. After repeated doses, increased amounts are found, although considering the relatively low molecular weight of this chemical and its metabolites, the amount found in bile of rats is never very high (Fig. 4). It could be that tumors induced by these chemicals in the duodenum proximate to the entrance of the bile ducts may relate to the presence of activated metabolites in the bile. However, on the basis of the studies on metabolism as well as the results obtained in germ-free animals, it would appear more

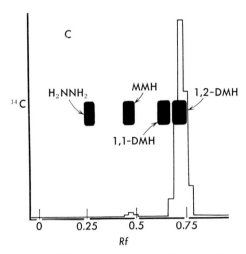

FIG. 2. Thin-layer chromatographic separation of hydrazine, monomethylhydrazine (MMH), 1,1-dimethylhydrazine (1,1-DMH), and 1,2-DMH on Avicel cellulose plates with 2-propanol-conc. HCl-water (130 : 30 : 40, v/v). The bands were detected using the Folin reagent (68). Also shown is a histogram representing a sample, run separately, of ^{14}C-labeled 1,2-DMH with a small amount of ^{14}C-MMH impurity.

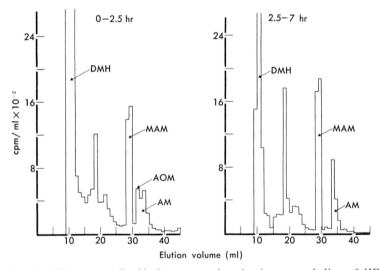

FIG. 3. High-pressure liquid chromatography of urinary metabolites of ^{14}C-1,2-DMH. A 0.1 ml aliquot of urine from a male Fischer rat obtained at 2.5 or 7 hr after ^{14}C-1,2-DMH administration (21 mg/kg, s.c.) was applied to an Aminex A-27 column eluted with 0.01 M sodium acetate, pH 5.6. Fractions of 1 ml were collected and the radioactivity was determined. Histogram peaks marked DMH, MAM, AOM, and AM correspond exactly to elution volumes of the respective synthetic standards which were run separately. Other technical details are given in Ref. 69.

likely that the process leading to the activated metabolites, and the ultimate carcinogen derived from DMH occurs in the colon mucosa. We are currently performing experiments to test this possibility directly by *in vitro* experiments. Similar

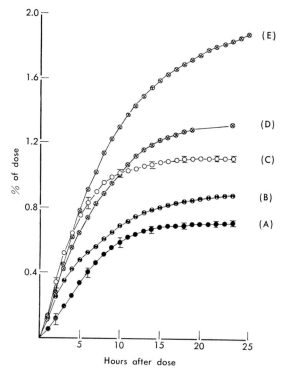

FIG. 4. Cumulative biliary excretion of radioactivity derived from ^{14}C-1,2-DMH by male Fischer rats after a variety of treatments. (A) Biliary excretion after a single 21 mg/kg dose of ^{14}C-1, 2-DMH at time 0 (4 animals). (B) Biliary excretion after a single 200 mg/kg dose of ^{14}C-1, 2-DMH (1 animal). (C) Rats pretreated 3 times with unlabeled 1, 2-DMH (21 mg/kg), once each week. A single 21 mg/kg dose of ^{14}C-1, 2-DMH was given the 4th week and biliary excretion was followed (2 animals). (D) and (E) animals (1 each) were pretreated with 90 mg/ kg phenobarbital 3 times (once daily), then with 200 mg/kg ^{14}C-1, 2-DMH on the fourth day. In all cases the necessary surgical procedures were performed on ether-anesthetized animals and bile was collected from fully conscious restrained animals with food and water available *ad libitum*.

procedures are being used to examine whether animals on a high-fat diet exhibited a higher capability to produce the active carcinogen metabolite in the colon mucosa.

In an indirect approach, similar to that used for our studies on carcinogens in the esophagus, DMH was administered while animals were fed diets containing the enzyme modifiers phenobarbital (PB), chrysene (CH), and β-naphthoflavone (NF). We found that PB and NF increased the multiplicity of tumors in the colon. PB increased both the multiplicity and incidence of tumors in the region of the colon 0–6 cm from the anus ("distal colon"). All three enzyme modifiers increased the incidence as well as the multiplicity of tumors in the duodenum (Table 7).

Wattenberg (72, 73) reported that disulfuram (DSF) exerted powerful inhibiting action on the carcinogenicity of DMH in the colon (see report at this Symposium). We found that this chemical inhibited the oxidation of azomethane (AM), and thus the metabolic conversion of DMH to ^{14}CO$_2$ (Fig. 5) (74, 75).

TABLE 7. Effects of PB, NF, and CH on the Carcinogenicity of DMH

Group[a]		Effective No. of rats	% animals with tumors		Mean No. of tumors per animal	
			Colon	Duodenum	Colon	Duodenum
DMH[b]	Adenomas	29	90	21	2.2	0.2
	Carcinomas	29	41	38	0.5	0.5
	Aden. and carc.	29	100	48	2.7	0.7
DMH and PB[b]	Adenomas	28	79	52	2.4	0.7
	Carcinomas	28	54	59	0.8	1.0
	Aden. and carc.	28	89	89	3.2	1.7
DMH and CH[b]	Adenomas	27	93	15	2.2	0.2
	Carcinomas	27	19	56	0.2	0.9
	Aden. and carc.	27	100	62	2.4	1.1
DMH and NF[b]	Adenomas	28	86	26	3.3	0.3
	Carcinomas	28	32	56	0.5	0.6
	Aden. and carc.	28	96	70	3.8	0.9

[a] Male Fischer rats, 4 weeks old, were conditioned on a semipurified diet for 1 week, then placed on the same diet containing enzyme modifiers. After 1 week, treatment with DMH (21 mg/kg, s.c., once a week) was begun. A total of 11 injections of DMH were given. After the last injection the animals remained on test diets one more week, then all animals were placed on semipurified diet without modifiers. After an additional 10 weeks, all rats were killed and autopsied, and the tissues studied microscopically. Control groups (30 animals each) were treated with diets as above but received no DMH. No tumors in any organs were found in these animals.   [b] PB, CH, and NF were fed in the diet at 500, 152, and 1,500 mg/kg diet, respectively (70).

Prevention of colon cancer

Considering the sound evidence that diets high in fat (and supported by less experimental or human evidence, a lack of fiber) are associated with a high risk for colon cancer, a view fully supported by studies in animal models, it seems indicated to recommend that the risk be lowered by decreasing the relative fat component of the diet. It would appear that a diet which is perhaps halfway between that consumed in Japan and that in the Western world, namely with approximately 27–30% of calories as fat, might present considerably lower risk. Studies in metabolic epidemiology, comparing the fecal composition of individuals on diets containing 45, 30, and 20% fat, for example, might have predictable value in validating such a recommendation without necessarily waiting for the many years required to see a decline in incidence of colon cancer. In view of the connection between fat level in the diet, and other chronic diseases such as cancer in the breast, prostate, pancreas, and also of coronary heart disease, adoption of such a modified diet would go a long way towards the reduction of these other main human premature killing diseases.

EPILOGUE

In addition to prevailing on individuals to adjust their way of life, especially as regards the intake of foods which present high risk for all of the diseases discussed here, it may also be possible to practice managerial prevention, namely to work

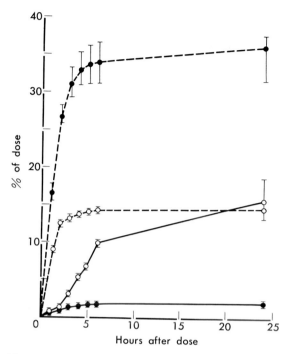

FIG. 5.   Cumulative excretion of ^{14}C-AM and $^{14}CO_2$ in the expired air of male Fischer rats and the effects of pretreatment with DSF. Open circles : animals (2 used) received 21 mg/kg ^{14}C-1, 2-DMH (s.c.) only. Filled circles : animals (3 used) received 1 g/kg DSF as a suspension in 0.4% starch, p.o., 2 hr prior to an s.c. dose of 21 mg/kg ^{14}C-1, 2-DMH. Methods used in the estimation of AM and CO_2 in the expired air are described in Ref. *71*. ●---● AM-DSF ; ○---○ AM-control ;   ○—○ CO_2-control ;   ●—● CO_2-DSF.

with the agricultural and food industries to improve the types of foods made available to the public from the point of view of disease prevention. National and international efforts in reducing the nitrite levels in foods have already begun to bear fruit. Efforts still need to be exerted to lower the fat component of key dietary constituents such as meats or dairy products. In some cases this is not only an agricultural or industrial question but also a legal and governmental problem. The scientific and medical community must exert every effort to continue research in this area so as to obtain detailed and, indeed, hopefully unambiguous evidence so that the various commercial, industrial, and political bodies and instruments will be readily convinced to alter the nature of foodstuff production as a preventive public health measure. Thus, it is hoped that individual and managerial prevention based on sound research will result in a reduction of cancers in the gastrointestinal tract.

ACKNOWLEDGMENTS

Research on the etiology of gastrointestinal cancer in our laboratory is supported by USPHS grants CA-14298, CA-15400, and CA-16382 (through the National Large Bowel Cancer Project) and contract CP-33208 from the National Cancer Institute. We are indebted to D. Bauersfeld and M. Mervis for editorial assistance.

REFERENCES

1. Shimkin, M. Some historical landmarks in cancer epidemiology. *In;* D. Schottenfeld (ed.), Cancer Epidemiology and Prevention, pp. 60–75, C. C. Thomas, Springfield, 1975.
2. Segi, M. and Kurihara, M. Cancer mortality for selected sites in 24 countries, #6 (1966–1967) Nagoya, Japan. Japan Cancer Society and Segi Institute of Cancer Epidemiology, 1972.
3. Cutler, S. J. and Devesa, S. S. Trends in cancer incidence and mortality in the U.S.A. *In;* R. Doll and I. Vodopija (eds.), Host Environmental Interactions in the Etiology of Cancer in Man, IARC Scientific Publications, No. 7, pp. 15–34, International Agency for Research on Cancer, Lyon, 1973.
4. Muir, C. S. Geographical differences in cancer patterns. *In;* R. Doll and I. Vodopija (eds.), Host Environmental Interactions in the Etiology of Cancer in Man, IARC Scientific Publications, No. 7, pp. 1–13, International Agency for Research on Cancer, Lyon, 1973.
5. Wynder, E. L. The epidemiology of large bowel cancer. Cancer Res., *35:* 3388–3394, 1975.
6. Correa, P. Comments on the epidemiology of large bowel cancer. Cancer Res., *35:* 3395–3397, 1975.
7. Wynder, E. L. Epidemiological contribution to the prevention of cancer. *In;* W. Nakahara, T. Hirayama, K. Nishioka, and H. Sugano (eds.), Analytic and Experimental Epidemiology of Cancer, pp. 3–29, University of Tokyo Press, Tokyo and University Park Press, Baltimore, 1974.
8. Schottenfeld, D. (ed.). Cancer Epidemiology and Prevention, pp. 1–574, C. C. Thomas, Springfield, 1975.
9. Nakahara, W., Hirayama, T., Nishioka, K., and Sugano, H. (eds.). Analytic and Experimental Epidemiology of Cancer, pp. 1–426, University of Tokyo Press, Tokyo and University Park Press, Baltimore, 1974.
10. Higginson, S. and Muir, C. S. Epidemiology. *In;* J. Holland and E. Frei, III (eds.), Cancer Medicine, pp. 241–306, Lea and Febiger, Philadelphia, 1973.
11. Wynder, E. L., Peters, J. A., and Vivona, S. (eds.). Symposium—Nutrition in the Causation of Cancer. Cancer Res., *35:* 3231–3550, 1975.
12. Pledger, R. A. (ed.), Symposium—Current Progress in Pancreatic Cancer Research. Cancer Res., *35:* 2226–2294, 1975.
13. Rauscher, F. J. and O'Connor, T. E. Virology. *In;* J. Holland and E. Frei, III (eds.), Cancer Medicine, pp. 15–44, Lea and Febiger, Philadelphia, 1973.
14. Gross, L. Oncogenic Viruses, 2nd. ed., Pergamon Press, London and New York, 1970.
15. Becker, F. F. Cancer, vols. 1 and 2, Plenum Press, New York and London, 1975.
16. Wynder, E. L. and Mabuchi, K. Etiological and preventive aspects of human cancer. Prev. Med., *1:* 300–334, 1972.
17. Day, N. E. Some aspects of the epidemiology of esophageal cancer. Cancer Res., *35:* 3304–3307, 1975.
18. Martinez, I., Torres, R., and Frias, Z. Cancer incidence in the United States and Puerto Rico. Cancer Res., *35:* 3265–3271, 1975.
19. Tuyns, A. J. Cancer of the oesophagus: Further evidence of the relation to drinking habits in France. Int. J. Cancer, *5:* 152–156, 1970.
20. Hormozdiari, H., Day, N. E., Aramesh, B., and Mahboubi, E. Dietary factors and

esophageal cancer in the Caspian littoral of Iran. Cancer Res., *35*: 3493–3498, 1975.

21. deJong, U. W., Breslow, N., Goh Ewe Hong, J., Sridharan, M., and Shanmugarat-nam, K.   Aetiological factors in oesophageal cancer in Singapore Chinese. Int. J. Cancer, *13*: 291–303, 1974.

22. The Coordinating Group for Research on Etiology of Esophageal Cancer in North China. The epidemiology and etiology of esophageal cancer in North China. A preliminary report. Chin. Med. J., *1*: 167–183, 1975.

23. Hoffmann, D., Hecht, S. S., Ornaf, R. M., and Wynder, E. L.   N′-Nitrosonornicotine in tobacco. Science, *186*: 265–267, 1974.

24. Hoffmann, D., Raineri, R., Hecht, S. S., Maronpot, R. R., and Wynder, E. L.   A study of tobacco carcinogenesis. XIV. Effects of N′-nitrosonornicotine and N′-nitrosoanabasine in rats. J. Natl. Cancer Inst., *55*: 977–979, 1975.

25. Wynder, E. L., Hultberg, S., Jacobsson, F., and Bross, J. B. Environmental factors in cancer of the upper alimentary tract: A Swedish study with special reference to Plummer-Vinson (Paterson-Kelly) syndrome. Cancer, *10*: 470–482, 1957.

26. Larsson, L. G., Sandström, A., and Westling, P.   Relationship of Plummer-Vinson disease to cancer of the upper alimentary tract in Sweden. Cancer Res., *35*: 3308–3316, 1975.

27. Druckrey, H.   Chemical carcinogenesis on N-nitroso derivatives. GANN Monogr. Cancer Res., *17*: 107–132, 1975.

28. Krüger, F. N.   New aspects in metabolism of carcinogenic nitrosamines. *In;* W. Nakahara, S. Takayama, T. Sugimura, and S. Odashima (eds.), Topics in Chemical Carcinogenesis, pp. 213–232, University of Tokyo Press, Tokyo and University Park Press, Baltimore, 1973.

29. Eisenbrand, G., Ivankovic, S., Preussmann, R., Schmähl, D., and Wiessler, M. Some recent results on the chemistry, formation and biological activity of N-nitroso compounds. GANN Monogr. Cancer Res., *17*: 133–143, 1975.

30. Japanese Cancer Association.   Experimental carcinoma of the glandular stomach. GANN Monogr., *8*: 1–396, 1969.

31. Bjelke, E.   Epidemiologic studies of cancer of the stomach, colon and rectum; with special emphasis on the role of diet. Scand. J. Gastroenterol., *9* (Suppl. 31): 1–253, 1974.

32. Sugimura, T. and Kawachi, T.   Experimental stomach cancer. *In;* H. Busch (ed.), Methods in Cancer Research, vol. 2, pp. 245–308, Academic Press, New York and London, 1973.

33. Bralow, S. P. and Weisburger, J. H. Experimental gastrointestinal carcinogenesis. Clin. Gastroenterol., 1976, in press.

34. Sander, J., Schweinsberg, F., LaBar, J., Bürkle, G., and Schweinsberg, E. Nitrite and nitrosable amino compounds in carcinogenesis. GANN Monogr. Cancer Res., *17*: 145–160, 1975.

35. Fassett, D. W.   Nitrates and nitrites. *In;* Toxicants Occurring Naturally in Foods, pp. 7–25, National Academy of Sciences, Washington, D.C., 1973.

36. Krol, B. and Tinbergen, B. J.   Proceedings of the International Symposium on Nitrite in Meat Products, p. 268, Center for Agricultural Publishing and Documentation, Wageningen, Netherlands, 1974.

37. Alexander, M. and Committee on Nitrate Accumulation. Accumulation of Nitrate, p. 106, National Academy of Sciences, Washington, D. C., 1972.

38. Binkerd, E. F. and Kolari, O. E.   The history and use of nitrate and nitrite in the curing of meat. Food Cosmet. Toxicol., in press.

39. Correa, P., Haenszel, W., Cuello, C., Tannenbaum, S., and Archer, M.   A model for gastric cancer epidemiology. Lancet, *ii*: 58–59, 1975.

40. Weisburger, J. H. and Raineri, R.   Dietary factors and the etiology of gastric cancer. Cancer Res., *35*: 3469–3474, 1975.

41. Mirvish, S. S.   Kinetics of nitrosamide formation from alkylureas, N-alkylurethanes, and alkylguanidines: Possible implication for the etiology of human gastric cancer. J. Natl. Cancer Inst., *46*: 1183–1193, 1971.

42. Endo, H., Takahashi, K., Kinoshita, N., Utsunomiya, T., and Baba, T.   An approach to the detection of possible etiologic factors in human gastric cancer. GANN Monogr. Cancer Res., *17*: 17–29, 1975.

43. Oiso, T.   Incidence of stomach cancer and its relation to dietary habits and nutrition in Japan between 1900 and 1975. Cancer Res., *35*: 3254–3258, 1975.

44. Tatematsu, M., Takahashi, M., Fukushima, S., Hananouchi, M., and Shirai, T. Effects in rats of sodium chloride on experimental gastric cancers induced by N-methyl-N'-nitro-N-nitrosoguanidine or 4-nitroquinoline-1-oxide J. Natl. Cancer Inst., *55*: 101–106, 1975.

45. Mirvish, S. S.   Blocking the formation of N-nitroso compounds with ascorbic acid *in vitro* and *in vivo*. Ann. N.Y. Acad. Sci., *258*: 175–180, 1975.

46. Raineri, R. and Weisburger, J. H.   Reduction of gastric carcinogens with ascorbic acid. Ann. N. Y. Acad. Sci., *258*: 181–189, 1975.

47. Weisburger, J. H., Reddy, B. S., and Joftes, D.   Colo-rectal Cancer. UICC Technical Report Series, No. 19, International Union against Cancer, Geneva, 1975.

48. Berg, J. W. and Howell, M. A.   The geographic pathology of bowel cancer. Cancer, *34*: 807–814, 1974.

49. Breslow, N. E. and Enstrom, J. E.   Geographic correlations between cancer mortality rates and alcohol-tobacco consumption in the United States. J. Natl. Cancer Inst., *53*: 631–639, 1974.

50. Reddy, B. S., Mastromarino, A., and Wynder, E. L.   Further leads on metabolic epidemiology of large bowel cancer. Cancer Res., *35*: 3043–3406, 1975.

51. Burkitt, D. P.   Large-bowel cancer: An epidemiological jigsaw puzzle. J. Natl. Cancer Inst., *56*: 441–442, 1976.

52. Narisawa, T., Magadia, N. E., Weisburger, J. H., and Wynder, E. L.   Promoting effect of bile acids on colon carcinogenesis after intrarectal instillation of N-methyl-N'-nitro-N-nitrosoguanidine in rats. J. Natl. Cancer Inst., *53*: 1093–1097, 1974.

53. Reddy, B. S., Narisawa, T., Weisburger, J. H., and Wynder, E. L.   Promoting effect of deoxycholic acid on colonic adenocarcinomas in germ-free rats. J. Natl. Cancer Inst., *56*: 441–442, 1976.

54. Chomchai, C., Bhadrachari, N., and Nigro, N. D.   The effect of bile on the induction of experimental intestinal tumors in rats. Dis. *Colon Rectum*, *17*: 310–312, 1974.

55. Nigro, N. D., Bhadrachari, N., and Chomchai, C.   A rat model for studying colonic cancer: Effect of cholestyramine on induced tumors. *Dis. Colon Rectum*, *16*: 438–443, 1973.

56. Laqueur, G. L. and Spatz, M.   Oncogenicity of cycasin and methylazoxymethanol GANN Monogr. Cancer Res., *17*: 189–204, 1975.

57. Zedeck, M. S. and Sternberg, S. S.   A model system for studies on colon carcinogenesis: Tumor induction by a single injection of methylazoxymethanol acetate. J. Natl. Cancer Inst., *53*: 1419–1421, 1974.

58. Matsumoto, H., Nagahama, T., and Larson, H. O. Studies on methylazoxymethan-

ol, the aglycone of cycasin: A synthesis of methylazoxymethyl acetate. Biochem. J., *95*: 13c–14c, 1965.

59. Narisawa, T., Wong, C. Q., and Weisburger, J. H.   Azoxymethane induces liver hemangiosarcomas but not colon cancer in inbred strain-2 guinea pigs. J. Natl. Cancer Inst., *56*: 453–654, 1976.

60. Narisawa, T., Nakano, H., Hayakawa, M., Sato, T., and Sakuma, A.   Tumors of the colon and rectum induced by N-methyl-N'-nitro-N-nitrosoguanidine. *In;* W. Nakahara (ed.), Topics in Chemical Carcinogenesis, pp. 145–158, University of Tokyo Press, Tokyo and University Park Press, Baltimore, 1972.

61. Narisawa, T., Wong, C. Q., and Weisburger, J. H.   Induction of carcinoma of the large intestine in guinea pigs by intrarectal instillation of N-methyl-N-nitrosourea. J. Natl. Cancer Inst., *54*: 785–787, 1975.

62. Homburger, F., Hsueh, S. S., Kerr, C. S., and Russfield, A. B.   Inherited susceptibility of inbred strains of Syrian hamsters by induction of subcutaneous sarcomas and mammary and gastrointestinal carcinomas by subcutaneous and gastric administration of polynuclear hydrocarbons. Cancer Res., *32*: 360–366, 1972.

63. Reddy, B. S., Weisburger, J. H., and Wynder, E. L.   Effects of dietary fat level and dimethylhydrazine on fecal acid and neutral steroid excretion and colon carcinogenesis in rats. J. Natl. Cancer Inst., *52*: 507–511, 1974.

64. Rogers, A. E. and Newberne, P. M. Dietary effects on chemical carcinogenesis in animal models for colon and liver tumors. Cancer Res., *35*: 3427–3431, 1975.

65. Newberne, P. M. and Rogers, A. E.   Nutritional modulation of carcinogenesis. This volume, pp. 15–40.

66. Reddy, B. S., Weisburger, J. H., Narisawa, T., and Wynder, E. L. Colon carcinogenesis in germ-free rats with 1, 2-dimethylhydrazine and N-methyl-N'-nitro-N-nitrosoguanidine. Cancer Res., *34*: 2368–2372, 1974.

67. Reddy, B. S., Narisawa, T., Wright, P., Vukusich, D., Weisburger, J. H., and Wynder, E. L.   Colon carcinogenesis with Azoxymethane and dimethylhydrazine in germ-free rats. Cancer Res., *35*: 287–290, 1975.

68. Fiala, E. S. and Weisburger, J. H. Thin-layer chromatography of some methylated hydrazines and detection by a sensitive spray reagent. J. Chromatogr., *105*: 189–192, 1975.

69. Fiala, E. S., Bobotas, G., Kulakis, C., and Weisburger, J. H. Separation of 1,2-dimethylhydrazine metabolites by high pressure liquid chromatography. J. Chromatogr., *117*: 181–185, 1976.

70. Fiala, E. S., Maronpot, R., Strebel, R., and Weisburger, J. H. Effect of phenobarbital, chrysene, or β-naphthoflavone on intestinal cancer induction by 1, 2-dimethylhydrazine. Unpublished.

71. Fiala, E. S., Kulakis, C., Bobotas, G., and Weisburger, J. H. Detection and estimation of azomethane in expired air of 1, 2-dimethylhydrazine-treated rats. J. Natl. Cancer Inst., in press.

72. Wattenberg, L. W.   Inhibition of dimethylhydrazine-induced neoplasia of the large intestine by disulfiram. J. Natl. Cancer Inst., *54*: 1005–1006, 1975.

73. Wattenberg, L. W.   Inhibition of chemical carcinogenesis by antioxidants. This volume, pp. 153–166.

74. Fiala, E. S. and Weisburger, J. H. *In vivo* metabolism of the colon carcinogen 1,2-dimethylhydrazine and the effects of disulfiram. Proc. Am. Assoc. Cancer Res., *17*: 58, 1976.

75. Fiala, E. S., Bobotas, G., Kulakis, C., and Weisburger, J. H. Inhibition of 1,2-dimethylhydrazine metabolism by disulfiram. Xenobitica, in press.

Discussion of Paper of Drs. Weisburger et al.

DR. HOZUMI: Is the promoting effect of bile acids in colon tumor formation specific for colon tumor? Is it also applicable to other kinds of tumors?

DR. WEISBURGER: This is a good question. Perhaps pancreas cancer may also involve bile acids or sterols as promoters by bile reflux into the pancreatic duct.

DR. WEBER: I have several questions regarding your elegant studies in rat colon cancer. How long does it take for colon cancer to develop and to detect in your system? What is the histology of your neoplasms? Can you transplant your primary tumors in inbred rats? Are these transplantable colon neoplasms available for biochemical studies in inbred rats?

DR. WEISBURGER: In the rat and mouse we can detect early colon cancer in about 10–15 weeks, in the guinea pig in 30–40 weeks. Dr. Narisawa can please comment on histology.

There are a number of transplantable colon cancers in rats and mice in the laboratory of Dr. E. Weisburger, U.S. Natl. Cancer Inst., Dr. J. Cole at Yale Univ., Dr. M. Martin in Dijon (France), Dr. T. H. Corbett at Southern Research Inst., Birmingham, U.S.A., Dr. R. E. Stowell in Davis, California, Prof. H. Sato, Sendai, and Prof. E. Cooper in Leeds (Gt. Britain). They are available from those laboratories.

DR. NARISAWA: We can detect rat colon tumors even of 1–2 mm in diameter by fiber endoscopy, and get biopsy specimens for histologic diagnosis (Am. J. Dig. Dis., *20*: 928, 1975). Generally, rat colon cancer induced by intrarectal administration of N-methyl-N'-nitro-N-nitrosoguanidine (MNNG) or methylnitrosourea (MNU), or by subcutaneous injection of dimethylhydrazine (DMH) or its derivatives are polypoid type and well-differentiated adenocarcinomas. Colon cancers induced by intrarectal instillation of MNNG or MNU in guinea pigs are infiltrative or constrictive type and moderately to poorly differentiated adenocarcinomas. Thus, it is hard to detect the early stage or small colon tumors in guinea pigs by endoscopic examination.

DR. MaCALLA: A recent issue of Science contained data on the county by county distribution of various cancers in the U.S.A. and suggested that there is a significant excess of certain types of tumors in the male population in centers having extensive manufacturing industry. Would you please comment on this in relation to your statement that there are only 5,000 new cases of occupational cancer per year in the U.S.A?

DR. WEISBURGER: The report of a concentration of cancer in various organs as a function of area of residence is interesting and these facts no doubt need careful consideration and evaluation. However, Japan has highly industrial complexes, yet their cancer pattern is quite different from the U.S.A. Workmen in the U.S.A. but not in Japan may take meats like hamburger for lunch. Thus, their diet and smoking habit, rather than place of employment seems more relevant in an overall consideration of causative situations as regards the main types of cancer.

DR. MAGEE: We have observed squamous carcinoma of the anal margin in mice given 1,2-dimethylhydrazine (1,2-DMH) by subcutaneous injection and this has also been reported by others. This might suggest that a carcinogen was present in the lumen of the bowel. Do you have evidence relating to the route of 1,2-DMH in the colon after subcutaneous injection and the possible metabolism of the compound by the colon?

DR. WEISBURGER: Squamous cancers in the anal region are seen in mice after treatment with 1,2-DMH. Dr. Narisawa has found such cancers also after intrarectal infusion of direct-acting MNU. This lesion is not usually seen in rats or in guinea pigs. As to the metabolism in the colon, we now believe that this class of colon carcinogens is metabolized to an active ultimate carcinogen by colon mucosa, on the basis of a number of lines of evidence, including the carcinogenicity of azoxy-methane in germ-free rats, as reported by Dr. Reddy in our laboratory.

DR. GELBOIN: Your elegant model system and analysis of the epidemiological data are so convincing that they may be misleading. Since we do not know the nature of the carcinogen in humans the model experiments may not be applicable. Furthermore, dietary habits unique in one component, for example high fat, no doubt are different in other factors as well. Thus, the other rather than the ex-amined factor may be relevant. I do not wish to detract from your attractive hypo-thesis, but merely to point out their hypothetical nature.

DR. WEISBURGER: It is true that we are guided by epidemiology in formulating hypotheses relative to environmental factors leading to cancer of the stomach, or the colon. The first, cancer of the stomach has been the subject of many ideas. The current approach, based on known nutritional factors such as low levels of micronutrients, plus the presence of high levels of nitrate-nitrite agrees with the established facts. The question to be studied is the substrate subject to nitrosation to form a local acting nitrosamide. The importance of the fat level in relation to colon cancer is based on population surveys in high- and low-risk areas, and has found support in the animal studies reported. The mechanisms must still be elucidated. However, as was recommended in connection with the prevention of coronary heart disease, it may be worth considering lowering the level of dietary fat even now.

FUNDAMENTALS IN CANCER PREVENTION, P. N. MAGEE ET AL. (EDS.),
UNIV. OF TOKYO PRESS, TOKYO / UNIV. PARK PRESS, BALTIMORE, PP. 143–151, 1976

Possibilities for Prevention of Large Bowel Cancer

R. E. O. Williams, M. J. Hill, and B. S. Drasar

Public Health Laboratory Service, Bacterial Metabolism Research Laboratory, Colindale Hospital, London, U.K.

Abstract: The wide differences in the incidence of cancer of the large bowel in different countries are most plausibly attributable to variations in diet or other associated factors. There is some evidence that dietary differences may operate by influencing the numbers of, and the substrates available to, the bacteria in the gut; bile steroids may be converted into carcinogens or cocarcinogens by a series of reactions attributable to *Bacteroides* and *Clostridium paraputrificum*.

This hypothesis suggests three ways in which the carcinogenic activity could be reduced: by reduction in the amount of bile steroids reaching the regions of the gut that are colonized by the relevant bacteria; by reduction in the action of the bacteria on the steroids; and by protection of the mucosa against their action. The hypothesis also forms the basis of a possible prognostic screening method.

Cancer of the large bowel is reported as having a lifetime attack rate of about 2% in England and about 5% in the United States; in Japan the mortality is far lower. The figures for incidence range from less than 1 case per 10,000 *per annum* (in the age group 35–64) in Uganda, through 5/10,000 in Japan, 19/10,000 in England and Wales, to over 30/10,000 in New Zealand and Scotland (*1*).

Numerous studies in the last 10 years have shown that these geographical differences cannot be attributed to genetic differences, and have pointed to some effect attributable to diet or associated environmental factors; and they have indicated that exposure to such factors over a relatively short period of years can suffice to bring migrant individuals from a low-risk to a high-risk category (*2*). It is difficult to obtain evidence to show whether the reverse is true, that individuals removed from exposure to the high-risk circumstances experience a lower incidence of the cancer. The reported low incidence in Seventh Day Adventists—a large proportion of whom are thought to be converts to their faith, which forbids meat eating—may be a pointer to such an effect (*3*).

Analysis of the statistics of cancer incidence and food intake in various countries points very strongly to an association of a high incidence of large bowel cancer with a high consumption of meat, fat, and "combined fat" (*i.e.*, fat constituting an integral part of other foodstuff, especially meat) (*4*). These results are supported by other analyses (*5, 6*). Recently Haenszel *et al.* (*7*) in a retrospective case-control study in migrant groups in Hawaii have pointed to an especially strong association with beef consumption, although this finding could not be confirmed in a small study in London by Meade *et al.* (personal communication, 1975).

Possible Role of Bacteria

Our group has been interested in the possibility that the dietary and geographical differences might operate by their effect on bacteria in the gut, and in particular that the gut bacteria might produce some carcinogen from bile steroids (*8*). This is an attractive hypothesis in that the amount of bile secreted into the gut is related to the amount of fat in the diet, and there is some evidence that some degradation products of bile steroids are cocarcinogens. Up to the present there are three lines of evidence supporting this hypothesis.

First, a succession of reactions can be demonstrated with different species of bacteria isolated from the gut that, *in vitro*, produce a partially desaturated steroid. The dehydrogenation reaction that is the last stage in this chain is effected only by a few varieties of clostridia particularly *Clostridium paraputrificum*, *Clostridium tertium*, and *Clostridium indolis* (*9*). In addition, gut bacteria are known to produce deoxycholic and lithocholic acids, which have been shown to act as cocarcinogens in rats treated with N-methyl-N'-nitro-N-nitrosoguanidine (MNNG) in the rectum (*10*).

Second, there is a very good correlation between the colon cancer incidence in a number of countries and the concentration of bile steroids in the faeces of samples of healthy people examined in those countries (*8*; Hill *et al.*, unpublished).

Third, patients with newly diagnosed large bowel cancer have been found to have in their faeces a higher concentration of bile steroids and a greater number of the nuclear dehydrogenating clostridia (NDC) demonstrated in the laboratory as able to produce the dehydrogenation reaction in the steroid nucleus, than control patients (*11*; Hill *et al.*, unpublished).

Possibilities for Prevention

In considering possibilities for the prevention of large bowel cancer, we propose to assume that the major factor in the etiology of the disease is the bacterial production of a carcinogen or cocarcinogen from bile acids. This is not, of course, yet firmly established and we have further long-term studies in which we are attempting to validate the hypothesis. Moreover there are suggestions that bacterial action on tryptophan or tyrosine in the gut might also liberate carcinogenic agents. Nevertheless it is of interest to consider what preventive possibilities would be open if the hypothesis is proved. We shall consider ways in which the production or activity of carcinogens derived from bile steroids might be reduced, or their effects mitigated. These ways may be grouped under four headings: (1) reduction in amount of bile steroids reaching those parts of the intestine that are colonized by bacteria able to produce the relevant reactions; (2) reduction in the extent to which bacteria attack the steroids; (3) protection of the colonic mucosa against the carcinogenic agent; (4) development of screening methods to detect individuals at specially high risk, so that they can be treated at a time when cure is possible.

Reduction in Steroid Concentration in Colon

The international comparisons reveal a strong correlation between reported national intake of fat and the faecal concentration of acid (biliary) steroids. In acute experiments, a reduction in the dietary fat intake results in a fall in faecal acid steroids (*12*). In principle, therefore, it should be possible to reduce the large bowel cancer incidence by reducing the habitual intake of fat, or meat-with-fat. How practical is this suggestion? In Britain the range of fat intake that was recorded in one study of a group of normal adults (civil servants) was from about 60 g/day to about 150 g/day. The regression line from the international studies suggests that a reduction from the highest intake to the lowest might be associated with a 70% reduction in cancer incidence. It is not, however, legitimate to extrapolate directly from international comparisons to the probable effect within one population, and in comparisons between individuals within Britain it has not been possible to demonstrate a clear relation between habitual fat intake and faecal steroid concentration. Indeed retrospective case-control studies have not indicated a higher fat intake in colon cancer patients than controls (*13*; Meade *et al.*, personal communication).

The prospects for a campaign to persuade people to eat less fat or less meat would require very convincing evidence to gain any support, and even with such support the techniques of mass dietary persuasion are probably quite inadequate to have any useful effect. The restriction is likely to come about on any scale only if a significant physical shortage of the relevant foods develops. The work of Haenszel *et al.* (*7*) suggests that, among meats, beef may have an especially potent effect in promoting the cancer. If this were the case, the necessary educational campaign might have a more limited aim, but one would be indeed an optimist to suppose that Americans, Britons, or Australians could readily be persuaded to eat less beef.

An alternative approach to the aim of reducing the steroid concentration in the gut is to attempt dilution. The consumption of some forms of vegetable "fibre," *e.g.*, bran, results in an increase in faecal volume, due to water retention, without increasing the total steroids lost, so there is some reduction in steroid concentration in the faeces. The maximum dilution effect observed in experimental work (*14–16*) was 40% using up to 100 g bran. Naive application of the "international" regression factor would suggest that this might possibly be associated with a 40% reduction in the cancer incidence. The nature of the vegetable fibre employed for this purpose is important and is not solely related to its water-holding ability, for with some, *e.g.*, bagasse, pectin, guar, there is binding of steroids, so that, although faecal volume is increased, the steroid concentration is unchanged and the total excretion increased.

In any case total faecal concentrations may be only marginally relevant; the concentration in the greater part of the colon may well be affected differently from that in faeces by the various fibre materials; and the availability of the steroids or their products to bacteria, and to the mucosa, may also be differentially affected.

Lastly, one might attempt to reduce the total steroid pool in the body in the hope that this would reduce the gut concentration. Clofibrate has been used for this purpose by workers studying the prevention of atheroma but it has the unacceptable side effect of producing bile that is supersaturated with cholesterol.

Protection of Bile Acids from Bacterial Action

Most of the bile steroids that are secreted into the gut are reabsorbed in the ileum unchanged or at most deconjugated by bacterial action. Only a small part suffers further bacterial attack and passes on to the colon. There can be relatively little bacterial action in normal individuals proximal to the terminal ileum, and any factor that favoured reabsorption in the mid-region should reduce the colonic concentrations. It is conceivable that individuals differ in their pattern of reabsorption; this might account for the observation of Rose et al. (17) who showed a negative correlation between serum cholesterol levels and colon cancer experience, in contrast to the positive correlation with coronary heart disease. In any case, we know of no way of encouraging ileal absorption at present.

Among the many virtues postulated at some time for fibre has been its capacity to bind bile steroids, with the implication that this protects them from bacterial attack. There is no evidence that this actually occurs. Another of the supposed actions of dietary fibre is its ability to accelerate the transit of intestinal contents, an action considered virtuous in that it might allow less time for the bacteria to attack the steroids, and less time for the supposed noxious products to remain in contact with the mucosa. However, in a short-term study in which volunteers consumed bagasse as a faecal-bulking agent, we found no evidence that the decreased transit time was associated with any reduction in the degree of degradation of steroids. There is certainly no reason to think that any regularly acceptable degree of intestinal hurry would deny the colonic bacteria the opportunity to attack the steroids. In a small number of subjects on a no-residue diet, who had a very long transit time, the degree of steroid degradation was very low. It seems to us that it is concentration of the noxious substances at the mucosa, rather than the speed with which individual molecules are travelling past, that should be important. It thus seems unlikely that dietary fibre has a simple effect on carcinogen production but there may be other ways in which it affects metabolism within the colon (18).

The bacterial action that we are postulating involves both bacteroides and clostridia. A regime that altered the numbers of these bacteria in the gut might offer a prophylactic method. There are indeed some indications that, in low-cancer countries, the bacteroides count of faeces may perhaps be lower than in high-cancer countries, so perhaps fewer bacteroides may be advantageous. But there is also some evidence that bacteroides, by producing volatile fatty acids in the gut, may have some protective effect against invasion by pathogenic bacteria. So a reduction in the bacteroides population might result in an increased frequency of bacterial diarrhoeal disease, and certainly many countries with a low incidence of large bowel cancer have a high incidence of diarrhoeal disease. The variation between individuals in Britain in the count of *C. paraputrificum* and other nuclear dehydrogenating clostridia, and the variation between the high- and low-cancer countries, is substantial. We know, as yet, of no benefit conferred by the carriage of these clostridia, and it is certainly possible that their elimination might reduce the cancer risk. Unfortunately we have no idea how this could be done.

Some recent work indicates that it might be possible so to alter the conditions within the colon as to affect the dehydrogenation activity of the clostridia. Vitamin K, which is produced by many gut bacteria, is a potent cofactor for this reaction. Perhaps there are ways in which vitamin K production might be reduced, or its effect neutralized. It is probable, too, that an alteration in the E_h within the colon might affect the dehydrogenation reaction since the relevant bacteria demand a low E_h for growth and in some cases an even lower E_h for enzyme production. Similarly a reduction in pH from 7 to 6 might inhibit many of the reactions. Whether either of these changes would be compatible with good health in other respects is not known.

Protection of Colonic Mucosa

We do not, of course, know the real nature of the carcinogen active on the colonic epithelium, nor whether it reaches the target cells directly from the gut lumen or indirectly by the blood stream, and we have no idea how the action of the carcinogen could be altered. Nevertheless there is some intriguing work now in progress on those bacteria that are intimately associated with the gut mucosa, and which have been shown, with certainty in animals and probably in man, to belong to different species from those found dominant in the luminal contents. The mucosa-associated bacteria may well play an important role in controlling the activities of the epithelium, and they would certainly be well placed to act on chemical substances liberated in the gut lumen before they reached the epithelial cells. Clearly, they could be carcinogen producers or carcinogen destroyers. There is need for a great deal of work on the nature and activity of mucosa-associated bacteria but the techniques for their study are difficult.

Screening Methods for Early Detection

The prognosis for surgical treatment of large bowel cancer, if detected early, is good, so that screening methods for early detection while not leading to prevention of the disease might reduce the mortality due to it. We are currently engaged in a prospective study that we hope will show whether the demonstration of a high level of acid steroids, or large numbers of the clostridia that have the dehydrogenating enzyme, in the faeces of healthy individuals, or both, can be used to predict the development of large bowel cancer. This study is in a very early stage and no results will be available for some years yet.

In the meanwhile there remain two recognized groups of patients known to be at high risk of developing large bowel cancer, namely those with long-standing ulcerative colitis and those with familiar polyposis. The carcinogenic mechanism in these conditions is not known but recent studies have indicated that the cancer developing in the polyposis patients is unlikely to be due to the same bacterial degradation process as we are postulating for large bowel cancers in other persons, since their gut bacteria show an extraordinary degree of inactivity in the metabolism of bile steroids (*19*).

CONCLUSIONS

In this paper we have sketched a number of ways in which the prevention of an important cancer could be envisaged, on the hypothesis that the disease is due to some carcinogen produced by bacterial action on biliary steroids. We should conclude by emphasizing that the hypothesis has yet to be proved. We hope that our current prospective studies may provide convincing evidence on its validity but we must wait some years for sufficient data to accumulate. Meanwhile it seems of some interest to speculate, as we have done in this paper, on what practical action could be recommended if the suggested mechanism is shown to be relevant, and to consider what research can usefully be initiated to develop methods that could be preventive.

REFERENCES

1. Doll, R.   The geographical distribution of cancer. Brit. J. Cancer, *23*: 1–8, 1969.
2. Haenszel, W. and Kurihara, M.   Studies of Japanese migrants. I. Mortality from cancer and other diseases among Japanese in the United States. J. Natl. Cancer Inst., *40*: 43–68, 1968.
3. Lemon, F. R., Walden, R. T., and Woods, R. W.   Cancer of the lung and mouth in Seventh-Day Adventists. Cancer Phila., *17*: 486–497, 1964.
4. Gregor, O., Toman, R., and Prušová, F.   Gastrointestinal cancer and nutrition. Gut, *10*: 1031–1034, 1969.
5. Drasar, B. S. and Irving, D.   Environmental factors and cancer of the colon and breast. Brit. J. Cancer, *27*: 167–172, 1973.
6. Armstrong, B. and Doll, R.   Environmental factors and cancer incidence and mortality in different countries, with special reference to dietary practices. Int. J. Cancer, *15*: 617–631, 1975.
7. Haenszel, W., Berg, J. W., Segi, M., Kurihara, M., and Locke, F. B. Large-bowel cancer in Hawaiian Japanese. J. Natl. Cancer Inst., *51*: 1765–1779, 1973.
8. Hill, M. J., Crowther, J. S., Drasar, B. S., Hawksworth, G., Aries, V., and Williams, R. E. O. Bacteria and aetiology of cancer of large bowel. Lancet, *i*: 95–100, 1971.
9. Goddard, P., Fernandez, F., West, B., Hill, M. J., and Barnes, P.   The nuclear dehydrogenation of steroids by intestinal bacteria. J. Med. Microbiol., *8*: 429–435, 1975.
10. Narisawa, T., Magadia, N. E., Weisburger, J. H., and Wynder, E. L.   Promoting effect of bile acids on colon carcinogenesis after intrarectal instillation of N-methyl-N′-nitro-N-nitrosoguanidine in rats. J. Natl. Cancer Inst., *53*: 1093–1097, 1974.

11. Hill, M. J., Drasar, B. S., Williams, R. E. O., Meade, T. W., Cox, A. G., Simpson, J. E. P., and Morson, B. C. Faecal bile-acids and clostridia in patients with cancer of the large bowel. Lancet, *i*: 535–539, 1975.

12. Hill, M. J. The effect of some factors on the faecal concentration of acid steroids, neutral steroids and urobilins. J. Pathol., *104*: 239–245, 1971.

13. Wynder, E. L. and Shigematsu, T. Environmental factors of cancer of the colon and rectum. Cancer Phila., *20*: 1520–1561, 1967.

14. Jenkins, D. J. A., Hill, M. S. [J.], and Cummings, J. H. Effect of wheat fibre on blood lipids, fecal steroid excretion and serum iron. Am. J. Clin. Nutr., *28*: 1975, in press.

15. Walters, R. L., McLean B. I., Davies, P. S., Hill, M. J., Drasar, B. S., Southgate, D. A. T., Green, J., and Morgan, B. Effects of two types of dietary fibre on faecal steroid and lipid excretion. Brit. Med. J., *2*: 536–538, 1975.

16. Eastwood, M. A., Kirkpatrick, J. R., Mitchell, W. D., Bone, A., and Hamilton, T. Effects of dietary supplements of wheat bran and cellulose on faeces and bowel function. Brit. Med. J., *4*: 392–394, 1973.

17. Rose, G., Blackburn, H., Keys, A., Taylor, H. L., Kannel, W. B., Paul, O., Reid, D. D., and Stamler, J. Colon cancer and blood-cholesterol. Lancet, *i*: 181–183, 1974.

18. Eastwood, M. A. Vegetable dietary fibre—Potent pith. Roy. Soc. Health J., *95*: 188–190, 1975.

19. Bone, E., Drasar, B. S., and Hill, M. J. Gut bacteria and their metabolic activities in familial polyposis. Lancet, *i*: 1117–1120, 1975.

Discussion of Paper of Drs. Williams et al.

DR. SUGIMURA: Do you have any comments on the case of familial polyposis of the colon, which is a distinct genetic disease? Are there any analytical data on bile acid excretion? Is there any information on bacterial flora in these patients?

Did anyone try to limit fat intake or to add bulk fiber to depress the transformation of polyps to malignant carcinoma?

I would like to call your attention to the presence of a rat strain which produces polyposis and adenocarcinoma in the colon. This rat mimics quite well the familial polyposis of man. At least two reports on this subject from Japan have appeared in J. Natl. Cancer Inst. (*55*: 1471, 1975; *56*: 651, 1976).

DR. WILLIAMS: The bacterial flora of polyposis patients is qualitatively quite similar to that of normal persons but there is a striking lack of degradation of steroids, so clearly the postulated etiology of cancer in those persons cannot apply in patients with congenital polyposis.

DR. WEISBURGER: Dr. Reddy of our staff, working with Dr. Lipkin of the Memorial Cancer Center in New York, has studied about 12 cases of familial polyposis. Confirming the microbiologic data of Prof. Williams, he found that such patients secrete more undegraded cholesterol and fewer metabolites such as coprostanone or coprostanol (Cancer, 1976, in press).

DR. BUTLER: Clinically patients with ulcerative colitis have a high incidence of colonic carcinoma. Is there any evidence of a change in either the flora or bile acid secretion in such patients?

DR. WILLIAMS: We have a study of ulcerative colitis patients in progress at present.

DR. FARBER: Dr. Williams, can you be certain that most of the metabolism of the bile acids is of bacterial origin, rather than due to the colon mucosa? If the bowel mucosa metabolizes bile acids, perhaps the patient with multiple polyposis may have a different mucosal metabolic effect, since the mucosal epithelial cells seem to be different in such patients.

DR. WILLIAMS: This is a very interesting suggestion. We have not investigated the possible mucosal contribution to bile acid metabolism nor that of the mucosal-associated bacteria.

DR. WATTENBERG: It is obviously very important to be conservative in any suggestions made to alter human diet. In the case of addition of fiber to the diet, the possibility would exist of adsorbing bile salts to the fiber, thus reducing free bile salt concentrations in the bowel lumen and possibly stimulating increased bile salt secretion in the bile.

There is a significant number of young people in the U.S.A. who have been treated over long periods of time for acne of the skin with broad spectrum antibiotics. Is there any information of what the effects of such treatment might be on the clostridia species which metabolize bile acids?

DR. WILLIAMS: I agree that good, direct evidence is very desirable before one advocates changes in diet. I have no information on any consequences that long-term tetracycline may have on gut bacteria and their effects on bile acids.

DR. WEBER: Professor Williams, I would value your comments on the possible role of extensive use of antibiotics. In view of the use of antibiotics in the past 20 years, also in premature infants, the possibility of an early damage, due to bacterial flora imbalance, may be of some relevance.

DR. WILLIAMS: I do not think there has been any change in the incidence of large-bowel cancer in the last 20 years that could correspond with the great increase in antibiotic usage during that period, so we cannot implicate antibiotics in the etiology of large bowel cancer.

DR. MAGEE: Earlier in this year there was a meeting at IARC (Lyon) to discuss the question of carcinogens in faeces. Do you think it would be worthwhile to make a serious effort to determine if any carcinogens are present in human faeces and to try to identify them?

DR. WILLIAMS: It would certainly be useful, if we knew what carcinogens we are looking for. Until we know that, all we can do is to try to define the more important substances present in different people and different circumstances.

DR. SUGIMURA: I would like to mention that Dr. Mower and Dr. Mandel in Honolulu are carrying out experiments on mutagens in faeces from Japanese people in Japan, Japanese immigrants in Hawaii, and Caucasians in Hawaii. This sort of experiment may be useful in understanding the different frequency of colon tumors among different groups of people.

FUNDAMENTALS IN CANCER PREVENTION, P. N. MAGEE ET AL. (EDS.),
UNIV. OF TOKYO PRESS, TOKYO / UNIV. PARK PRESS, BALTIMORE, PP. 153–166, 1976

Inhibition of Chemical Carcinogenesis by Antioxidants and Some Additional Compounds

Lee W. WATTENBERG

Department of Laboratory Medicine and Pathology, University of Minnesota, Minneapolis, Minnesota, U.S.A.

Abstract: Current data indicate that environmental carcinogens are involved as causative factors in a substantial proportion of all cancers occurring in man. Geographic differences in the incidence of cancer of a particular organ as well as variations in incidence over a period of time are generally attributed to changes in the magnitude of exposure to cancer-producing compounds. It is possible that in some instances an alternative situation exists; namely, that changes in factors inhibiting carcinogens are present. In support of this possibility, data will be presented showing that a number of antioxidants and some additional compounds occurring in the environment have the capacity to inhibit the neoplastic effects of chemical carcinogens.

A considerable amount of work has been done with the carcinogen-inhibiting properties of phenolic antioxidants. Two of these, butylated hydroxyanisole and butylated hydroxytoluene are widely used as food additives. Carcinogens shown to be inhibited by one or both of these compounds include polycyclic aromatic hydrocarbons, diethylnitrosamine, 4-nitroquinoline-N-oxide, uracil mustard, urethane, N-2-fluorenylacetamide, and *p*-dimethylaminoazobenzene.

Several sulfur-containing antioxidants, *i.e.*, tetraethylthiuram disulfide (disulfiram, Antabuse), diethyldithiocarbamate, and dimethyldithiocarbamate have been studied in a more limited way. They inhibit neoplasia resulting from administration of polycyclic aromatic hydrocarbons. Disulfiram and diethyldithiocarbamate have been studied for their inhibitory capacities against dimethylhydrazine-induced neoplasia of the large intestine and have been found to be remarkably effective.

In addition to the antioxidants, benzyl isothiocyanate and to a lesser extent benzyl thiocyanate, two naturally occurring plant constituents, inhibit the neoplastic effects of polycyclic aromatic hydrocarbons.

Major deficiencies in our present knowledge are a paucity of information as to the range of compounds which inhibit chemical carcinogenesis and a lack of understanding as to precise mechanisms of inhibition. Ultimately, information in both of these areas could provide a basis for more accurately evaluating epidemiological data bearing on the occurrence of neoplasia and for consideration of the potential role of inhibitors of chemical carcinogenesis as a protective device for man.

Studies of the occurrence of cancer of specific organ sites in man have shown considerable geographical variations. It also has been found that the incidence of a particular neoplasm may change markedly over a period of time. Thus in the U.S.A., cancer of the lung and pancreas has been increasing and cancer of the stomach decreasing. Since considerable evidence indicates that environmental carcinogens are involved as causative factors in a substantial proportion of all cancers occurring in man, differences in cancer incidence in geographical areas and population groups, or changes in incidence with time have been generally attributed to alterations in the magnitude of exposure to external carcinogenic agents. However it is possible that in some instances, the observed differences may be due, at least in part, to alterations in the level of protection against carcinogenic agents. This presentation will describe a variety of inhibitors of chemical carcinogenesis, some of which are found in the environment. Particular emphasis will be given to antioxidants.

Historical

Experiments on inhibition of chemical carcinogenesis date back to 1929. At that time Berenblum published a paper in which it was shown that dichloroethyl sulfide inhibited skin tumor formation resulting from repeated painting of mouse skin with a carcinogenic tar (1). Subsequently, a number of other compounds were found to have similar effects on epidermal neoplasia in mice (2). These can be divided into four main classes: hydrolyzing halogen compounds such as valeryl chloride or benzene sulfochloride; compounds which are metabolized to mercapturates such as bromobenzene (3); the anhydrides of α, β-unsaturated dicarboxylic acids such as maleic anhydride and citraconic anhydride; and several low molecular weight aromatic hydrocarbons such as phenanthrene. In experiments with these compounds it was possible to retard and in some instances prevent the appearance of neoplastic lesions of the mouse skin.

Inhibition of epidermal neoplasia is an unusual situation in allowing for high local concentrations of inhibitors. In addition, toxicity problems are generally less as compared to systemic administrations. These early studies of inhibition of chemical carcinogenesis were followed by a more diverse group of experiments based on an increasing amount of information concerning the chemistry and metabolism of chemical carcinogens and biochemistry in general. Of enormous importance was the data indicating that carcinogens have a common reactive form; namely, a positively charged electrophilic species which binds to macromolecules. Many carcinogens are metabolized to this active form *via* the microsomal mixed function oxidase system, some by other metabolic pathways, and a significant group requires no enzyme activation (4).

The existence of these common features has provided the stimulus for more recent lines of investigation into inhibition of chemical carcinogenesis. One of these, which is very active at the present time, entails protection against chemical carcinogens by altering the microsomal mixed function oxidase system (2, 5, 6). A second mechanism of protection involves the use of noncarcinogenic compounds structurally related to specific carcinogens in order to obtain competitive inhibition (2). A third series of investigations has been based on the use of antioxidants. These will be discussed in detail subsequently. A fourth line of investigation has employed protease inhibitors (7, 8). An additional area of exploration for means of inhibiting carcinogenesis which is quite distinctive from the above is aimed at reversing the early phases of neoplasia. At present, a major emphasis in this approach entails use of vitamin A and related compounds (9, 10).

Inhibition of Chemical Carcinogenesis by Antioxidants and Some Additional Compounds

The use of antioxidants as possible inhibitors of the chemical carcinogens is based in general on the concept that the antioxidants will exert a scavenging effect on the reactive species of carcinogens thus protecting cellular constituents from attack. In early studies, wheat germ oil and α-tocopherol were employed. Experiments showing positive and negative results have been published (11). Confirmatory reports on the positive experiments have not appeared so that the implications of this work are not clear. Our own experience with α-tocopherol has not shown it to be inhibitory (11). However it is quite possible that under appropriate conditions, an inhibitory effect might be obtained.

During the past several years, studies have been carried out with other antioxidants. Several of these have been found to inhibit the effects of a substantial variety of chemical carcinogens (Fig. 1 and Table 1). The most extensive work of this type has been done with phenolic antioxidants; in particular, butylated hydroxyanisole (BHA) and butylated hydroxytoluene (BHT). Inhibition occurs

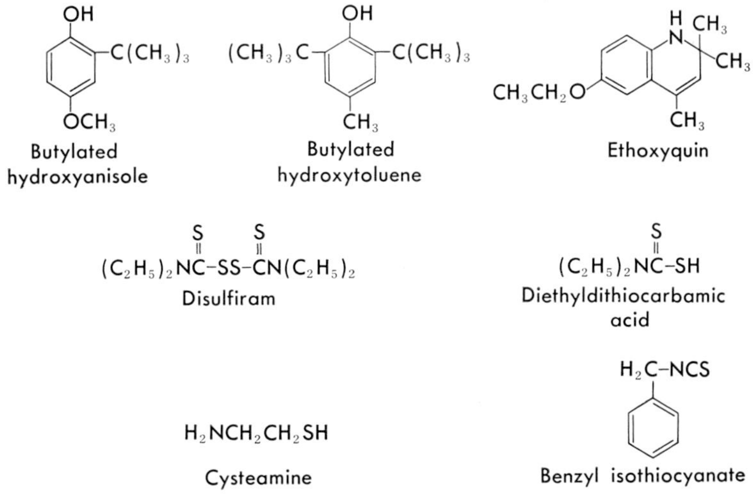

FIG. 1. Compounds inhibiting chemical carcinogenesis.

TABLE 1.   Inhibition of Carcinogen-induced Neoplasia by Antioxidants and Some Additional Compounds

Carcinogen	Antioxidant	Species	Site of neoplasm inhibited	Reference
BP	BHA	Mouse	Forestomach, lung	11, 12
BP	Disulfiram, benzyl isothiocyanate	Mouse	Forestomach	13, 14
DMBA	BHA, BHT, ethoxyquin	Mouse	Forestomach, lung	11, 12
DMBA	BHA, BHT, ethoxyquin	Rat	Breast	11
DMBA	Disulfiram, dimethyldithio-carbamate, benzyl isothiocyanate, benzyl thiocyanate, cysteamine hydrochloride	Rat	Breast	13–15
7-Hydroxymethyl-12-methyl-benz(a)anthracene	BHA	Mouse	Lung	12
Dibenz(a, h)anthracene	BHA	Mouse	Lung	12
Diethylnitrosamine	BHA, ethoxyquin	Mouse	Lung	16
4-Nitroquinoline-N-oxide	BHA, ethoxyquin	Mouse	Lung	16
Uracil mustard	BHA	Mouse	Lung	12
Urethane	BHA	Mouse	Lung	12
FAA	BHT	Rat	Liver	17
N-OH-FAA	BHT	Rat	Liver, breast	17
p-Dimethylaminoazobenzene	BHT	Rat	Liver	18
DMH	Disulfiram, diethyldithiocarbamate	Rat	Large intestine	14, 19

FAA, N-2-fluorenylacetamide; N-OH-FAA, N-hydroxy-N-2-fluorenylacetamide; DMH, dimethylhydrazine.

under a number of experimental conditions. It has been found in situations where the route of administration results in direct contact of carcinogen with the target tissue, $i.e.$, neoplasia of the forestomach in mice fed benzo(a)pyrene (BP) or 7,12-dimethylbenz(a)anthracene (DMBA). Comparable suppression of neoplasia is also obtained in experiments in which the carcinogen is acting at a site remote from that of administration, $i.e.$, inhibition of mammary tumor formation in rats given DMBA orally. Of particular interest for those concerned with gastric neoplasia are a number of experiments in which the BHA or BHT were added to diets containing polycyclic aromatic hydrocarbon carcinogens. In these studies the target tissue in which neoplasia occurred was the forestomach. Those animals that received BHA or BHT in the diet along with the carcinogen showed pronounced suppression of neoplasia at this site.

BHA and BHT are of interest because of their extensive use as food additives. Of the two compounds, BHA is preferable, since it is less toxic than BHT. However, both compounds can be employed at very high doses before eivdence of toxicity appears (20, 21). In studies in which BHA or BHT were added to the diet along with BP, it was found that at a concentration of either antioxidant of 5 mg/g diet, inhibition of the carcinogenic effect on the forestomach of the mouse of a concentration of BP of 1 mg/g diet occurs (11). In the United States, the human consumption of these phenolic antioxidants is of the order of magnitude of several milligrams a day. Assuming that the results of the animal experiments hold for man, this amount of the antioxidants could be of importance in inhibiting the effects of chronic exposure to low doses of carcinogens, the type of exposure which is most likely to occur in human populations.

In addition to BHA and BHT, inhibition of polycyclic hydrocarbon-induced carcinogenesis of the forestomach has been brought about by antioxidants with different chemical structures. One of these is 6-ethoxy-1,2-dihydro-2,2,4-trimethyl-quinoline(ethoxyquin), an antioxidant which is widely used as an additive in commercial animal diets, but not in food for human consumption. More recently several sulfur-containing antioxidants have been studied for their carcinogen-inhibiting capacities. Four of these are effective inhibitors. These are tetraethyl-thiuram disulfide (disulfiram, Antabuse), diethyldithiocarbamate, dimethyldithio-carbamate, and cysteamine (Table 1). Disulfiram and dimethyldithiocarbamate have been employed in studies of polycyclic hydrocarbon-induced neoplasia of the forestomach. Both compounds are potent inhibitors (13). Several sufur-containing antioxidants inhibit mammary tumor formation resulting from administration of DMBA. These include disulfiram, dimethyldithiocarbamate, and cysteamine. The former two compounds were studied under conditions in which the antioxidants were administered orally and the DMBA by the same route (13). In the case of cysteamine, the antioxidant was administered intraperitoneally and the DMBA intravenously (15).

Disulfiram has been used in experiments in which cancer of the large bowel was produced by multiple subcutaneous injections of DMH. Under these conditions, disulfiram caused total inhibition of neoplasia of the large bowel (19). More recently diethyldithiocarbamate, the reduction product of disulfiram, has been employed in a comparable study. This compound also produced complete inhibition of neoplasia of the large bowel (Table 2).

Along with the study of the inhibitory capacities of the various sulfur-containing antioxidants, benzyl thiocyanate and benzyl isothiocyanate, two naturally occurring compounds were included. It has been found that these compounds can inhibit neoplasia resulting from exposure to polycyclic aromatic hydrocarbon carcinogens (13, 14). Of the two compounds, benzyl isothiocyanate is more potent and more versatile as an inhibitor than the corresponding thiocyanate. Both compounds will inhibit mammary tumor formation in the rat when administered in the diet for one week or when given by oral intubation 4 hr prior to administration

TABLE 2.   Effects of Disulfiram and Diethyldithiocarbamate on Tumor Formation in the Large Intestine of Female CF_1 Mice Given Sixteen Doses of DMH Subcutaneously[a]

Additions to the diet[b]	No. of mice at risk	Mice with tumors of the large intestine		
		No.	%	No. of tumors/mouse
None	20	18	90	4
Disulfiram: 5 mg/g	20	0	0	0
Sodium diethyldithiocarbamate: 7.5 mg/g	18	0	0	0

[a] Nine-week-old female CF_1 mice were given subcutaneous injections of 0.4 mg DMH in 0.2 ml 0.001 M EDTA brought to pH 6.5 with sodium bicarbonate in the cervical area once a week for 16 weeks and sacrificed 14 weeks after the last administration (19).   [b] Experimental diets consisting of powdered Purina Rat Chow with the indicated additions or without additions were started 11 days before the initial administration of DMH and were continued until 4 days after the last administration (19).

TABLE 3.   Effects of Benzyl Isothiocyanate and Benzyl Thiocyanate on DMBA-induced Mammary Tumor Formation in Female Sprague Dawley Rats

Material administered[a]	No. of rats	Body weight (g)		Mammary tumors[b]		
		At 7 weeks	At 23 weeks	No. of rats with tumors	% of rats with tumors	No. of tumors per rat
Olive oil	14	149	308	14	100	2.2
Benzyl isothiocyanate	14	149	289	2	14	0.14
Benzyl thiocyanate	14	149	279	5	36	0.43

[a] Olive oil 1 ml or 0.33 mmoles of inhibitor in 1 ml olive oil were administered by oral incubation 4 hr prior to oral administration of 12 mg of DMBA in 1 ml olive oil. Rats were 7 weeks of age (11).   [b] Mammary tumors occurring 16 weeks after administration of the DMBA.

of a carcinogenic dose of DMBA. An experiment with this latter dose schedule is shown in Table 3. If benzyl isothiocyanate is added to a diet containing BP, it will inhibit the occurrence of tumors of the forestomach and lung resulting from this carcinogen. Benzyl thiocyanate is ineffective as an inhibitor under these conditions. Sodium thiocyanate is inactive as an inhibitor in all systems which have been studied.

Inhibition of chemical carcinogenesis by selenium salts has been reported by Shamberger. In an initial paper, the experimental system employed consisted of initiation of epidermal neoplasia with DMBA followed by promotion with croton oil. Sodium selenide added to the croton oil suppressed the development of skin tumors (22). In a subsequent paper repeated applications of methylcholanthrene were employed. Again, addition of sodium selenide inhibited epidermal neoplasia. In a further experiment mice were placed on a selenium-deficient diet (Torula yeast) without supplements or with added sodium selenide or sodium selenite. BP was applied to the skin daily to produce epidermal neoplasia. Under these conditions, a slight inhibition was found with both of the selenium salts (23). Shamberger has also cited evidence that there is an inverse relationship between selenium occurrence in soil and forage crops and human cancer death rates in the United States and Canada in 1965 and between human blood levels of selenium and human cancer death rates in several cities (24).

Mechanism(s) of Inhibition of Chemical Carcinogens by Antioxidants

The mechanism or mechanisms by which the antioxidants inhibit carcinogen-induced neoplasia has not been established and may differ for various antioxidants. Several possibilities exist which can be divided into two major categories. The first involves some type of direct interaction between antioxidant and reactive species of carcinogen. The second possibility is that the antioxidant is acting in an indirect manner. Of primary interest in this regard is alteration of enzyme activity. Both types of mechanisms are currently under investigation.

The original rationale for use of antioxidants in inhibiting chemical carcino-genesis was based on the premise that they might react with active species of carcinogens and thus protect tissue constituents from attack. However, direct proof of this type of protective mechanism is difficult to produce *in vivo*. Solution chemistry in which *in vitro* demonstration of an interaction of antioxidant and active form of the carcinogen is found is not sufficient since *in vivo* conditions may be very different. At the moment, definitive studies showing a direct interaction *in vivo* between antioxidant and carcinogen have not been reported.

Two studies in which cells in culture systems have been employed to investigate inhibition of effects of antioxidants on chemical carcinogens have been published. In one of these, leukocyte cultures were incubated with DMBA in the presence or absence of added antioxidants. Chromosome breaks were quantitated. Under these conditions, BHT, ascorbic acid, α-tocopherol, and sodium selenite reduced the number of breaks as compared to cultures lacking the antioxidants (25). In a second investigation, the effect of added cysteamine-HCl on transformation of mouse fibroblasts (M2 line) by DMBA was determined. Cysteamine-HCl reduced the number of transformed foci (15). While inhibitory effects were observed in both of the cell culture studies, neither provided evidence of a direct interaction of antioxidant and carcinogen.

Antioxidants have been found to alter the properties of a number of biological systems (20, 21). Thus the possibility exists that they protect against carcinogens by some indirect mechanism. In a study of this type, the effect of BHT on the metabolism of FAA and N-OH-FAA was investigated in rats. Administration of BHT led to excretion in urine of a increased amount of both carcinogens chiefly accounted for as glucuronic acid conjugates. Forty-eight hours after administration of the labelled carcinogens, lower levels of radioactivity were found in blood, liver and bound to DNA of liver in the animals given BHT as compared to controls. Data were interpreted as indicating that BHT enhanced detoxification of FAA and N-OH-FAA by increasing glucuronide conjugation (26).

A series of studies have been initiated to determine the mechanism of inhibition of BP carcinogenesis by BHA. BP is metabolized by the microsomal mixed function oxidase system which acts upon a wide variety of xenobiotic compounds including polycyclic aromatic hydrocarbons (27). Reactive metabolites as well as detoxification products are produced (28–30). The phenolic metabolites of individual polycyclic aromatic hydrocarbons can be quantitated as a group. This catagory of reaction is designated aryl hydrocarbon hydroxylase (AHH). Some phenolic antioxidants induce increased activity of microsomal mixed function oxidase activity towards several of the substrates metabolized by the microsomal mixed function oxidase system (31, 32). While BHA was inactive or at most weakly active as an inducer for those reactions reported, the early work had not included metabolism of BP or other polycyclic aromatic hydrocarbons. Accordingly, the possibility existed that this antioxidant might alter the microsomal metabolism of BP.

The effects of BHA on BP metabolism were subsequently studied in an experimental system employing conditions under which BHA inhibits neoplasia due to this carcinogen. Female A/HeJ mice were used. Oral administrations of BP to these mice results in pulmonary tumor formation. However if the mice are fed a diet containing BHA 5 mg/g, inhibition of pulmonary neoplasia occurs (12). The

TABLE 4.   Microsomal AHH Activity and Binding of BP Metabolites to DNA in Livers of Mice Fed BHA and Corresponding Controls

Expt. No.	AHH activity (units/mg wet wt.)[a]		Binding of BP metabolites to DNA[b]			
	BHA-fed	Control	μCi/80 μg BP added to reaction mixture	BHA-fed (dpm/mg DNA)	Control (dpm/mg DNA)	Ratio of BHA/control
1	4.2	4.8	0.25	162	279	0.58
2	9.8	9.1	0.25	288	683	0.42
3	8.5	9.0	0.25	221	564	0.39
4	8.0	7.9	0.25	306	701	0.44

[a] One unit=fluorescence equivalent to 0.1 ng 3-hydroxybenzo(a)pyrene/min.   [b] Binding of BP metabolites to calf thymus DNA in a reaction mixture also containing ^{14}C-BP, liver microsomes, and NADPH (33).

biochemical studies described below were carried out on female A/HeJ mice fed BHA 5 mg/g of diet for 2 weeks and corresponding controls maintained under the same conditions but lacking the BHA in the diet.

AHH activity of microsomes from BHA-fed mice and controls was determined (33). No significant difference was found (Table 4). The AHH procedure measures petroleum ether-alkaline extractable hydroxylated metabolites of BP as a group. The main contribution of the results from the AHH procedure is that it gives an index of the overall microsomal metabolism of this compound. However, the data are limited in that distinctions between various hydroxylated metabolites of BP are not made nor are other metabolites identified. Thus while BHA did not change AHH activity, studies of other parameters showed that BHA had altered the microsomal system metabolizing BP. Incubation of BP and DNA with microsomes from BHA-fed mice resulted in significantly less binding of BP metabolites to DNA than with control microsomes (Table 4). There is approximately one-half the binding of BP metabolites to DNA in the presence of microsomes from BHA-fed mice as compared to controls. Microsomes from control or BHA-fed mice incubated without cofactor produced no counts bound to DNA above background levels (33).

In addition to changes in binding of BP metabolites to DNA, other characteristics of the liver microsomes were altered by BHA feeding. If α-naphthoflavone (ANF) was added to the microsomal reaction mixture, less of this compound was required to produce inhibition of AHH with microsomes from BHA-fed mice than from control microsomes (33). Cytochrome P-450 was determined by its carbon monoxide binding spectrum. In microsomes from BHA-fed mice, increases in concentration over control levels were seen per milligram of microsomal protein and per gram of liver. Microsomal protein content per gram of liver was not changed. In the BHA-fed mice, liver weight was significantly increased over controls. This increase in liver weight is similar to that observed by others in rats given BHA by oral administration (31, 32).

The ethyl isocyanide binding spectra at pH 7.4 were measured to see if any other forms of P-450, such as P_1-450, might have been produced by BHA feeding. The peak at 430 nm was the same in control and treated animals. However, the peak at 455 nm was lower in the microsomes from BHA-fed mice than from controls (33). This resulted in a ratio of the maxima at 455 nm : 430 nm that was significantly different in BHA-fed mice as compared to the controls. The effects of pH on the alteration of the heights of the two maxima were determined. The pH at which the two maxima are of equal magnitude is termed the "pH intercept" and is used as a parameter for characterizing the form of cytochrome P-450 present. The pH intercept for the cytochrome P-450 from the liver of mice fed BHA was 8.49 whereas that from that of the control animals was 8.27 (34).

In further work, a study was made of cytochrome P-450 reductase. This was determined without added microsomal substrate or in the presence of BP, BHA, or ethylmorphine. No difference in reductase activity between control and BHA-fed mice was found in the absence of added substrate or in the presence of BP or BHA. However in the presence of ethylmorphine a lower reductase activity was found in the BHA-fed animals as compared to the controls (34).

The results which have been obtained thus far show that consumption of a diet containing BHA results in an increased cytochrome P-450 in the liver and an alteration in the microsomal mixed function oxidase system of that organ. Four parameters reflect this alteration. (1) The microsomal AHH system shows an increased sensitivity to inhibition by ANF although the level of AHH activity is not altered. (2) The ethyl isocyanide difference spectra shows significant change. (3) Cytochrome P-450 reductase activity in the presence of ethylmorphine differs from that found in the control mice. (4) Microsomal incubation of BP in the presence of added DNA shows a decreased binding of BP metabolites to the DNA.

Studies of the mechanism(s) of inhibition of polycyclic aromatic hydrocarbon carcinogenesis by benzyl thiocyanate and benzyl isothiocyanate have not been carried out thus far. Some work relating to disulfiram does exist. Work of Schmähl and Krüger presented in this conference series in 1972 showed that methylation of macromolecules following administration of dimethylnitrosamine was inhibited by disulfiram. However, evidence of inhibition of neoplasia was not found (35). More recently in investigations of the metabolism of DMH, Fiala and Weisburger have found that the oxidation of this carcinogen is markedly inhibited in animals fed disulfiram in the diet (36).

DISCUSSION

Probably the single most important aspect of the material presented is that it demonstrates that a considerable variety of compounds have the capacity to inhibit chemical carcinogenesis. Major deficiencies in our present knowledge are the paucity of information as to the range of chemical structures which result in inhibition and precise information as to mechanisms of inhibition. Knowledge concerning mechanism would obviously be of importance in the search for additional inhibitors and in the design of more potent inhibitors than are currently known.

At the present time, we do not know whether any of the inhibitors that have been studied actually exert an inhibitory effect on human exposures to carcinogens. BHA and BHT which are widely used as food additives might have such an effect.

Likewise, selenium levels might be of importance. However it is very possible that naturally occurring compounds which are much more potent or for other reasons are more important inhibitors of carcinogenesis exist, and that we simply have not identified them yet. Obviously these data would be important for epidemiological studies of neoplasia. In addition, it would seem probable that synthetic compounds of high inhibitory potency and low toxicity could be produced when adequate information as to mechanisms of inhibition become known. Ultimately, a firm knowledge of naturally occurring and synthetic inhibitors would provide a basis for consideration of their use as a protective device for man. It is too early to know whether this has any plausibility. However if we are unable to rid our environment of chemical carcinogens, which should be the prime objective of cancer research, efforts at diminishing their impact would have merit.

ACKNOWLEDGMENT

Investigations included in this presentation were supported by Public Health Service Contract No. NO-1-CP-33364 and Public Health Service Grants No. 14146 and 15638, all from the National Cancer Institute.

REFERENCES

1. Berenblum, I. The modifying influence of dichloroethyl sulfide on the induction of tumours in mice by tar. J. Pathol. Bacteriol., *32*: 425–434, 1929.
2. Wattenberg, L. W. Chemoprophylaxis of carcinogenesis: A review. Cancer Res., *26*: 1520–1526, 1966.
3. Crabtree, H. G. Influence of bromobenzene on the induction of skin tumours by 3, 4-benzpyrene. Cancer Res., *4*: 688–693, 1944.
4. Miller, E. C. and Miller, J. A. Biochemical mechanisms of chemical carcinogenesis. *In;* H. Busch (ed.), The Molecular Biology of Cancer, pp. 377–402, Academic Press, New York, 1974.
5. Wattenberg, L. W. and Leong, J. L. Inhibition of the carcinogenic action of benzo-(a)pyrene by flavones. Cancer Res., *30*: 1922–1925, 1970.
6. Wattenberg, L. W., Loub, W. D., Lam, L. K., and Speier, J. L. Dietary constituents altering the responses to chemical carcinogens. Fed. Proc., *35*: 1327–1331, 1975.
7. Troll, W., Kassen, A., and Januff, A. Tumorigenesis in mouse skin. Inhibition by synthetic inhibitors of proteases. Science, *169*: 1211–1213, 1971.
8. Hozumi, M., Ogawa, M., Sugimura, T., Takeuchi, T., and Umezawa, H. Inhibition of tumorigenesis in mouse skin by leukopeptin, a protease inhibitor from *Actinomycetes*. Cancer Res., *32*: 1725–1728, 1972.
9. Saffiotti, U., Montesano, R., Sellakumar, A. R., and Borg, S. A. Experimental cancer of the lung. Inhibition by vitamin A of the induction of tracheobronchial squamous metaplasia and squamous cell tumors. Cancer, *20*: 857–864, 1967.
10. Sporn, M. D. Inhibition of chemical carcinogenesis by vitamin A. Fed. Proc., *34*: 1975, in press.
11. Wattenberg, L. W. Inhibition of carcinogenic and toxic effects of polycyclic hydrocarbons by phenolic antioxidants and ethoxyquin. J. Natl. Cancer Inst., *48*: 1425–1430, 1972.

12. Wattenberg, L. W. Inhibition of chemical carcinogen-induced pulmonary neoplasia by butylated hydroxyanisole. J. Natl. Cancer Inst., *50*: 1541–1544, 1973.

13. Wattenberg, L. W. Inhibition of carcinogenic and toxic effects of polycyclic hydrocarbons by several sulfur-containing compounds. J. Natl. Cancer Inst., *52*: 1583–1587, 1974.

14. Wattenberg, L. W. Unpublished.

15. Marquardt, H., Sapozink, M., and Zedeck, M. Inhibition by cysteamine-HCl of oncogenesis induced by 7, 12-dimethylbenz(a)anthracene without affecting toxicity. Cancer Res., *34*: 3387–3390, 1974.

16. Wattenberg, L. W. Inhibition of carcinogenic effects of diethylnitrosamine and 4-nitroquinoline-N-oxide by antioxidants. Fed. Proc., *31*: 633, 1972.

17. Ulland, B., Weisburger, J., Yamamoto R., and Weisburger, E. Antioxidants and carcinogenesis: Butylated hydroxytoluene, but not diphenyl-*p*-phenylenediamine, inhibits cancer induction by N-2-fluorenylacetamide and by N-hydroxy-N-2-fluorenylacetamide in rats. Food Cosmet. Toxicol., *11*: 199–207, 1973.

18. Frankfurt, O., Lipchina, L., and Bunto, T. The influence of 4-methyl-2, 6-*tert*-butylphenol (Ionol) on the development of hepatic tumors in rats. Bull. Exp. Biol. Med., *8*: 86–88, 1967.

19. Wattenberg, L. W. Inhibition of dimethylhydrazine-induced neoplasia of the large intestine by disulfiram. J. Natl. Cancer Inst., *54*: 1005–1006, 1975.

20. Hathaway, D. Metabolic fate in animals of hundred phenolic antioxidant function. *In;* Advances in Food Research, pp. 1–56, Academic Press, New York, 1966.

21. Pascal, G., Chichester, C., Mrak, E., and Stewart, G. (eds.). Physiological and metabolic effects of antioxidant food additives. World Rev. Nutr. Diet., *19*: 237–299, 1974.

22. Shamberger, R. J. Protection against cocarcinogenesis by antioxidants. Experientia, *22*: 116, 1966.

23. Shamberger, R. J. Relationship of selenium to cancer. V. Inhibitory effect of selenium on carcinogenesis. J. Natl. Cancer Inst., *44*: 931–936, 1970.

24. Shamberger, R. and Willis, C. Selenium distribution and human cancer mortality. Clin. Lab. Sci., *2*: 211–221, 1971.

25. Shamberger, R. J., Baughman, F. F., Kalchert, S. L., Willis, C. E., and Hoffman, G. C. Carcinogen-induced chromosomal breakage decreased by antioxidants. Proc. Natl. Acad. Sci. U.S., *70*: 1461–1463, 1973.

26. Grantham, P., Weisburger, J., and Weisburger, E. Effect of the antioxidant butylated hydroxytoluene on the metabolism of the carcinogens N-2-fluorenylacetamide and N-hydroxy-N-2-fluorenylacetamide. Food Cosmet. Toxicol., *11*: 209–217, 1973.

27. Mannering, G. Microsomal enzyme systems which catalyze drug metabolism. *In;* B. N. La Du, H. G. Mandel, and E. L. Way (eds.), Fundamentals of Drug Metabolism and Drug Disposition, pp. 206–252, Williams & Wilkins, Baltimore, 1971.

28. Selkirk, J., Croy, R., Roller, P., and Gelboin, H. V. High-pressure liquid chromatographic analysis of benzo(a)pyrene metabolism and covalent binding and the mechanism of action of 7,8-benzoflavone and 1,2-epoxy-3, 3, 3-trichloropropane. Cancer Res., *34*: 3474–3480, 1974.

29. Holder, G., Yagi, H., Dansette, P., Jerina, D., Levin, W., Lu, A., and Conney, A. Effects of inducers of epoxide hydrase on the metabolism of benzo(a)pyrene by liver microsomes and a reconstituted system: Analysis by high-pressure liquid chromatography. Proc. Natl. Acad. Sci. U.S., *71*: 4356–4360, 1974.

30. Ts'o, P., Caspary, W., Cohen, B., Leavitt, J. C., Lesko, S. A., Lorentzen, R. J., and Schechtman, L. M.   Basic mechanisms in polycyclic hydrocarbon carcinogenesis. *In;* P.Ts'o and J. A. DiPaolo (eds.), Chemical Carcinogenesis, pp. 113–148, Marcel Dekker, New York, 1974.

31. Gilbert, D., Martin, A., Gargolli, S. Abraham, R., and Golberg, L.   The effect of substituted phenols on liver weights and liver enzymes in the rat: Structure-activity relationships. Food Cosmet. Toxicol., *7*: 603–619, 1969.

32. Martin, A. and Gilbert, D.   Enzyme changes accompanying liver enlargement in rats treated with 3-*tert*-butyl-4-hydroxyanisole. Biochem. J., *106*: 22 p, 1968.

33. Speier, J. and Wattenberg, L.   Alteration in microsomal metabolism of benzo(a)-pyrene in mice fed butylated hydroxyanisole. J. Natl. Cancer Inst., *55*: 469–472, 1975.

34. Wattenberg, L. W., Speier, J., and Kotake, A.   Effects of antioxidants on metabolism of aromatic polycyclic hydrocarbons. *In;* G. Weber (ed.), Advances in Enzyme Regulation, vol. 14, Pergamon Press, New York, 1975, in press.

35. Schmähl, D. and Krüger, F. W.   Influence of disulfiram (tetraethylthiuram disulfide) on the biological actions of N-nitrosamines.   *In;* W. Nakahara, S. Takayama, T. Sugimura, and S. Odashima (eds.), Topics in Chemical Carcinogenesis, pp. 199–211, University of Tokyo Press, Tokyo and University Park Press, Baltimore, 1972.

36. Fiala, E. S. and Weisburger, J. H. Personal communication.

Discussion of Paper of Dr. Wattenberg

DR. BUTLER: Is there any evidence that antioxidants may be considered to be carcinogens?

DR. WATTENBERG: I am not aware of any antioxidant, comparable to those used in the present study, which by itself is carcinogenic.

DR. SATO: What kind of tumor did you induce in the forestomach of the mice by DMBA? Is the *in vivo* binding of ^{14}C-benzo(a)pyrene to DNA also reduced when you administer butylated hydroxyanisole (BHA) to the animals?

DR. WATTENBERG: There is a range of tumors varying from squamous cell papillomas to infiltrating, metastasizing squamous cell carcinomas. This experiment has not been done with BHA.

DR. LIEBERMAN: Can you distinguish between the effects of antioxidants on metabolic activation and their scavenger effects by using a direct-acting carcinogen such as β-propiolactone or 7-bromomethyl-12-methylbenz(a)anthracene on mouse skin?

DR. WATTENBERG: These experiments are somewhat difficult because applications of carcinogens and antioxidants to the skin entail relatively high, brief exposures of an unphysiological type.

DR. KURODA: (1) Have you any information on the pre- and post-treatment effects of antioxidants on carcinogen-induced tumors? (2) Do the effects of antioxidants depend on their concentrations? (3) Have you any information on the effect of antioxidants on *in vitro* transformation of cultured mammalian cells?

DR. WATTENBERG: (1) Antioxidants administered after the carcinogen do not give protection against neoplasia. (2) Yes, under the experimental conditions employed, relatively high doses of antioxidants are used in order to obtain protection. With decreasing doses of antioxidant, proportionally less inhibition is obtained. (3) Work of this nature has been done by others and is summarized in the manuscript.

DR. OKADA: In simplifying the mode of action of antioxidants, they may act (1) to make the target cells less susceptible to a carcinogen; (2) to make a carcinogen less reactive to target cells and (3) to inhibit "promotion" of precancerous cells to become cancer cells. Cysteamine, in the case of radiation, does act on (2): could you tell us at what step "antioxidants" act?

DR. WATTENBERG: At the present time we have only incomplete knowledge as to the mechanism of action of BHA. The available data indicate that the carcinogen is made less reactive to target sites (your mechanism number 2). Mechanism number 1 is possible but we cannot answer this question at the moment. Since administration of BHA after exposure to carcinogens does not protect against neoplasia, it appears unlikely that it affects the course of events once the carcinogen has already reacted with target sites.

DR. MAGEE: Following the suggestion of Dr. Lieberman, it might be interesting to test N-methylnitrosamides by intrarectal administration in the same mouse strain that you used in your experiments on the inhibitory effect of disulfiram on colon carcinogenesis by 1,2-dimethylhydrazine, since N-methylnitrosourea is believed to be a direct-acting carcinogen.

DR. WATTENBERG: We have done a study of this nature in which the carcinogen employed was methylazoxymethanol acetate. This carcinogen was administered intrarectally. Prior administration of disulfiram, also intrarectally, did not have a significant inhibitory effect against neoplasia of the large bowel resulting from the exposure to methylazoxymethanol acetate.

FUNDAMENTALS IN CANCER PREVENTION, P. N. MAGEE ET AL. (EDS.), UNIV. OF TOKYO PRESS, TOKYO / UNIV. PARK PRESS, BALTIMORE, PP. 167–190, 1976

Benzo(a)pyrene Metabolism: Enzymatic and Liquid Chromatographic Analysis and Application to Human Tissues

Harry V. Gelboin, Takao Okuda, James K. Selkirk, Nobuo Nemoto, Shen K. Yang, Herbert J. Rapp, and Robert C. Bast, Jr.

Chemistry and Biology Branches, National Cancer Institute, Bethesda, Maryland, U.S.A.

Abstract: We have developed different methods for assessing the capacity and variability of tissues to metabolize benzo(a)pyrene (BP). These include the use of high-pressure liquid chromatography (HPLC) for the quantitative separation and analysis of polycyclic aromatic hydrocarbon metabolites, the assay of BP-4,5-oxide hydratase and the assay for glutathione-S-BP-4,5-oxide transferase as well as the assay for aryl hydrocarbon hydroxylase (AHH). These techniques are applicable to the analysis of small amounts of human tissue and may be useful in assessing the role of metabolism in carcinogen susceptibility. The relationship of metabolism to carcinogenesis can also be probed by the use of inducers and inhibitors of the involved enzyme systems. Thus induction by either polycyclic hydrocarbons or phenobarbital and inhibition by 7,8-benzoflavone (7,8-BF) or trichloropropylene oxide (TCPO) have unique and differential effects on various pathways of BP metabolism. The 7,8-BF inhibits the formation of each of 8 metabolites to about the same degree. TCPO completely inhibits dihydrodiol formation and has little effect on quinone formation. Induction by 3-methylcholanthrene changes the metabolic profile. AHH is highly inducible in both human lymphocytes and monocytes and the metabolic profile has been measured by HPLC. Five new metabolite peaks have been detected in human lymphocytes.

The initial biological receptors for the polycyclic aromatic hydrocarbons are the microsomal mixed function oxygenases. The polycyclic aromatic hydrocarbons (PAH) are initially oxygenated by this enzyme system and subsequent metabolism of the products involves either further oxygenation by the same oxygenases, hydration of the epoxide intermediates to dihydrodiols or conjugation of the oxygenated intermediates to water-soluble products. The carcinogenic potential of the hydrocarbon may be either diminished or enhanced by the metabolic activity of these enzyme systems (*1–3*) and thus it is possible that variation in the activity of these enzyme systems are directly related to the variability in the carcinogenic effects of

167

the PAH in each individual. Heterogeneity in the activities of these enzymes may thus be an important factor in the heterogeneity of individuals to carcinogen susceptibility. It is thus important to develop methods that can describe the profiles of these enzyme activities in individuals. In this report we present various methods for the study of PAH metabolism. A combination of these approaches may yield a systematic analysis with which the relationship of metabolism and carcinogen susceptibility of an individual might be assessed.

PAH are a large class of chemicals common to the environment (4) and are present in the atmosphere (5), waterways and oceans, soil (6), marine life and in the food chain (4).

Major sources of PAH include emissions from transportation, heat and power generation, refuse burning, industrial processes and oil contamination by effluent disposal or oil spills into waterways (4). Epidemiological studies indicate that the environment is a significant determinant (4) in the incidence of human cancer (7) although many of the specific causal agents have yet to be identified. One major causal agent is known. Inhalation of smoke by cigarette smokers is clearly a major factor in the high incidence of lung cancer among smokers (8). Many of the PAH present in smoke are powerful carcinogens in experimental animals and are thus logical suspects as the carcinogens causing lung cancer in humans. Since the PAH are also common environmental pollutants, they are also suspect of contributing to cancer at other organ sites.

In this study we have examined benzo(a)pyrene (BP) as a prototype PAH. BP is a powerful carcinogen (9), a most common hydrocarbon in the environment (4), its metabolism has been extensively studied (10–14) and the strong fluorescence of its phenolic metabolites has been the basis for a very sensitive assay of a PAH microsomal cytochrome P-450 type mixed-function oxygenase, the aryl hydrocarbon (BP) hydroxylase (AHH) (15). The oxidative metabolism of polycyclic hydrocarbons is catalyzed by the "mixed-function oxygenases" which are part of the endoplasmic reticulum and consist of a terminal cytochrome (P-450) and an electron transport chain. The microsomal oxygenases are present in most tissues of mammals (16). They metabolize and are inducible by a wide spectrum of xenobiotics (17) which include pesticides, drugs, food additives, and PAH (2) and by some endogenous substrates such as steroids (18).

The detoxification role of the microsomal mixed function oxygenases and related enzymes has been well established and reviewed (1, 2, 18). It is clear that oxygenation of the PAH at several sites results in detoxified inactive metabolites and the induction of this enzyme system parallels in several cases a marked inhibition of tumorigenesis. An example is that of the pretreatment of rats with small amounts of polycyclic hydrocarbons which decreases tumor formation in the mammary gland induced by subsequently administered polycyclic hydrocarbons (19). Another report showed that the intraperitoneal injection of the enzyme inducer 5,6-benzoflavone (5,6-BF) inhibited 7,12-dimethylbenz(a)anthracene (DMBA)-induced tumorigenesis in the lung and mammary gland of rodents (1). One possible explanation for these results is that prior treatment of the animals with these enzyme inducers causes an increase in mixed-function oxygenase activity in the liver, the major site of metabolism, and this in turn may lower the concentration of the carcinogen in the target tissue, in the latter cases, the lung and mammary gland. Another possibility is that the induced enzyme catalyzes the reactions of the detoxification pathway of metabolism to a greater extent than those of the carcinogen activation pathway (see below).

Although the mixed function oxygenases clearly serve a detoxification role, the evidence is also clear that some of the polycyclic hydrocarbons are metabolically activated to cytotoxic and carcinogenic intermediates by these enzymes. The evidence for the role of the mixed function oxygenases in carcinogen activation is as follows: (a) microsomal NADPH-requiring oxygenases catalyze the formation of hydrocarbon-DNA complexes (20–22); (b) the cellular level of AHH activity is positively correlated with the cytotoxic effects of polycyclic hydrocarbons in a variety of different cells (23, 24); (c) inhibition of enzyme activity by 7,8-BF inhibits polycyclic hydrocarbon toxicity, metabolism, and macromolecule binding in cell culture (25); (d) inhibition of AHH reduces the covalent binding of DMBA to nucleic acids and protein of mouse skin (26); (e) inhibition of AHH by 7,8-BF inhibits tumorigenesis by DMBA in mouse skin (26). In the latter study, the 7,8-BF had either no effect or a stimulatory effect on BP tumorigenesis indicating that the role of the microsomal hydroxylases may be unique for different hydrocarbons. All of the latter effects clearly relate to the activity of the NADPH-dependent mixed-function oxygenases, but may also be influenced by the action of the related enzymes in hydrocarbon metabolism (see below).

Microsomal AHH is present and inducible in a variety of tissues of different species. It also varies in different mouse strains (16, 27) and is affected by age, developmental stage, sex, and hormonal balance (16). The microsomal oxygenases are also present, as measured by the AHH in human tissues. Thus AHH has been found in human liver (28), placenta (29, 30), lymphocytes (31, 32), monocytes (33, 34), and lung macrophages (35).

BP Metabolism—Analysis by High-pressure Liquid Chromatography (HPLC)

A new and most promising technique for metabolite analysis, HPLC, has been developed (14, 36, 37). This technique is far superior to thin-layer chromatography (TLC) and permits a clean and quantitative separation of at least 8 BP metabolites. Our current research indicates that further development of the appropriate conditions will enable a comprehensive and quantitative separation of most if not all hydrocarbon metabolites. Figure 1 shows a typical separation of a number of BP metabolites and shows the distinct peaks formed by each compound. There are three distinct diol peaks, two phenol peaks, and a quinone region.

In a more recent study (38) we found that an HPLC system using a recycling procedure was able to separate ten of the 12 BP phenols. With this system we were able to identify the 3-OH-BP, 9-OH-BP, 1-OH-BP, and 7-OH-BP as metabolic products of BP. Figure 2a shows the separation of 10 isomeric phenols by recycle HPLC and Figure 2b shows the separation of 4 phenol metabolites by this technique.

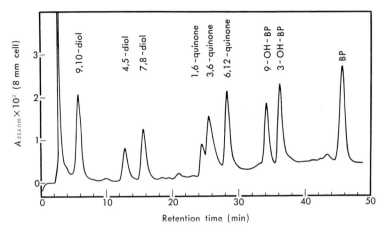

FIG. 1. HPLC separation of BP metabolites.

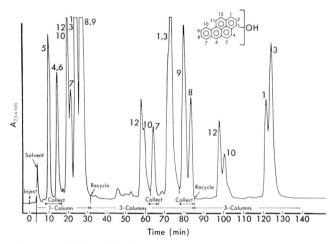

FIG. 2a. HPLC of BP phenols.

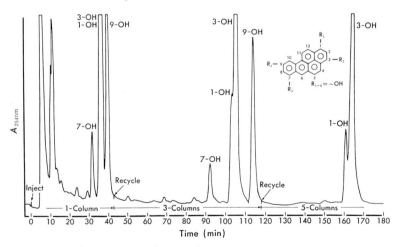

FIG. 2b. HPLC of BP phenol metabolites.

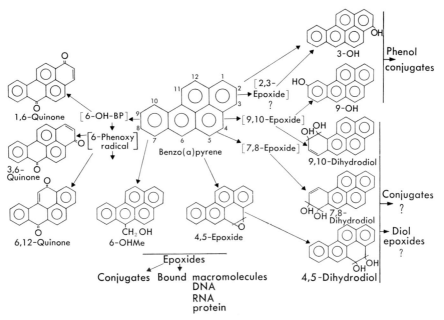

Fig. 3.   BP metabolism.

Figure 3 shows some of the known and suspected metabolites of BP. Upon incubation of BP with cells or tissue preparations, various metabolites have been isolated (13, 39–42). Those separated by HPLC include 3 dihydrodiols, the 7,8-dihydrodiol, 9,10-dihydrodiol, and 4,5-dihydrodiol, 2 phenols, the 3-OH and the 9-OH and 3 quinones, the 1,6-quinone, 3,6-quinone, and 6,12-quinone (14, 36). Under special conditions the BP-4,5-oxide can be isolated (43). There has been one report that 6-OH-Me-BP is also formed during BP metabolism (44). With preparations containing the soluble fraction of cell proteins or with whole cells, unidentified water-soluble metabolites are also produced (45). In several reports recently reviewed (39) the K-region epoxide was suggested to be the active intermediate of BP. In an earlier report (46) evidence was presented that the 7,8-diol was the metabolite most active in the binding to DNA catalyzed by the mixed-function oxygenases. Thus it appeared that a further metabolite of the 7,8-diol may be a very active species in respect to DNA binding. A recent report has suggested that the BP-7,8-diol is converted to a 7,8-dihydrodiol-9,10-epoxide-BP and this compound is very active in the binding to DNA (12).

In a recent study (47) we found that the 7,8-diol-9,10-oxide was several thousandfold more mutagenic than any of the other metabolites tested which included a variety of phenols and simple epoxides. The 7,8-diol-9,10-oxide was directly mutagenic to V-79 cells at both a ouabain resistance locus and a 8-azaguanine resistance locus (Table 1a). We also found that the 7,8-diol was the most active compound requiring conversion to the mutagenic form by the hydroxylating enzymes (Table 1b). Thus of 12 potential metabolites tested, the 7,8-diol-9,10-oxide was the most mutagenic and its presumed precursor, the 7,8-diol was the

TABLE 1 a.   Direct Mutagenicity of BP and Derivatives in V79 Cells

Hydrocarbon	Conc. (μM)	Ouabain resistant/10^6	8-Azaguanine resistant/10^5
BP, 1-OH, 3-OH, 6-OH, 7-OH, 8-OH, 9-OH, 6-CH$_3$, 6-CH$_2$OH, 4, 5-diol, 7, 8-diol	4.0	0.9–1.4	6–19
4, 5-Epoxide	0.7	1.5	15
	4.0	6.2	36
	11.0	162.0	467
	17.0	794.0	1,236
7, 8-Diol-9, 10-oxide	0.1	30.0	10
	0.3	167.0	261
	0.7	3,050.0	4,050

TABLE 1 b.   Cell-mediated Mutagenicity of BP and Derivatives in V79 Cells

Hydrocarbon	Conc. (μM)	Ouabain resistant/10^6	8-Azaguanine resistant/10^5
1-OH, 3-OH, 6-OH, 7-OH, 8-OH, 9-OH, 6-CH$_3$, 6-CH$_2$OH, 4,5-diol	3.6–3.8	0.7–3.8	6–37
BP	0.1	1.5	14
	0.4	8.0	44
	1.2	20.0	79
	4.0	108.0	321
7. 8-Diol (*trans*)	0.07	9.0	55
	0.2	54.0	109
	0.4	116.0	487
	0.7	182.0	806

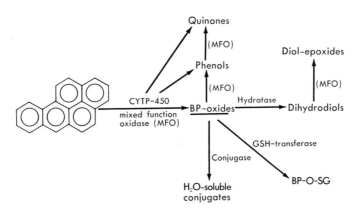

Fig. 4.   Enzymatic reactions of BP.

most active in the presence of the mixed-function oxygenase enzyme systems.

Figure 4 shows the enzyme systems and Table 2 the several assays for the enzymes that are involved in the formation of the various metabolites shown in Fig. 3. The sequence of enzyme action is as follows: the initial oxygenation is catalyzed by the microsomal mixed-function oxygenases which contain multiple

TABLE 2.   Assays for BP Metabolism

Method	Enzyme measured	Substrate	Products
AHH	Mixed-function oxidase (P-450)	BP	Phenols equivalent to 3-OH-BP and 9-OH-BP
Hydratase	BP-4, 5-oxide hydratase	^{3}H-BP-4, 5-oxide	^{3}H-BP-4, 5-dihydrodiol
GSH-transferase	Glutathione-S-BP-4, 5-oxide transferase	^{3}H-BP-4, 5-oxide	^{3}H-BP-4, 5-O-glutathione
HPLC	1) Mixed-function oxidase	^{3}H-BP	Phenols
	2) Hydratase		Dihydrodiols
	3) Nonenzymatic reactions		Quinones
			Hydroxymethyl-BP
			Diol-epoxides
			Epoxides
			Unknown metabolites
Water-soluble product formation	1) Mixed-function oxidase	^{3}H-BP	Water-soluble conjugates
	2) Hydratase		
	3) Transferases (GSH), Gluc(?)SO$_4$(?)		
Covalent binding	1) Mixed-function oxidase	^{3}H-BP	^{3}H-BPX-DNA
	2) Hydratase		^{3}H-BPX-RNA
	3) Transferases (GSH), Gluc(?)SO$_4$(?)		^{3}H-BPX-protein

forms of cytochrome P-450. This results in the formation of oxides in at least the 4,5-, 7,8-, and 9,10-positions. The most stable of these, the 4,5-oxide, has been isolated under special conditions and the 7,8- and 9,10-oxides as well as the 4,5-oxide are likely intermediates (43). Their formation can be deduced from the presence of all 3 of the corresponding dihydrodiols. These are presumably formed by the action of arene oxide hydratase on the oxide intermediates. Further evidence that this mechanism prevails is the finding that a hydratase inhibitor 1,1,1-tri-chloropropylene oxide (TCPO) completely eliminates dihydrodiol formation (14), and the re-addition of a partially purified hydrase results in the appearance of the dihydrodiols (37). The phenols and quinones can be either formed nonen-zymatically from the oxide intermediate or be the result of a direct oxygenation by the mixed-function oxidase. That a mechanism of oxygenation independent of arene oxide intermediacy is operative, is suggested by the finding that activation of the BP and oxygenation occurs at the 6-position (41) with quinone formation at the 1,6-, 3,6-, and 6,12-positions. The 6-position oxygenation does not sterically permit an oxide intermediate and thus we may conclude that not all of the oxy-genated products are formed solely through oxide intermediates.

Mixed-function Oxygenase—AHH

The primary catalytic attack on the PAH is by the microsomal mixed-function oxygenase P-450-containing enzyme systems. Enzyme purification studies have shown that this system is composed of at least 4 forms of the enzyme (48). With dif-ferent steroid and biphenyl substrates the various forms of the cytochrome P-450 show preferential hydroxylation at specific positions. In collaboration with the latter group we have found that the various forms of P-450 have different catalytic activity with respect to the formation of the different BP metabolites. Thus the

TABLE 3.   Effect of MC Pretreatment on Metabolite Formation

Metabolite	Specific activity[a]		Specific activity ratio[b]
	Control	MC-induced	
BP-9, 10-diol	16	404	25.2
BP-4, 5-diol	37	132	3.5
BP-7, 8-diol	10	198	19.8
BP-quinones[c]	117	309	2.6
9-OH-BP	29	140	4.8
3-OH-BP	272	956	3.5
Total	481	2,139	4.4

[a] Specific activities (pmoles/min/mg protein) determined at 0.14 microsomal protein per ml of incubation mixture. About 10% errors are estimated to be associated with these determinations.   [b] Specific activity ratio for each metabolite varies with the amount of microsomes used in the *in vitro* incubations (see text for discussion).   [c] Containing 1,6-quinone, 3,6-quinone, and 6,12-quinone. From Yang *et al.* (in press).

specific form of the cytochrome P-450 may be uniquely relevant to either the detoxification or activation pathways of metabolisms. The different forms of the cytochrome P-450 are also preferentially induced by different inducers of the mixed function oxygenases such as methylcholanthrene (MC) or phenobarbital and the different forms of the enzyme can also be preferentially inhibited. Thus 7,8-BF inhibits the MC-induced enzyme in rat liver but does not inhibit the uninduced control rat liver (49). Thus induction or inhibition may alter the balance or metabolic pathways (13, 50). An example of altered metabolism after induction (51) is shown in Table 3. The relative amounts of the 9,10-diol and 7,8-diol to the other metabolites are greatly increased after enzyme induction by MC pretreatment. This may be due to the induction of a specific form of cytochrome P-450 or to an altered ratio of mixed-function oxygenases and the arene oxide hydratase which results in an altered profile of metabolites. The ratios of mixed-function oxygenase to hydratase can be altered in different ways by pretreatment with either phenobarbital or MC (52), the former having its major effect as an increase in the hydratase while the latter having its major effect as an increase in the oxygenase.

BP-4,5-oxide Hydratase

A second major enzyme system involved in PAH metabolism is arene oxide hydratase. This class of enzymes has recently been reviewed (53). An assay for this enzyme using ³H-BP-4,5-oxide as the substrate has recently been developed (52). The assay measures the formation of the product, BP-4,5-dihydrodiol. Product formation is linear with time and protein concentration (Fig. 5) and product formation is stoichiometric with substrate disappearance. This enzyme is likely similar or identical with the epoxide hydrase that has been studied using styrene oxide as the substrate (53). The K-region oxide of BP is a product of BP metabolism and thus may be more useful in assessing the properties and activity of the hydratase system in polycyclic hydrocarbon metabolism and carcinogenesis. This enzyme is inducible by phenobarbital but is only slightly effected by hydrocarbons and

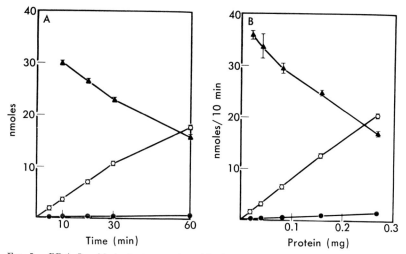

FIG. 5.   BP-4, 5-oxide hydratase.   A : with time.   B : with protein concentration.   ▲ oxide disappearance ;   □ diol formation ;   ● water soluble.

under certain conditions the AHH can be induced by MC while the hydratase remains unchanged (52). The hydratase can also be inhibited by TCPO which completely eliminates diol formation (14).

Glutathione S-Arene Oxide Transferase

Other enzyme systems involved in BP metabolism are those engaged in the conversion of the BP-oxygenated intermediates to water-soluble conjugates. One of these is the glutathione-S-arene oxide transferase. We have developed an assay using BP-4,5-oxide for glutathione-S-BP oxide transferase (54). This enzyme system may be related to that reported for the conjugation of naphthalene oxide (55). This assay can utilize either radioactive glutathione or the ^{3}H-labelled BP-4,5-oxide as the substrate marker for conjugate formation. Figure 6 shows the linearity of conjugate formation with time and protein concentration by this enzyme system. Several highly purified forms of glutathione transferase have been described that

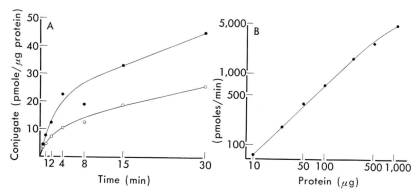

FIG. 6.   Glutathione-S-BP-4, 5-oxide transferase.

TABLE 4. Specific Activity of Homogeneous Rat and Human Glutathione-S Transferases

Enzyme		BP-4, 5-oxide	Alkyl epoxide (nmole/min/mg)	Bromosulfo-phthalein
Rat liver transferase	A	100	100	530
	B	14	0	6
	C	127	0	18
	E	51	6,100	0
	AA	8	0	4
Human liver transferase	β	25	0	10
	δ	33	0	1

conjugate a variety of substrates including halide and oxide compounds (56). In collaboration with Dr. Jakoby's laboratory, we have examined these purified homogeneous preparations and have found that there are at least 7 forms of the glutathione-S-BP-4,5-oxide transferase, 5 from rat liver and 2 from human liver, that have differing activity toward BP-4,5-oxide and 2 non-PAH substrates, an alkyl epoxide and bromosulfophthalein (57). Table 4 shows that each of these purified forms of the transferase has a unique specificity towards BP-4,5-oxide. This specificity and the amount of each enzyme present in a given tissue of an individual may affect the efficiency of the detoxification of the arene oxides of PAH and thus may be important keys in the removal of carcinogenic intermediates.

In addition to the above enzyme systems there are many reports of the presence of different BP conjugates in the urine and bile. It is suggested that these may be glucuronides or sulfates but a final characterization or identification of the enzymatic basis for their formation has not been made.

Table 2 shows some of the assays applicable to the enzyme systems described. The chart is largely self-explanatory. Each assay has both advantages as well as disadvantages. The chief virtues of the AHH fluorescence assay is its extraordinary sensitivity (15). The sensitivity is sufficient to detect as little as one pmole of phenols equivalent to one of the major phenol products, 3-OH-BP, and thus this assay permits the analysis of minute amounts of tissue. The chief advantage of the HPLC (14) system is its ability to yield a more complete picture of BP metabolism. Thus it accomplishes a separation and quantification of the different known metabolites and has already achieved the separation of new unknown metabolites which have yet to be characterized (see below).

The hydratase and glutathione (GSH)-transferase assays relate quite specifically to well defined reactions in which a single substrate and product is defined. The BP-4,5-oxide is converted to the BP-4,5-dihydrodiol by the action of the hydratase and is conjugated with GSH by the action of the glutathione transferases. These enzymes may also have different specificities toward the various BP intermediates. The assay for water-soluble product formation gives an indication of the total sequential reactions involved in the metabolism of the BP by the cell. Its disadvantages are largely that it gives no insight into the nature of each product nor to the relative levels of each of the enzymes involved in the complete pathway of BP metabolism.

An additional assay which has potential for use in detecting reactive intermediates of carcinogens is their binding to macromolecules. This can be done *in vitro* and the macromolecule receptor can be either DNA or RNA protein (*20–22, 46, 58*). This technique has the potential of detecting reactive species formed by the preparation without assaying for the individual enzymes. Its reliability as a predictive assay however depends on the degree of similarity between the *in vitro* system and the *in vivo* reality.

Analyses of BP-metabolizing Activity in Human Tissues—Monocytes and Lymphocytes

In assessing the level of enzymes of BP metabolism in human tissues, two conditions must prevail. The tissue must be easily obtainable and the level of the reaction must be of sufficient magnitude to be readily measured. The most sensitive of all the methods described is the AHH assay. We found that this enzyme system is present and inducible in mitogen-stimulated human lymphocytes (*31*). At the same time, the AHH method was utilized by Busbee *et al.* (*32*) to analyze the inducibility of AHH in lymphocytes obtained from small amounts of blood from human donors.

Subsequent reports (*59*) showed a high reproducibility of the AHH assay with human lymphocytes within a given individual and a trimodal distribution of inducibility values among the population surveyed (*60*). These studies indicated that the AHH in families followed strictly Mendelian inheritance in respect to enzyme inducibility and the values of the children followed the pattern predicted by the AHH levels of their parents. An additional report indicated that lung cancer patients showed an abnormally high distribution of high AHH inducibility (*61*). Since these exciting reports the same laboratory has indicated an inability to reproduce some of these results (Shaw, personal communications) and there are conflicting new reports on the reproducibility of the assay as well as on the trimodal distribution of AHH inducibility in the population (*62, 63*). Many laboratories are presently engaged in studies designed to clarify this situation.

None of the solid human tissues in which AHH has been detected can be readily obtained for clinical and epidemiological study. Detection of AHH in macrophages of the human lung, rat liver (*35*), and guinea pig peritoneum (*64*) suggested that peripheral blood monocytes might also contain the enzyme. AHH is present and highly inducible in monocytes from human peripheral blood (*64*) and the enzyme inducibility is much greater in monocytes than in lymphocytes. The advantage of monocytes is that both the degree of induction is much greater than in lymphocytes and monocytes do not require prior stimulation with mitogens. Their disadvantages reside mainly in the requirement for greater amounts of blood from the donor. A set of duplicate assays for control and induced levels require approximately 50–100 ml of blood as compared with only 10 ml for the lymphocyte assay. Table 5 shows typical results on the reproducibility of AHH values in monocytes and lymphocytes from 6 different individuals who were examined on 3 different occasions. The mean of the inducibility is approximately 18-fold with monocytes and only slightly more than 2-fold with lymphocytes. Furthermore in our laboratory the reproducibility of the AHH values is considerably greater with mono-

TABLE 5.   Reproducibility and Comparability of AHH in Human Monocytes and Lymphocytes

Donor No.	Monocytes			Lymphocytes		
	Control	BA-treated	BA-treated / Control	Control	BA-treated	BA-treated / Control
1739	0.27±0.09	4.64±0.49	13.4±3.8	1.12±0.26	1.96±0.77	1.64±0.27
2781	0.36±0.04	5.20±0.12	14.6±1.4	1.40±0.37	3.23±1.57	2.09±0.49
2798	0.33±0.04	7.46±1.06	23.2±4.3	0.46±0.12	1.22±0.44	2.42±0.42
1970	0.40±0.05	6.35±0.81	16.9±3.9	0.54±0.17	1.15±0.16	2.35±0.34
2827	0.32±0.01	5.44±0.63	17.2±2.1	0.31±0.05	0.73±0.10	2.35±0.04
3085	0.27±0.05	5.83±1.53	21.7±3.4	0.31±0.02	1.10±0.47	3.72±1.32
Mean	0.32	5.82	17.8	0.69	1.56	2.16
$\frac{S.E.}{Mean} \times 100$ (%)	13.1	12.0	14.2	21.6	32.7	18.1

cytes. Thus the variability in lymphocytes is more than twice that observed with monocytes. For monocytes the standard error (S.E.)/mean ×100 was 13.1, 12.0, and 14.2 for control, induced, and induced/control, respectively. The corresponding values with lymphocytes was 21.6, 32.7, and 18.1, respectively. Figure 7 shows the distribution of control and induced AHH values in monocytes obtained from different individuals. The control values range in AHH specific activity, in units per million cells, from less than 1 to 3 and induced values range from 2 to 13. The inducibility ranges from a low of 6-fold to a high of 37-fold. In a few cases we

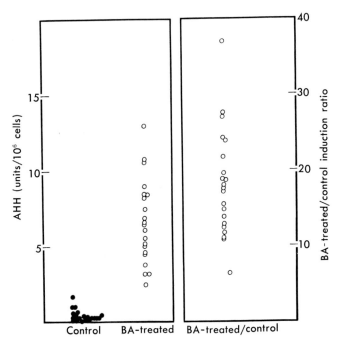

FIG. 7.   AHH in monocytes from different individuals.

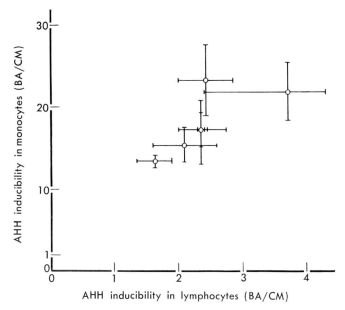

FIG. 8.   AHH inducibility in human monocytes and lymphocytes.

observed an even higher inducibility. We observe no distinct grouping or any evidence of a trimodal distribution in the more than 25 individuals we have examined. Figure 8 suggest that there may be some positive relationship between inducibility in monocytes and lymphocytes. In these individuals examined, the inducibility in monocytes ranged from 12- to 24-fold and the range of inducibility in lymphocytes ranged from 1.8- to 3.8-fold with a large clustering around 2.2-fold. Thus Fig. 8 shows that, within limits, there seems to be a positive relationship between the activities in the two cell types. Thus the AHH values in the two cells show some parallel although the lymphocyte values are more than twice as variable as the monocyte values. This can be seen by the two wide horizontal lines relative to the vertical lines which signify the range of values for a given individual. It seems clear that there are significant and reproducible differences in the AHH values in different individuals in monocytes and although the variability is greater in lymphocytes the evidence suggests that inducibility in lymphocytes also varies among different individuals. We have not found evidence suggesting a trimodal distribution and we are now examining individuals with lung cancer.

BP Metabolism in Human Liver, Lymphocytes, and Monocytes—Analyses by HPLC

The profile of metabolites of BP formed by rat liver microsomal metabolism of BP is seen in the dashed line in Fig. 9. A small unidentified peak elutes first and is followed by 3 glycols, *viz.*, the 9,10-dihydrodiol, 4,5-dihydrodiol, and 7,8-dihydrodiol; 3 quinones, *viz.*, 1,6-quinone, 3,6-quinone, and 6,12-quinone; and 2 phenols peaks which contain 9-OH-BP and 3-OH-BP, respectively. Although each of these metabolite peaks contain primarily the indicated metabolite, they may possibly

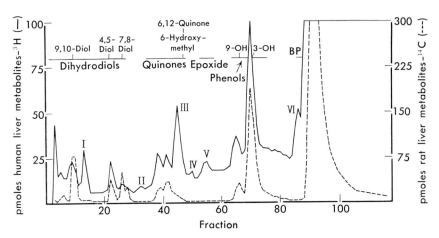

FIG. 9.   Pattern of BP metabolites formed by incubation with human liver microsomes.

also contain small amounts of other unidentified metabolites. A comparison between the metabolism of BP by microsomes from human liver and rat liver is shown in Fig. 9. A large number of metabolites are formed by human liver microsomes which are not formed by rat liver microsomes. In the diol region, a large peak (I) appears just after the 9,10-dihydrodiol (Fractions 13–15), and a small peak (II) appears after the 7,8-dihydrodiol (Fractions 31–34). The quinone region indicates a major peak (III) at the region of 6,12-quinone. However we have found that 6-hydroxymethyl-BP cochromatographs with 6,12-quinone in this system and peak III may correspond to the former compound which has been reported as a BP metabolite (44). A smaller peak (IV) follows immediately after (Fractions 49–51) with a peak in the region where BP-4,5-epoxide migrates (43). The relative activity of hydratases in human liver may determine the lifetime of the epoxide and the identity of this peak remains to be clarified.

The high background in Fractions 31–80 results from small quantities of ³H-BP leaching from the column and occurs when the ratio of metabolites to ³H-BP is very low. The background of ³H-BP can be reduced by prior removal of the ³H-BP by TLC. This was done prior to the HPLC shown in Fig. 11. The formation of the BP metabolites by human lymphocytes during a 30-min period is seen in Fig. 10. This pattern is quite different than that from rat liver and has characteristics that are quite similar to that of human liver. The patterns of human liver and lymphocytes, however, are not identical and show some distinct differences. None of the three dihydrodiols appeared after a 30-min incubation of ³H-BP with lymphocytes. The metabolites I, III, V, VI migrate identically as those observed with human liver (Fig. 9) and the small peaks II and IV are absent. In the lymphocytes the relative amount of Peak III in the quinone region was reduced, and the ratio of the 3-OH-BP peak to the 9-OH-BP was considerably reduced. Also there was a relatively larger amount of peak VI compared to all the other metabolites.

The profile in Fig. 11 shows the metabolites formed during a 24-hr incubation of ³H-BP with lymphocytes in culture. In contrast to the absence of diol formation

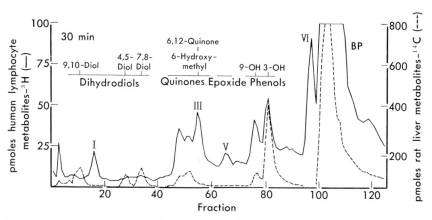

Fig. 10.   Pattern of BP metabolites by human lymphocytes for 30 min.

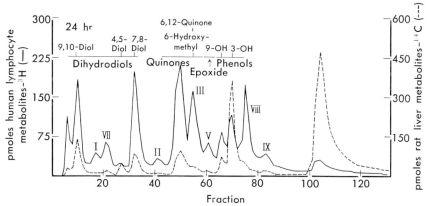

Fig. 11.   HPLC of BP metabolites by human lymphocytes for 24 hr. The balk of BP was removed by TLC prior to HPLC.

during a 30-min incubation, all three dihydrodiols are formed with the 7,8-di-hydrodiol as the major peak. This result agrees with the report that diols are formed by lymphocytes (65) although the methods used in the latter reports are inadequate for the separation of the individual diols, phenols or quinones, and the new metabolites. The lymphocytes form metabolites which migrate as peaks I, III, and V corresponding to the new metabolites formed by human liver. Peak IV which is observed in human liver (Fig. 9) does not appear but may possibly be hidden between peaks III–V. The bulk of BP was removed prior to HPLC by TLC chromatography in the preparation shown in Fig. 11. Thus Peak VI which is seen in the human metabolites in Figs. 9 and 10 may have been removed during the TLC.

In addition to the peaks I–VI, several additional new peaks are formed during the longer incubation period of BP with lymphocytes. This may reflect a further metabolism of some of the primary metabolites by the mixed-function oxygenase system. There is an additional peak in the dihydrodiol region (VIII), and two more peaks in the phenol region labelled VIII and IX. Thus, our data shows that human lymphocytes incubated with BP for 24 hr form many metabolites that

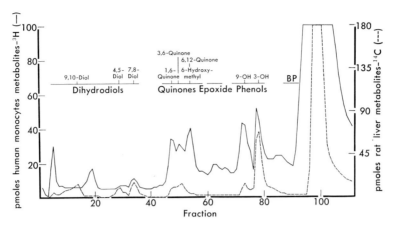

Fig. 12.   Metabolism of BP by human monocytes.

migrate identically to those formed by human liver. There are however additional peaks formed by the lymphocytes and the ratios of metabolites observed in lymphocytes differ from those in liver.

Figure 12 shows the HPLC pattern of metabolites obtained upon incubation of human monocytes and ^{3}H-BP followed by an HPLC separation. The monocytes form three unidentified new peaks which correspond to those observed with human liver and lymphocytes. The ratios of metabolites are quite different than those observed with human liver. There is no detectable 9,10-diol or 4,5-diol, low levels of the 7,8-diol and a relatively large amount of the 9-OH phenol peak. The variation in metabolite profile in each tissue examined is likely a reflection of the type of or ratio of the different mixed-function oxygenases present and the relative amounts of the hydratase, GSH transferases and other conjugases.

CONCLUSIONS

We have developed various methods and enzyme assays that can be used in examining BP metabolism in human tissues. These techniques can be easily modified for application to the metabolism of other polycyclic hydrocarbons. It is now possible to assess the activities of: mixed-function oxidases by the AHH fluorescent assay, BP-4,5-oxide hydratase and glutathione S-BP-4,5-oxide transferase by radio-assays, and to perform an analysis by HPLC of metabolites formed by easily obtainable human tissues. Some of the results obtained in the studies are: (1) HPLC has also been used to separate 10 synthetic BP phenols and to isolate 4 as metabolites, the 3-OH-BP, 9-OH-BP, 1-OH-BP, and 7-OH-BP. (2) The BP-7,8-diol-9,10-oxide was the most mutagenic of a large number of BP derivatives tested in a mammalian mutagenesis system. Other findings from these studies are: (3) enzyme induction by MC results in an altered pattern of metabolites. (4) Five homogeneous rat liver and two human liver enzymes show unique glutathione S-BP-4,5-oxide transferase activity. (5) The inducibility of AHH ranges from about 2- to 4-fold in lymphocytes from different individuals. (6) The metabolic activity of human liver, lymphocytes, and monocytes has been studied by HPLC. The human tissues form 5 new metabolites which are unidentified. Each of the human tissues form metabolic profiles of BP that are different from the profiles formed by rat liver and are somewhat different from each other.

Further development of the described method may permit the analysis of various human populations for the enzyme activities and metabolites related to polycyclic hydrocarbon action. This may yield information on the relationship between metabolism and the heterogeneity in human susceptibility to carcinogenesis induced by PAH.

NOTE ADDED IN PROOF

We have recently found (E. Huberman, L. Sachs, S. K. Yang, and H. V. Gelboin, Identification of the mutagenic metabolites of benzo(a)pyrene in mammalian cells. Proc. Natl. Acad. Sci. U.S., *73*: 607–611, 1976) that the predominant form of diol epoxide made by rat liver microsomes is the *r*-7, *t*-8-dihydroxy-*t*-9, 10-oxy-7,8,9,10-tetrahydrobenzo(a)pyrene and that this form has a very much higher mutagenic activity than any known benzo(a)pyrene metabolite. This suggests that this compound may be the ultimate carcinogenic form of benzo(a)pyrene.

REFERENCES

1. Wattenberg, L. W. and Leong, J. L. Inhibition of the carcinogenic action of 7,12-dimethylbenz(a)anthracene by beta-naphthoflavone. Proc. Soc. Exp. Biol., *128*: 940–943, 1968.
2. Gelboin, H. V. Carcinogens, enzyme induction, and gene action. Adv. Cancer Res., *10*: 1–81, 1967.
3. Gelboin, H. V., Kinoshita, N., and Wiebel, F. J. Microsomal hydroxylases: Induction and role in polycyclic hydrocarbon carcinogenesis and toxicity. Fed. Proc., *31*: 1298–1309, 1972.
4. National Academy of Science Reports, U.S.A. Particulate Polycyclic Organic Matter. Committee on Biologic Effects of Atmospheric Pollutants, Division of Medical Sciences, National Research Council, Washington, D.C., 1972.
5. Andelman, J. B. and Suess, N. J. Polynuclear aromatic hydrocarbons in the water environment. Bull. WHO, *43*: 479–508, 1970.
6. Shabad, L. M., Cohan, Y. L., Illnitsky, A. P., Khesina, A. Y., Sherbak, N. P., and Smirnov, G. A. The carcinogenic hydrocarbon benzo(a)pyrene in the soil. J. Natl. Cancer Inst., *47*: 1179–1191, 1971.
7. Haenzel, W. and Traeuber, K. E. Lung cancer mortality as related to residence and smoking histories. II. White females. J. Natl. Cancer Inst., *32*: 803–838, 1964.
8. U. S. Department of Health, Education, and Welfare. Smoking and Health. Report of the Advisory Commitee to the Surgeon General of the Public Health Service Publication 1103, U.S. Government Printing Office, Washington, D. C., 1964.
9. Hartwell, J. L. and Shubik, P. Survey of Compounds Which Have Been Treated for Carcinogenic Activity. Public Health Service Publication 149, 2nd ed., U.S. Government Printing Office, Washington, D.C., 1951.
10. Conney, A. H., Miller, E. C., and Miller, J. A. Substrate-induced synthesis and

other properties of benzpyrene hydroxylase in rat liver. J. Biol. Chem., *228*: 753–766, 1957.

11. Sims, P. The metabolism of benzo(a)pyrene by rat liver homogenates. Biochem. Pharmacol., *16*: 613–618, 1968.

12. Sims, P., Grover, P. L., Swaisland, A., Pal. K., and Hewer, A. Metabolic activation of benzo(a)pyrene proceeds by a diol-epoxide. Nature, *252*: 326–328, 1974.

13. Kinoshita, N., Shears, B., and Gelboin, H. V. K-region and non-K-region metabolism of benzo(a)pyrene by rat liver microsomes. Cancer Res., *33*: 1937–1944, 1973.

14. Selkirk, J. K., Croy, R. G., Roller, P. P., and Gelboin, H. V. High-pressure liquid chromatographic analysis of benzo(a)pyrene metabolism and covalent binding and the mechanism of action of 7,8-benzoflavone and 1,2-epoxy-3,3,3-trichloropropane. Cancer Res., *34*: 3474–3480, 1974.

15. Nebert, D. W. and Gelboin, H. V. Substrate-inducible microsomal aryl hydroxylase in mammalian cell culture. I. Assay and properties of induced enzyme. J. Biol. Chem., *243*: 6242–6249, 1968.

16. Nebert, D. W. and Gelboin, H. V. The *in vivo* and *in vitro* induction of aryl hydrocarbon hydroxylase in mammalian cells of different species, tissues, strains, and developmental and hormonal states. Arch. Biochem. Biophys., *134*: 76–89, 1969.

17. Conney, A. H. and Burns, J. J. Metabolic interactions among environmental chemicals and drugs. Science, *178*: 576–586, 1972.

18. Conney, A. H. Pharmacological implications of microsomal enzyme induction. Pharmacol. Rev., *19*: 317–366, 1967.

19. Huggins, C., Grand, L., and Fukunishi, R. Aromatic influences on the yields of mammary cancers following administration of 7,12-dimethylbenz(a)anthracene. Proc. Natl. Acad. Sci. U.S., *51*: 737–742, 1964.

20. Gelboin, H. V. A microsome-dependent binding of benzo(a)pyrene to DNA. *In;* E. D. Bergmann and B. Pullman(eds.), Physico-Chemical Mechanisms of Carcinogenesis, The Jerusalem Symposia on Quantum Chemistry and Biochemistry, vol. 1, pp. 175–187, 1968.

21. Grover, R. L. and Sims, P. Enzyme-catalyzed reactions of polycyclic hydrocarbons with deoxyribonucleic acid and protein *in vitro*. Biochem. J., *110*: 159–160, 1968.

22. Gelboin, H. V. A microsome-dependent binding of benzo(a)pyrene to DNA. Cancer Res., *29*: 1272–1276, 1969.

23. Gelboin, H. V., Huberman, E., and Sachs, L. Enzymatic hydroxylation of benzpyrene and its relationship to cytotoxicity. Proc. Natl. Acad. Sci. U.S., *64*: 1188–1194, 1969.

24. Belitskii, G. A., Vasil'ev, Ir. M., Ivanova, O. Iu., Lavrova, N. A., Progoshina, E. L., Samoilina, N. L., Stavrovskaya, A. A., Khesina, A. Ya., and Shabad, L. M. Metabolism of benzo(a)pyrene by cells of different mammals *in vitro* and toxic effect of polycyclic hydrocarbons on the cells. Vop. Onkol., *16*: 53, 1970.

25. Diamond, L. and Gelboin, H. V. Alpha-naphthoflavone: An inhibitor of hydrocarbon cytotoxicity and microsomal hydroxylase. Science, *166*: 1023–1025, 1969.

26. Kinoshita, N. and Gelboin, H. V. Aryl hydrocarbon hydroxylase in 7, 12-dimethylbenz(a)anthracene skin tumorigenesis: On the mechanism of 7,8-benzoflavone inhibition of tumorigenesis. Proc. Natl. Acad. Sci. U.S., *69*: 824–828, 1973.

27. Gielen, J. E., Goujon, F. M., and Nebert, D. W. Genetic regulation of aryl hydrocarbon hydroxylase induction. II. Simple Mendelian expression in mouse tissue *in vivo*. J. Biol. Chem., *24*: 1125–1137, 1972.

28. Kuntzman, R., Mark, L. C., Brand, L., Jacobson, M., Levin, W., and Conney, A. H. Metabolism of drugs and carcinogens by human liver enzymes. J. Pharmacol. Exp. Ther., *152*: 151–156, 1966.

29. Welch, R. M., Harrison, Y.E., Gommi, B. W., Poppers, P. T., Ernster, M., and Conney, A. H. Stimulatory effect of cigarette smoking on the hydroxylation of 3, 4-benzpyrene and the N-demethylation of 3-methyl, 4-mono-methyl amino-azobenzene by enzymes in human placenta. Clin. Pharmacol. Ther., *10*: 100, 1969.

30. Nebert, D. W., Winker, J., and Gelboin, H. V. Aryl hydrocarbon hydroxylase activity in human placenta from cigarette smoking and non-smoking women. Cancer Res., *29*: 1763–1769, 1969.

31. Whitlock, J. P., Jr., Cooper, H. L., and Gelboin, H. V. Aryl hydrocarbon (benzo(a)-pyrene) hydroxylase is stimulated in human lymphocytes by mitogens and benz(a)-anthracene. Science, *177*: 618–619, 1972.

32. Busbee, D. L., Shaw, C. R., and Cantrell, E. T. Aryl hydrocarbon hydroxylase induction in human leukocytes. Science, *178*: 315–316, 1972.

33. Bast, R. C., Jr., Whitlock, J. P., Jr., Miller, H., Rapp, H. J., and Gelboin, H. V. Aryl hydrocarbon benzo(a)pyrene hydroxylase in human peripheral blood monocytes. Nature, *250*: 664–665, 1974.

34. Ptashne, K., Brothers, L., Axline, S. G., and Cohen, S. N. Aryl hydroxylase induction in mouse peritoneal macrophages and blood-derived human macrophages. Proc. Soc. Exp. Biol. Med., *146*: 585–589, 1974.

35. Cantrell, E. T., Warr, G. A., Busbee, D., and Martin, R. R. Induction of aryl hydrocarbon hydroxylase in human pulmonary alveolar macrophages by cigarette smoking. J. Clin. Invest., *52*: 1881–1884, 1973.

36. Selkirk, J. K., Croy, R. G., and Gelboin, H.V. Benzo(a)pyrene metabolites: Efficient and rapid separation by high-pressure liquid chromatography. Science, *184*: 169–171, 1974.

37. Holder, G., Yagi, H., Dansette, P., Jerina, D. M., Levin, W., Lu, A. Y. H., and Conney, A. H. Effects of inducers and epoxide hydrase on the metabolism of benzo-(a)pyrene by liver microsomes and a reconstituted system: Analysis by high pressure liquid chromatography. Proc. Natl. Acad. Sci. U.S., *71*: 4356–4369, 1974.

38. Croy, R. G., Selkirk, J. K., Harvey, R. G., Engel, J. F., and Gelboin, H. V. Separation of ten benzo(a)pyrene phenols by recycle high pressure liquid chromatography and identification of four phenols as metabolites. Submitted to Biochem. Pharmacol.

39. Sims, P. and Grover, P. L. Epoxides in polycyclic aromatic hydrocarbon metabolism and carcinogenesis. Adv. Cancer Res., *18*: 165–274, 1974.

40. Ts'o, P. O. P., Caspary, W. J., Cohen, B. I., Levitt, J. C., Lesko, S. A., Jr., Lorentzen, R. J., and Schechtman, L. M. Basic mechanism in polycyclic hydrocarbon carcinogenesis. *In;* P. O. P. Ts'o and J. A. Di Paolo (eds.), Chemical Carcinogenesis, part A, p. 113, Marcel Dekker, Inc., New York, 1974.

41. Nagata, C., Tagashira, Y., and Kodama, M. Metabolic activation of benzo(a)-pyrene: Significance of the free radical. *In;* P. O. P. Ts'o and J. A. Di Paolo (eds.), Chemical Carcinogenesis, part A, pp. 87–111, Marcel Dekker, Inc., New York, 1974.

42. Jerina, D. M. and Daly, J. W. Arene oxides: A new aspect of drug metabolism. Science, *184*: 573–582, 1974.

43. Selkirk, J. K., Croy, R. G., and Gelboin, H. V. Isolation and characterization of benzo(a)pyrene-4,5-epoxide as a metabolite of benzo(a)pyrene. Arch. Biochem. Biophys., *168*: 322–326 1975.

44. Flesher, J. W. and Sydnor, K. L.   Possible role of 6-hydroxy methyl benzo(a)pyrene as a proximate carcinogen of benzo(a)pyrene and 6-methyl benzo(a)pyrene. Int. J. Cancer, *11*: 433–437, 1973.

45. Diamond, L.   Metabolism of polycyclic hydrocarbons in mammalian cell cultures. Int. J. Cancer, *8*: 451–462, 1971.

46. Borgen, A., Darvey, H., Castagnoli, N., Crocker, T. T., Rasmussen, R. E., and Wang, I. Y. Metabolic conversion of benzo(a)pyrene by Syrian hamster liver microsomes and binding of metabolites to deoxyribonucleic acid. J. Med. Chem., *16*: 502–504, 1973.

47. Huberman, E., Sachs, L., and Gelboin, H. V. Identification of the mutagenic metabolites of benzo(a)pyrene in mammalian cells. Submitted to Proc. Natl. Acad. Sci. U.S.

48. Haugen, D. A., Van Der Heoven, T. A., and Coon, M. J.   Purified liver microsomal cytochrome P-450. Separation and characterization of multiple forms. J. Biol. Chem., *250*: 3567–3570, 1975.

49. Wiebel, F. J., Leutz, J. C., Diamond, L., and Gelboin, H. V.   Aryl hydrocarbon (benzo(a)pyrene) hydroxylase in microsomes from rat tissues: Differential inhibition and stimulation by benzoflavones and organic solvents. Arch. Biochem. Biophys., *144*: 78–86, 1971.

50. Rasmussen, R. E. and Wang, I. Y.   Dependence of specific metabolism of benzo-(a)pyrene on the inducer of hydroxylase activity. Cancer Res., *34*: 2290–2295, 1974.

51. Yang, S. K., Selkirk, J. K., Plotkin, E., and Gelboin, H. V.   Kinetic analysis of the quinones by high-pressure liquid chromatography: Effect of enzyme induction. Cancer Res., *35*: 3642–3650, 1975.

52. Leutz, J. C. and Gelboin, H. V.   Benzo(a)pyrene-4,5-oxide hydratase: Assay, properties, and induction. Arch. Biochem. Biophys., *168*: 722–725, 1975.

53. Oesch, F.   Mammalian epoxide hydrases: Inducible enzymes catalyzing the inactivation of carcinogenic and cytotoxic metabolites derived from aromatic and objective compounds. Xenobiotica, *3*: 305–340, 1972.

54. Nemoto, N. and Gelboin, H. V.   Assay and properties of glutathione-S-benzo(a)-pyrene-4,5-oxide transferase. Arch. Biochem. Biophys., *170*: 739–742, 1975.

55. Hayakawa, T., Lemahieu, R. A., and Udenfriend, S.   Studies on glutathione S-arene oxidase. Transferase-A sensitive assay and partial purification of the enzyme from sheep liver. Arch. Biochem. Biophys., *162*: 223–230, 1974.

56. Habig, W. H., Pabst. M. J., and Jakoby, W. B.   Glutathione S-transferases. J. Biol. Chem., *249*: 7130–7139, 1974.

57. Nemoto, N., Gelboin, H. V., Habig, W. H., Ketley, J. N., and Jakoby, W. B. K-region benzo(a)pyrene-4,5-oxide is conjugated by homogeneous glutathione S-transferases. Nature, *255*: 512, 1975.

58. Gelboin, H. V., Miller, J. A., and Miller, E. C.   The *in vitro* formation of protein-bound derivatives of aminoazo dyes by rat liver preparations. Cancer Res., *19*: 975, 1959.

59. Kellermann, G., Cantrell, E., and Shaw, C. R.   Variation in extent of aryl hydrocarbon hydroxylase induction in cultured human lymphocytes. Cancer Res., *33*: 1654–1656, 1973.

60. Kellermann, G., Luyten-Kellermann, M., and Shaw, C. R.   Genetic variation of aryl hydrocarbon hydroxylase in human lymphocytes. Am. J. Hum. Genet., *25*: 327–331, 1973.

61. Kellermann, G., Shaw, C. R., and Luyten-Kellermann, M.   Aryl hydrocarbon

hydroxylase inducibility and bronchogenic carcinoma. New Engl. J. Med., *289*: 934–937, 1973.

62. Kouri, R. E., Ratrie, H., III, Atlas, S. A., Niwa, A., and Nebert, D. W. Aryl hydro-carbon hydroxylase induction in human lymphocyte cultures by 2,3,7,8-tetrachloro-dibenzo-*p*-dioxide. Life Sci., *15*: 1585–1595, 1974.

63. Kellermann, G., Luyten-Kellermann, M., Horning, M. G., and Stafford, M.   Cor-relation of aryl hydrocarbon hydroxylase activity of human lymphocyte cultures and plasma elimination rates for antipyrine and phenylbutazone. Drug Metab. Dispos., *3*: 47–50, 1975.

64. Bast, R. C., Jr., Shears, B. W., Rapp, H. J., and Gelboin, H. V.   Aryl hydrocarbon (benzo(a)pyrene) hydroxylase in guinea pig peritoneal macrophages: Benz(a)anthra-cene-induced increase of enzyme activity *in vivo* and in cell culture. J. Natl. Cancer Inst., *51*: 675–678, 1974.

65. Booth, J., Keysall, G. R., Kalyani, P. L., and Sims, P.   The metabolism of polycyclic hydrocarbons by cultured human lymphocytes. FEBS Lett., *43*: 341–344, 1974.

Discussion of Paper of Drs. Gelboin et al.

DR. WEISBURGER: Regarding the technically elegant procedures of Dr. Gelboin we have shown even prior to the isolation of cytochrome P-450 by R. Sato of Osaka University that there might be several forms of oxidases when we studied the metabolism of 2-acetylaminofluorene in several species (Science, *125*: 503, 1957). Have you studied metabolism of polycyclic aromatic hydrocarbons (PAH) in the forestomach which is sensitive to cancer induction as shown by Dr. Wattenberg, or in newborn rat liver? These are 2 organs to PAH in mice. Adult rat liver maybe has mainly detoxification metabolites.

DR. GELBOIN: We have not studied the metabolism in the forestomach. We do not know the basis for tissue specificity of carcinogens. It may be due to differences in the metabolism of carcinogens, different steady state levels of active carcinogenic intermediates, or their lack of proximity to key receptor sites. These tissue differences may also be due to other postcarcinogen activation processes such as the stability of the gene-action system, efficiency of repair processes such as DNA repair, or promotion differences. We simply don't know the answer at the present time.

DR. RAJEWSKY: Could you say a few words about what is presently known of the type and site of binding to DNA of, *e.g.*, the benzo(a)pyrene (BP)-derived 7,8 diol-9,10-oxide?

DR. GELBOIN: Many groups are examining this problem. Both Brooks in England and Weinstein in the U.S.A. think that this compound gives similar binding to that formed *in vivo* from BP. The binding is covalent.

DR. FARBER: This is a very important and elegant study that will obviously give us a new foundation for understanding PAH carcinogenesis. An obvious question concerns the possible differences between different tissues in the same species and between the same tissue in different species.

DR. GELBOIN: There are marked and distinct differences between human, rat, and hamster tissues. The livers of each give very different patterns. The human liver, lymphocytes, and monocytes all show 5 peaks that are not observed in rat liver. Within a species the differences are not as marked but can be very dependent on whether whole cells, homogenates, microsomes, or purified enzymes are used. In

just different forms the enzymes yield different products (F. J. Wiebel, J. K. Selkirk, H. V. Gelboin, D. A. Haugen, T. A. van der Hoeven, and M. J. Coon, Proc. Natl. Acad Sci. U.S., *72*: 3917–3920, 1975.). A very important but difficult question is to analyze the pattern formed *in vivo*. The steady state concentration of metabolites is so low that this becomes a difficult task.

DR. HOZUMI: How about the stability of metabolic patterns of BP in cultured cells? I am interested in this problem in connection with the susceptibility of tissue culture cells and *in vitro* transformation by BP during long-term cell cultures.

DR. GELBOIN: With cells in culture we see a preponderance of water-soluble conjugated metabolites. This is especially true when low levels of hydrocarbons are used. The time of incubation is also relevant. For example, lymphocytes incubated for 24 hr with BP show a very different pattern than after incubation for only 20 min. We are about to examine the nature of the water-soluble metabolites.

DR. TAKEBE: Can you correlate your data of high mutagenic activity of 7,8-diol-9,10-oxide of BP to carcinogenic activity? We have ample quantitative data on mutagenic activity of carcinogens in bacteria, but very few in mammalian cells. Also, do you have any data on chemicals other than derivatives of BP?

DR. GELBOIN: My collaborators, Drs. Huberman and Sachs are now examining the *in vitro* transforming activity of the diol epoxide. To my knowledge this has not yet been completed. We are also presently measuring the activity of this compound in *in vivo* tumorigenesis. We have not studied compounds other than polycyclic hydrocarbon derivatives.

DR. MAHER: I feel sure that this technical question on the mutagenicity data you presented is better addressed to Dr. E. Huberman but I question the frequencies of mutants obtained with the diol-epoxide. You showed 0.7 μM gives 4,050 AG (8-azaguanine)-resistant mutants per 100,000 survivors. This is 4%, an incredibly high frequency. In addition, the dose response was quite unusual; 0.1 μM gave 10 per 100,000, 0.3 μM gave 260 per 100,000, and 0.7 μM gave 4,050 per 100,000, *i.e.*, a 7-fold increase in compound administered yielded a 400-fold increase in frequency of mutations in this V79 system.

DR. GELBOIN: I do not know the explanation for the question you posed. The details of the procedures and the results will be published shortly in the Proc. Natl. Acad. Sci. U.S., *73*: 607–611, 1976.

DR. SATO: Could you please tell me the stabilities of metabolites of BP which are made by incubation with liver homogenates?

DR. GELBOIN: Our procedure including the high-pressure liquid chromatography (HPLC) is as short as 1–2 hr. Sometimes we store the metabolites we isolate before we do the HPLC. The metabolites we isolate are of course sufficiently stable. There may, however, be others that undergo oxidation. This may make some derivatives at the 6-position and possibly some epoxides. We can only isolate the BP-4,5-oxide with specially treated columns.

FUNDAMENTALS IN CANCER PREVENTION, P. N. MAGEE ET AL. (EDS.
UNIV. OF TOKYO PRESS, TOKYO / UNIV. PARK PRESS, BALTIMORE, PP. 191–215, 1976

Overlapping of Carcinogens and Mutagens

Takashi Sugimura,[*1] Shigeaki Sato,[*1] Minako Nagao,[*1] Takie
Yahagi,[*1] Taijiro Matsushima,[*2] Yuko Seino,[*1] Mieko Takeuchi,[*1]
and Takashi Kawachi[*1]

*National Cancer Center Research Institute, Tokyo, Japan[*1] and Institute of Medical Science, University
of Tokyo, Tokyo, Japan[*2]*

Abstract: The importance of identifying suspected carcinogens as mutagens is
emphasized. This is evident from the chronological increase in the numbers of
compounds identified as both carcinogenic and mutagenic. Recent results supporting the correlation between the carcinogenic and mutagenic effects of compounds are reported. An improved method for detecting mutagenic compounds
by using microbes is described. This method can be applied to the identification of
ultimate forms of carcinogens.

The mutagenicity of a food additive, AF-2 which is carcinogenic to mice
was demonstrated by this mutagenic test. A derivative of this compound was
found to bind to DNA.

Confirmation of the hazardous carcinogenic effect of cigarette smoke condensate by its strong mutagenic effect on microbes is described. The discrepancy
between the estimated content of mutagens and that of known carcinogens in
cigarette smoke condensate is discussed.

One of the most important problems in cancer research is to find causative
agents of cancer. Irradiation, viruses, and thousands of chemical compounds are
known to cause cancer in many species of animals, and these agents are also supposed to be responsible for human cancer. The exact relations of these agents to
human cancer are difficult to establish. However, among these factors humans are
most likely to be exposed to chemical compounds, so these are probably the most
important cause of human cancer, and in fact this has been demonstrated by
epidemiological surveys (1–5). Actually, many chemical compounds in our environment have been shown to be carcinogenic to experimental animals. The suscep-
tibilities of various animal species to these carcinogenic compounds vary greatly,
and the actual amounts of these compounds to which humans are exposed are
much less than those tested in animal experiments. However, it seems very likely
that these carcinogenic chemical compounds are somehow related to human cancer.

Accordingly, it is very important and urgent to find out which compounds are carcinogenic to animals and whether they really exist in our environment.

Animal experiments provide definite evidence of carcinogenicity, but such experiments are time-consuming and laborious. Thus, it would be better to use some other methods which are easier and quicker. One possible method is to detect carcinogens as mutagens. The relation between carcinogens and mutagens has long been postulated and the mechanism of carcinogenesis has even been explained in terms of gene mutations. The mechanism of carcinogenesis is not yet clear, but a close relation between carcinogens and mutagens has been clearly demonstrated recently by methods for detection of mutagens using microbes (6) combined with a liver microsomal system which converts many chemicals to mutagenic derivatives (7) and by extensive surveys of the carcinogenic effects of many compounds on animals.

This article stresses the relationship between mutagens, demonstrated with microbial assay systems, and carcinogens. Results obtained in our laboratory on many compounds are introduced and a modified method for detecting mutagens is presented.

Relation between Carcinogens and Mutagens

Figure 1 shows the chronological increase in evidence of the correlation between representative carcinogens and mutagens. Chemicals identified as carcinogens and mutagens, respectively, are shown in the circles on the left and right, and those shown to be both carcinogenic and mutagenic in the overlapping area of the circles. As can be seen the number of compounds in the overlapping area has increased year by year. For example, 4-nitroquinoline 1-oxide (4NQO) was shown to be mutagenic in 1955, and proved to be carcinogenic in 1957 (8). However, the mutagenicities of well-known carcinogens such as N,N-dimethylnitrosamine (DMN), N,N-dimethyl-4-aminoazobenzene (DAB), 2-acetylaminofluorene (AAF), and benz(a)anthracene (BA) were not demonstrated until 1960. DMN was proved to be mutagenic in 1962 (9), AAF in 1968 (10), BA in 1972 (11), and DAB in 1975 (12). Butyl-N-(4-hydroxybutyl)nitrosamine (BBN) was shown to be carcinogenic in 1964 (13) and proved to be mutagenic 11 years later. On the other hand, the carcinogenicity of N-methyl-N'-nitro-N-nitrosoguanidine (MNNG) was demonstrated in 1966 (14–16), 6 years after detection of its mutagenicity (17). The mutagenicity of AF-2, 2-(2-furyl)-3-(5-nitro-2-furyl)acrylamide, a food preservative once used in Japan, was first demonstrated in 1973 (18, 19), and within 1 or 2 years, its carcinogenicity was proven (20, 21), as discussed later. Recently, once a compound has been found to be carcinogenic, its mutagenicity has usually been demonstrated soon afterwards, and *vice versa*. This is due to the establishment of new and sensitive methods for detecting mutagenicity and to careful and extensive experiments on carcinogenicity. However, even in 1975, some carcinogens have still not been shown to be mutagenic, and *vice versa*. In the future, it is possible that all carcinogens may be shown to be mutagens and all mutagens to be carcinogens. This needs further investigation. However, Fig. 1 shows that detection of com-

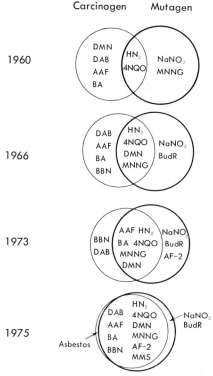

Carcinogen   Mutagen

1960

1966

1973

1975

FIG. 1.   Chronology of overlapping of carcinogens and mutagens. Abbreviations are specified in the text. BudR, bromodeoxyuridine; MMS, methyl methanesulfonate.

pounds as mutagens is strong evidence that they are carcinogens. This is useful because tests on mutagenicity in bacteria are much less laborious and quicker than tests on carcinogenicity in animals.

A Simple Method to Detect Mutagens

Ames (6, 7, 22) developed a method to detect the mutagenicity of chemicals by reverse mutation of an auxotroph for histidine of *Salmonella typhimurium*. This method as modified in our laboratory (12, 23) is briefly as follows.

An activating system (S-9 Mix) is prepared by injecting polychlorinated biphenyl (KC-500) or phenobarbital into male Sprague-Dawley rats to induce drug-metabolizing system, separating the postmitochondrial fraction of their livers and mixing it with NADPH, NADH, glucose-6-phosphate, and glucose-6-phosphate dehydrogenase. The test substance dissolved in dimethylsulfoxide (DMSO) is incubated with S-9 Mix and the tester strain of bacteria for 20 min at 37°C. Then, soft agar is added and the mixture is poured onto minimal-glucose agar containing a limited amount of L-histidine in a Petri dish. The number of revertant colonies per plate is counted after incubating the plate at 37°C for 2 days. The tester strains usually used are *S. typhimurium* TA100 and TA98, derived from TA1535 and TA 1538, respectively, by introduction of R-factor plasmids (24).

Figure 2 shows results of a mutagenicity test on *o*-aminoazotoluene (*o*-AT) using strain TA100. The carcinogenicity of this compound in the liver was first demonstrated by Yoshida (*25*) and its mutagenicity has been reported on TA1538

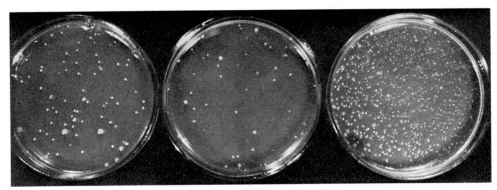

Fig. 2. Revertant colonies of *S. typhimurium* TA100 observed after treatment by *o*-aminoazotoluene with and without S-9 Mix. Left: none. Middle: *o*-AT 50 μg, −S-9 Mix. Right: *o*-AT 50 μg, +S-9 Mix.

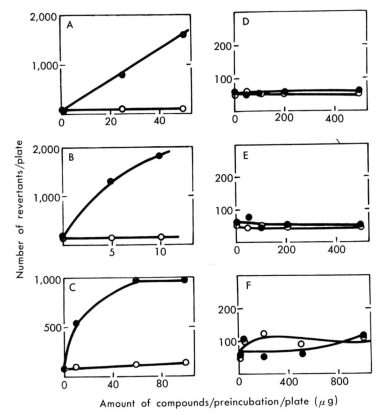

Fig. 3. Numbers of revertants of *S. typhimurium* TA100 obtained after incubation with various amounts of chemicals. A, 4-dimethylamino-stilbene; B, benzo (a) pyrene; C, 7,12-dimethylbenz (a) anthracene; D, stilbene; E, pyrene; F, anthracene. ● +S-9Mix; ○ −S-Mix.

strain cells with S-9 Mix (7). As shown in Fig. 2 revertant colonies were only observed when o-AT had been incubated with the activation system. Thus o-AT itself was not mutagenic but some derivatives, such as the N-hydroxyamino derivative formed by the activating system of rat liver microsomes, were assumed to be mutagenic.

Results on the mutagenicities of several other compounds demonstrated with the same strain of bacteria are shown in Fig. 3. 4-Dimethylaminostilbene, benzo-(a)pyrene, and 7,12-dimethylbenz(a)anthracene, which are known to be strong carcinogens, were all mutagenic only after activation by the liver microsomes. However, stilbene, pyrene, and anthracene were not mutagenic before or after incubation with S-9 Mix. So far they have not been shown to be carcinogenic.

When testing the mutagenicity it is important to check the dose-dependent mutagenic effect of a compound. The mutagenic substances in Fig. 3 showed clear dose-dependent effects with the activation system. However, some chemicals show dose-dependent mutagenic activity only up to a certain concentration, and above this their mutagenic activity decreases. This may be due to the lethal effect of a high concentration of the test compound on the tester strain. In our laboratory only compounds which show clear dose-dependent effects are regarded as mutagenic.

As shown above, the mutagenicity test system using S. typhimurium in combination with the liver microsomal activating system can detect the mutagenicities of substances which are not themselves mutagenic but which are converted to mutagenic compounds in vivo. By comparing the mutagenic effects of a compound with and without the activating system it is possible to deduce what form of the compound is carcinogenic in vivo. This is discussed again later.

Relation of the Mutagenicities and Carcinogenicities of the Compounds Tested in This Laboratory

The mutagenicities or DNA-damaging activities of more than 250 compounds have been tested in our laboratory using several bacterial systems. Results on 240 compounds, mutagenicities of which wese tested and listed alphabetically, are shown in Table 1 together with the data on their carcinogenicities. The carcinogenicities of these compounds correlated well with results of tests on their mutagenicities and the best correlation was obtained using S. typhimurium TA100.

Out of 240 compounds listed in Table 1, 146 compounds have been tested so far for carcinogenicity. The correlation between the carcinogenicities and mutagenicities of these compounds is shown schematically in Fig. 4. The upper part of the abscissa shows numbers of carcinogens and lower part numbers of non-carcinogens. The right side of the ordinate shows numbers of mutagens and left side numbers of non-mutagens. The compounds tested in our laboratory were thus classified into 4 groups on the basis of their carcinogenicities and mutagenicities. As clearly demonstrated in the figure, there was a very high correlation between the carcinogenic activities and mutagenic activities of these compounds, shown by the fact that values for almost 86% of the compounds were in the upper right and lower left quadrants of the figure. This high correlation between carcinogenicity and

TABLE 1.   Mutagenicities of Compounds Tested in This Laboratory and Their Correlations to Carcinogenicities

		TA1535[a]	TA1536	TA1537	TA1538	TA100	TA98	WP-2	Carcinogenicity
1	AB-206 (Nalidixic acid derivative)	—*[b]			—*	—*			
2	AC-5-AC' (Indanone derivative)	—	—	—	—				
3	5-Acetamido-3-(5-nitro-2-furyl)-6H-1,2,4-oxadiazine	—	—	—	—	+	+		+
4	Acetanilide				—*	—*			—
5	N-Acetoxy-2-acetylaminofluorene	—	—	—	+				+
6	N-Acetoxy-N-methyl-4-aminoazobenzene					+	+		
7	4-Acetylaminobiphenyl	—*	—*	—*	—*	+*	+*		+
8	2-Acetylaminofluorene	—*	—*	—*	+*	+*			+
9	2-Acetylamino-4-[2-(5-nitro-2-furyl)vinyl]-1,3-thiazole	—	—	—	—	+		+	
10	Acetylsalicylic acid					—*	—*	—	—
11	Acid violet 6B					—*	+*		+
12	Acriflavine	—	—	+	—				—
13	Adriamycin					—*	+		+
14	Amaranth (Red No. 2)					—*	—*	—	—
15	4-Aminoazobenzene	—*	—*	—*	—*	+*	+*	—*	+
16	o-Aminoazotoluene					+*	+*		+
17	p-Aminobenzoic acid ethyl ester					—*	—*	—	
18	4-Aminobiphenyl	—*	—*	—*	+*	+*	+*	—*	+
19	2-Amino-5-[2-(5-nitro-2-furyl)-1-(2-furyl)-vinyl-1-]-1,3,4-oxadiazole	—	—	—	—			+	
20	2-Amino-4-(5-nitro-2-furyl)thiazole	—	—	—	—	+		+	+
21	2-Amino-4-[2-(5-nitro-2-furyl)vinyl]-1,3-thiazole	—	—	—	—	+		+	
22	4-Aminoquinoline 1-oxide·HCl					+*	+*		—
23	N-Amyl-N-(3-carboxypropyl)nitrosamine	+							
24	N-Amyl-N-(4-hydroxybutyl)nitrosamine	+*							+
25	Aniline·HCl					—*	—*		—
26	Anthracene	—*	—*	—*	—*	—*	—*	—*	—
27	Anthranilic acid					—*	—*		—
28	Aryl benzene sulfonate (Na salt)					—*	—*	—	—
29	Azoxymethane	+*				+*			+
30	β-Benzene hexachloride					—*	—*		—
31	γ-Benzene hexachloride					—*	—*		+
32	Benzo(a)pyrene					+*	+*		+
33	Benzo(a)pyrene-4,5-oxide					+	+		+
34	N-Benzoyloxy-N-methyl-4-aminoazobenzene					+	+		+
35	N-n-Butyl-N-n-amylnitrosamine					+*	—*		+
36	Butylbutanolamine	—*	—*	—*	—*	—*	—*		
37	N-Butyl-N-(2-carboxyethyl)nitrosamine	+							+
38	N-Butyl-N-(carboxymethyl)nitrosamine	—							
39	N-Butyl-N-(3-carboxypropyl)nitrosamine	+							+
40	N-tert-Butyl-N-(3-carboxypropyl)nitrosamine	—							
41	N-Butyl-N-(2,4-dihydroxybutyl)nitrosamine	+*							
42	N-Butyl-N-(3-glycylcarboxypropyl)nitrosamine	—							

Continued . . .

TABLE 1.   Continued.

	TA1535[a]	TA1536	TA1537	TA1538	TA100	TA98	WP-2	Carcino-genicity
43 N-Butyl-N-(2-hydroxybutyl)nitrosamine	+*							
44 N-Butyl-N-(3-hydroxybutyl)nitrosamine	+*							−
45 N-Butyl-N-(4-hydroxybutyl)nitrosamine	+*							+
46 N-tert-Butyl-N-(4-hydroxybutyl)nitrosamine	−*							−
47 N-Butyl-N-(2-hydroxy-3-carboxypropyl)-nitrosamine	−							
48 N-Butyl-N-(2-hydroxyethyl)nitrosamine	+*							+
49 N-Butyl-N-(3-hydroxypropyl)nitrosamine	+*							−
50 N-Butyl-N-(3-oxobutyl)nitrosamine	+*							+
51 N-Butyl-N-(2-oxopropyl)nitrosamine	+*							+
52 N-n-Butyl-N′-nitro-N-nitrosoguanidine	+	−	−	−	+			+
53 N-iso-Butyl-N′-nitro-N-nitrosoguanidine	+	−	−	−	+			+
54 Butylnitrosourea					+	−*	+	+
55 N-n-Butyl-N-nitrosourethane					+	+		+
56 Butylurea					−*	−*		−
57 N-n-Butylurethane					+*	+*		
58 ε-Caprolactone					−*	−*		
59 Carboxymethyl cellulose					−*	−*	−	−
60 5-Chloro-8-hydroxyquinoline					−*	−*		
61 2-Chloroquinoline					−*	−*		−
62 Cortisone acetate					−*	−*		
63 Crystal violet	−	−	−	−				
64 Cycasin					−			+
65 Daunomycin·HCl					+	+		+
66 Dechlorogriseofulvin					−*	−*		
67 Dextrane					−*	−*		−
68 4,6-Diamino-2-(5-nitro-2-furyl)-s-triazine	−	−	−	−	+		+	+
69 N,N-Di-n-amylnitrosamine					+*	−*		+
70 5,7-Dibromo-8-hydroxyquinoline					−*	−*		
71 N,N-Di-n-butylamine					−*	−*		
72 N,N-Di-n-butylnitrosamine					+*	−*		+
73 5,7-Dichloro-8-hydroxyquinoline					−*	−*		
74 4,7-Dichloroquinoline					+*	+*		
75 Diethylcarbamazine	−*	−*	−*	−*	−*	−*	−*	
76 N,N-Diethylnitrosamine					+*	+*		+
77 N,N-Di-(4-hydroxybutyl)nitrosamine	−*							−
78 2,4-Dihydroxyquinoline·Na					+*	+*		
79 N,N-Dimethylamine·HCl					−*	−*	−	−
80 N,N-Dimethyl-4-aminoazobenzene					+*	+*		+
81 trans-2-[(Dimethylamino)methylimino]-5-[2-(5-nitro-2-furyl)vinyl]-1,3,4-oxadiazole	−	−	−	−	+		+	+
82 4-Dimethylaminostilbene					+*	+*		+
83 7,12-Dimethylbenz[a]anthracene	−*	−*	+*	−*	+*	+	−*	+
84 2-(2,2-Dimethylhydrazino)-4-(5-nitro-2-furyl)thiazole	−	−	−	−	+		+	+
85 N,N-Dimethylnitrosamine	+*				+*	−*		+

Continued . . .

TABLE 1. Continued.

	TA1535[a]	TA1536	TA1537	TA1538	TA100	TA98	WP-2	Carcinogenicity
86 N,N-Diphenylnitrosamine					−*	−*		−
87 N,N-Di-n-propylnitrosamine					+*	−*		+
88 Erythrosine					−*	−*	−	−
89 D-Ethionine					−*		−*	
90 L-Ethionine					−*		−*	+
91 N-Ethyl-N-(3-carboxypropyl)nitrosamine	+							+
92 N-Ethyl-N-(4-hydroxybutyl)nitrosamine	+*							+
93 N-Ethyl-N-(2-hydroxyethyl)nitrosamine	+*							+
94 N-Ethyl-N-(3-hydroxypropyl)nitrosamine	+*							−
95 N-Ethyl-N′-nitro-N-nitrosoguanidine	+	−	+	−	+			+
96 Ethynylestradiol					−*	−*		
97 F30066 (nitrofuran derivative)					+	−		
98 Fluorene	−*	−*	−*	−*	−*	−*	−*	−
99 Fluorescein sodium					−*	−*		−
100 Formic acid 2-[4-(5-nitro-2-furyl)-2-thiazolyl]hydrazide			−	−	+		+	+
101 2-Formylamino-4-[2-(5-nitro-2-furyl)vinyl]-1,3-thiazole			−	−	+		+	
102 2-Formylamino-4-(4-nitrophenyl)thiazole					+	+		+
103 Furaltadine			−	−			+	
104 2-(2-Furyl)-3-(5-nitro-2-furyl)acrylamide			−	−	+	+	+	+
105 Gallic acid					−*	−*		
106 Griseofulvin					−*	−*		+
107 H18 (Nitrofuran derivative)	−	−	−	−	+	+	+	
108 H34 („ „)	−	−	−	−	+	+	+	
109 H36 („ „)	−	−	−	−	+	+	+	
110 H59 („ „)	−	−	−	−	+	+	+	
111 N-n-Hexyl-N′-nitro-N-nitrosoguanidine	+	−	−	−	+			
112 Hycanthone	−	−	+	+	+	+	−	+
113 2-Hydrazino-4-(4-aminophenyl)thiazole					+	+*		+
114 2-Hydrazino-4-(4-nitrophenyl)thiazole					+	+		+
115 5-Hydroxyacenaphthene					−*	−*		−
116 N-Hydroxy-2-acetylaminofluorene	−	−	−	+				+
117 N-Hydroxy-4-aminoazobenzene					+*	+*		+
118 4-Hydroxyaminoquinoline 1-oxide	−	−	+	+				+
119 3-Hydroxyanthranilic acid					−*	−*		+
120 p-Hydroxybenzoic acid n-propyl ester					−*	−*	−	−
121 N-(2-Hydroxyethyl)-N-(4-hydroxybutyl)-nitrosamine	+*							
122 N-(3-Hydroxypropyl)-N-(4-hydroxybutyl)-nitrosamine	−*							−
123 N-Hydroxy-N-methyl-4-aminoazobenzene					+*	+		
124 8-Hydroxyquinoline					+*	+*		
125 8-Hydroxyquinoline-5-sulfonic acid					+*	−*		
126 N-Hydroxyurethane						+*		+
127 IA-3 (Chloroindazole analogue of lucanthone)	−	−	−	−	+*	+*	−	
128 IA-3 N-oxide	−	−	−	−	+*	+*	−	

Continued . . .

TABLE 1. Continued.

		TA1535[a]	TA1536	TA1537	TA1538	TA100	TA98	WP-2	Carcino-genicity
129	IA-4 (Chloroindazole analogue of hycanthone)	—	—	—	—	+	+*	—	
130	IA-4 N-oxide	—	—	—	—	+*	+*	—	
131	IA-10 (Chloromethylpiperazinyl analogue of lucanthone)	—	—	—	—	+*	—*	—	
132	IA-10 N-oxide	—	—	—	—	+*	—*	—	
133	IA-11 (Chloromethylpiperazinyl analogue of hycanthone)	—	—	—	—	+*	+*	—	
134	Indene	—	—	—	—				
135	Isoquinoline					—*	—*		
136	Kanamycin	—	—	—	—				
137	D-Methionine					—*	—*		—
138	L-Methionine					—*	—*		—
139	3-Methoxy-4-aminoazobenzene					+*	+*		+
140	4'-Methoxycarbonyl-N-acetoxy-N-methyl-4-aminoazobenzene					+	+		
141	4'-Methoxycarbonyl-N-benzoyloxy-N-methyl-4-aminoazobenzene					+	+		
142	4'-Methoxycarbonyl-N-hydroxy-N-methyl-4-aminoazobenzene					+*	+		
143	4'-Methoxycarbonyl-N-methyl-4-aminoazo-benzene					—*	—*		
144	2-Methoxy-5-nitrotropone	—*	—*	—*	—*	+*	+*		+
145	N-Methyl-4-aminoazobenzene					+*	+*		+
146	Methylazoxymethanol acetate	+				+	—*		+
147	Methyl benzoquate	—*			—*	—*			
148	N-Methyl-N-benzylnitrosamine					+*	—*		+
149	N-Methyl-N-n-butylnitrosamine					+*	—*		+
150	N-Methyl-N-(3-carboxypropyl)nitrosamine	+							+
151	2-Methyl-4-dimethylaminoazobenzene					+*	+*		+
152	3'-Methyl-4-dimethylaminoazobenzene	—*	—*	—*	—*	+*	+*	—*	+
153	N-Methyl-N-n-dodecylnitrosamine					+*	—*		+
154	N-Methyl-N-(4-hydroxybutyl)nitrosamine	+*							+
155	4-Methyl-1-[(5-nitrofurfurylidene)amino]-2-imidazolidene	—	—	—	—	+		+	+
156	2-Methyl-4-(5-nitro-2-furyl)thiazole	—	—	—	—	+		+	+
157	N-Methyl-N'-nitroguanidine	—	—	—	—	—			—
158	N-Methyl-N'-nitro-N-nitroguanidine	—	—	—	—	—		—	
159	N-Methyl-N'-nitro-N-nitrosoguanidine	+	—	+	—	+		+	+
160	N-Methyl-N-nitrosourea					+	—*		+
161	3-Methylisoquinoline					—*	—*		
162	4-Methylquinoline					+*	+*		
163	6-Methylquinoline					+*	+*		
164	7-Methylquinoline					+*	+*		
165	8-Methylquinoline					+*	+*		
166	Methyltestosterone					—*	—*		
167	Methylurea					—*	—*		
168	Metrifonate	—	—	—	—	+	—*	—	
169	Metronidazole	—	—	—	—	+	—*	+	+

Continued . . .

TABLE 1. Continued.

		TA1535[a]	TA1536	TA1537	TA1538	TA100	TA98	WP-2	Carcino-genicity
170	Nalidixic acid	—*			—*	—*			
171	α-Naphtol					—*	—*		—
172	β-Naphtol					—*	—*		—
173	α-Naphthylamine					+*	—		—
174	β-Naphthylamine					+*	+*		+
175	Nifuroxime	—	—	—	—			+	
176	Niridazole	—	—	—	—	+	+	+	+
177	5-Nitroacenaphthene					+	+		+
178	5-Nitro-2-furamidoxime	—	—	—	—	+		+	—
179	Nitrofurantoin	—	—	—	—	+		+	—
180	5-Nitro-2-furaldehyde diacetate	—	—	—	—			+	
181	Nitrofurazone	—	—	—	—	+	+	+	+
182	2-(5-Nitro-2-furfurylidene)amino ethanol	—	—	—	—	+		+	
183	2-(5-Nitro-2-furfurylidene)amino ethanol N-oxide	—	—	—	—	+		+	
184	5-Nitro-2-furoic acid	—	—	—	—	+		—	
185	3-(5-Nitro-2-furyl)acrylamide	—	—	—	—	+		+	
186	5-Nitro-2-furyl acrylic acid	—	—	—	—	+		+	
187	N-{[3-(5-Nitro-2-furyl)-1,2,4-oxadiazol-5-yl]methyl}acetamide	—	—	—	—	+		+	+
188	5-Nitro-2-furyl propionic acid	—	—	—	—			+	
189	5-Nitro-2-furyl propiolic acid ester	—	—	—	—			—	
190	N-[5-(5-Nitro-2-furyl)-1,3,4-thiadiazol-2-yl]-acetamide	—	—	—	—	+		+	+
191	4-(5-Nitro-2-furyl)thiazole	—	—	—	—	+		+	+
192	N-[4-(5-Nitro-2-furyl)-2-thiazolyl]acetamide	—	—	—	—	+		+	+
193	N-[4-(5-Nitro-2-furyl)-2-thiazolyl]formamide	—	—	—	—	+		+	+
194	4-Nitropyridine 1-oxide	—	—	—	+			+	+
195	4-Nitroquinoline	—	—	—	+			+	+
196	6-Nitroquinoline					+	+		
197	8-Nitroquinoline					+	+		
198	4-Nitroquinoline 1-oxide	—	—	—	+	+	+		+
199	NSC3424 (Quinacrine mustard)	—	+	+	+				
200	NTH-1 (Nitrothiazole derivative)					+	—*		
201	NTH-2 („ „)					+	+		
202	NTH-3 („ „)					+	—*		
203	Penicillic acid					—*	—*		+
204	N-n-Pentyl-N'-nitro-N-nitrosoguanidine	+	—		—	+			+
205	Phenacetine					—*	—*		
206	N-Phenyl-N-(4-hydroxybutyl)nitrosamine	—*							
207	2-(2-Phenyl)-3-(5-nitro-2-furyl)acrylamide	—	—	—	—	+		+	
208	Phloxine					—*	—*		—
209	Polychlorinated biphenyl (KC-300)					—*	—*	—	—
210	Polychlorinated biphenyl (KC-500)					—*	—*	—	+
211	Potassium 1-methyl-7-[2-(5-nitro-2-furyl)-vinyl]-4-oxo-1,4-dihydro-1,8-naphthyridine-3-carboxylate	—	—	—	—	+		+	+

Continued . . .

TABLE 1.   Continued.

		TA1535[a]	TA1536	TA1537	TA1538	TA100	TA98	WP-2	Carcinogenicity
212	Propane sultone					+	−*		+
213	β-Propiolactone					+	−*		+
214	N-n-Propyl-N-n-butylnitrosamine					+*	−*		+
215	N-Propyl-N-(3-carboxypropyl)nitrosamine	+							+
216	N-Propyl-N-(4-hydroxybutyl)nitrosamine	+*							+
217	N-Propyl-N'-nitro-N-nitrosoguanidine	+	−	−	−	+			+
218	Pteroside A	−	−	−	−				
219	Pteroside B	−	−	−	−				
220	Pynacianol	−	−	−	−				−
221	Pyrene					−*	−*		−
222	Pyrogallol					+			
223	Quinoline					+*	+*		+
224	Quinoline-2-carboxylic acid					−*	−*		
225	Quinoline-N-oxide·H₂O					+*	+*		
226	Quinoline-8-sulfonyl chloride					−*	−*		
227	Rubratoxin B					−*	−*		
228	Saccharine sodium				−*	−*	−*		−
229	Salicylic acid					−*	−*	−	−
230	Shikimic acid	−*			−*	−*	−*		+
231	Sodium nitrite	+				+	−	−	−
232	SQ18,506 (trans-5-amino-3-[2-(5-nitro-2-furyl) vinyl]1,2,4-oxadiazole)	−	−	−	−	+	+	+	
233	Sterigmatocystin					+	+		+
234	Stilbene					−*	−*		−
235	Streptomycin	−	−	−	−				
236	Testosterone propionate					−*	−*		−
237	2,2,2-Trifluoro-N-[4-(5-nitro-2-furyl)-2-triazolyl]acetamide	−	−	−	−	+		+	+
238	Tween 60					−*	−*	−	
239	Tween 80					−*	−*	−	
240	UK4271 (6-hydroxymethyl-2-isopropylamino-methyl-7-nitro-1,2,3,4-tetrahydroquinoline)	−	−	−	−	+	−*		

[a] TA series are *S. typhimurium* strains (6). WP-2 is *E. coli* strain.   [b] +, positive without S-9 Mix;   +*, positive with S-9 Mix;   −, negative without S-9 Mix;   −*, negative with and without S-9 Mix.

mutagenicity also shows the usefulness of the mutagenicity test with the bacterial system in screening for carcinogens.

A few compounds showed carcinogenicity but not mutagenicity and others mutagenicity but not carcinogenicity, as also shown in Fig. 1. Further extensive tests on animals are required to examine the possible carcinogenic effects of the substances which appear to be mutagenic but not carcinogenic. At the same time more sensitive methods are needed to examine the possible mutagenicities of chemicals, including those which have proved carcinogenic but not mutagenic in several systems.

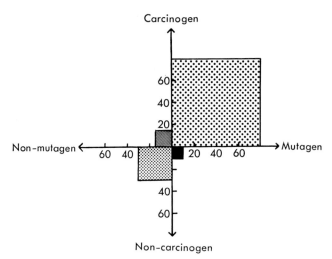

FIG. 4. Numbers of mutagens and non-mutagens tested in our laboratory and their correlation to carcinogenic activities.

Noteworthy Cases of Mutagenicities of Carcinogens

Recently tests in our laboratory by the modified mutation test system revealed the mutagenicities of many compounds (*12, 23*). The mutagenicities of several of these are very interesting in relation to their carcinogenicities. One group of these compounds became mutagenic on activation by microsomes. This group includes many azo dyes such as DAB, N-methyl-4-aminoazobenzene (MAB), 3′-methyl DAB, 2-methyl-DAB, 4-aminoazobenzene (AB), and 3-methoxy-AB (*7, 12*), which have long been known to be carcinogenic but had not previously been shown to be mutagenic. Dialkylnitrosamines, such as DMN, N,N-diethylnitrosamine (DEN), N,N-di-*n*-butylnitrosamine, N,N-di-*n*-propylnitrosamine, N,N-di-*n*-amylnitrosamine, N-methyl-N-*n*-butylnitrosamine, N-*n*-propyl-N-*n*-butylnitrosamine, N-methyl-N-*n*-dodecylnitrosamine, and N-*n*-butyl-N-*n*-amylnitrosamine were also proved to be mutagenic. All these compounds are known to be carcinogenic (*13, 26–29*). BBN, which is known to induce bladder tumors specifically (*13*) was also proved to be mutagenic when treated with S-9 Mix. Azoxymethane and N-hydroxyurethane, which are carcinogenic compounds, were also found to be mutagenic.

It is also interesting that quinoline was found to be mutagenic with the activation system, because Hirano *et al.* (*30*) recently showed that it was carcinogenic in the liver, so that its mutagenicity is well correlated with its carcinogenicity.

All the above compounds were mutagenic when incubated with the microsomal enzyme system. However, we recently found the second group of compounds which were mutagenic without activation. This group includes N-acetoxy-MAB, 4′-methoxycarbonyl-N-acetoxy-MAB, and 4′-methoxycarbonyl-N-benzoyloxy-MAB. N-Benzoyloxy-MAB was also proved to be mutagenic without activation. Its carcinogenicity was demonstrated on rats (*31*). Mutagenicity without activation was also found on α-acetoxy-dialkylnitrosamines like N-butyl-N-(1-acetoxybutyl)-

nitrosamine (*32*). N-Butyl-N-(carboxypropyl)nitrosamine (BCPN), one of the metabolites of BBN, which is also carcinogenic in the bladder was found to be mutagenic without S-9 Mix. This compound may be the proximate carcinogen of BBN as discussed later.

Another interesting compound which is mutagenic without activation is pyrogallol. It was found to be definitely mutagenic on TA100. Pyrogallol has not yet been shown to be carcinogenic and further extensive studies are required on this possibility.

Ultimate Carcinogens and Mutagens

Many carcinogenic compounds are metabolized *in vivo* to some form which can interact with macromolecules in the cells. The interaction of activated compounds with intracellular macromolecules, such as DNA, is thought to be the primary event in malignant transformation of cells. The metabolites of carcinogens which interact with cellular components and which are thought to induce tumors are called ultimate or direct carcinogens, whereas compounds which can induce tumors when administered to animals but which cannot react directly with intracellular macromolecules are called procarcinogens. The intermediate metabolites of procarcinogens which are not reactive but produce tumors when they are metabolized further are called proximate carcinogens (*33*). For example, AAF itself is thought to be a procarcinogen; its metabolite, N-hydroxy-AAF (N-OH-AAF), which is also carcinogenic but which does not react with macromolecules, is a proximate carcinogen; its esterified product, N-acetoxy-AAF, can bind to intracellular components and is carcinogenic, so it is an ultimate carcinogen (*33, 34*).

It is difficult to clarify the metabolic pathways of carcinogens from the results of *in vivo* experiments only. Even when some metabolites are detected and shown to be carcinogenic these metabolites cannot be concluded to be ultimate forms of carcinogens. To confirm that the metabolites are ultimate carcinogens, their interaction with DNA or other cellular components should be demonstrated. Usually, intermediate metabolites of chemicals formed *in vivo* are rather unstable or have high turn-over rates and they are sometimes difficult to obtain in sufficient amounts to characterize.

Based on the high correlation between the carcinogenicities and mutagenicities of compounds and on the fact that mutagenicity results from the interaction of a chemical with DNA, we can deduce what forms of compounds are ultimate carcinogens from results of mutation tests on bacteria with and without the activation system from liver microsomes. For example, the carcinogen AAF was mutagenic on bacteria with, but not without, the activating system (*7, 35*), whereas its metabolites, such as N-OH-AAF and N-acetoxy-AAF were mutagenic without the activating system (*35, 36*). N-OH-AAF turns out to be a more potent mutagen with S-9 Mix. On the other hand, N-acetoxy-AAF is inactivated with S-9 Mix. These facts strongly support the idea that N-OH-AAF is the proximate form of AAF and N-acetoxy-AAF is the ultimate one.

As shown previously, azo dyes, including DAB, 3'-methyl-DAB, MAB, and

AB were recently found to be mutagenic only when they were activated by S-9 Mix. This implies that these carcinogenic compounds require activation *in vivo* before they can react with intracellular components and induce malignant transformation or mutation. Thus, in this sense, they may be regarded as procarcinogens or promutagens. However, their derivatives like N-hydroxy-MAB and 4'-methoxy-carbonyl-N-hydroxy-MAB were mutagenic on *S. typhimurium* TA98 with or without S-9 Mix, but mutagenic on TA100 only with S-9 Mix (*12*), indicating that they require further metabolism to induce mutation of TA100 cells. N-Acetoxy-MAB and N-benzoyloxy-MAB were mutagenic to both strains of bacteria even without activation system (*12*). In fact, these 2 compounds have been shown to interact directly with amino acids (*31, 37*), protein (*31*), and nucleic acids (*31*) *in vitro*. Thus, N-acetoxy-MAB and N-benzoyloxy-MAB can be considered as ultimate carcinogens or ultimate mutagens.

Similar results were obtained on dialkylnitrosamines: DBN was only mutagenic when it was activated with S-9 Mix, whereas its derivative, N-butyl-N-(1-acetoxy-butyl)nitrosamine was strongly mutagenic without activation (*32*). Accordingly, the latter compound seems to be the ultimate mutagen or ultimate carcinogen of the former, as suggested by Okada *et al.* (*32*).

BBN was shown to be mutagenic with the activation system, but its metabolite BCPN, which is the main product excreted in the urine when BBN is administered to animals, was mutagenic without S-9 Mix. However, BCPN is a rather stable compound and may require further metabolism before reacting with intracellular components. In this sense, BCPN may be considered as a proximate carcinogen of BBN.

Benzo(a)pyrene is mutagenic with the activation system but not without S-9 Mix, as shown in Figs. 3 and 9. However, its derivatives such as 7,8-dihydroxy-9,10-epoxy-7,8,9,10-tetrahydrobenzo(a)pyrene is strongly mutagenic without S-9 Mix, and is supposed to be the ultimate form of benzo(a)pyrene (*38, 39*).

All these findings show that the mutation test on bacteria is a very good method not only for rapid screening for carcinogenic compounds but also for elucidating their ultimate or direct forms.

Carcinogenicity and Mutagenicity of the Food Additive, AF-2, and Its Interaction with DNA

One example of a compound which was present in our environment until it was recently proved to be a mutagen and true carcinogen, is the food additive named AF-2 commercially. This compound, with the structure 2-(2-furyl)-3-(5-nitro-2-furyl) acrylamide has been widely used as a food preservative for the last 9 years in Japan. The mutagenic activity of this compound was tested on *S. typhimurium* TA100. As shown in Fig. 5, it had a clear dose-dependent mutagenic effect on these cells (*40*). The mutagenicity of AF-2 was also demonstrated on the same strain bacteria (*24*) and on other systems (*18, 19, 41–44*).

The mutagenicity of this food additive strongly suggested its carcinogenicity and the risk of its use as a food additive. Within 1 or 2 years after the discovery of its mutagenicity, the actual carcinogenic effect of this chemical on mice was

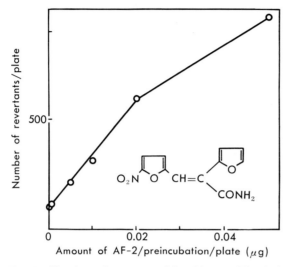

FIG. 5.   Numbers of revertants of *S. typhimurium* TA100 obtained after incubation with various doses of AF-2 without S-9 Mix. Structure of AF-2 is also shown.

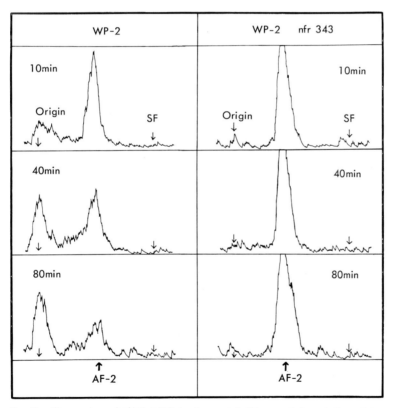

FIG. 6.   Conversion of $[^{14}C]$-AF-2 to the metabolite remaining at the origin on thin-layer chromatography after incubation for various times with cell suspensions of *E. coli* wild (WP-2) and nitrofuran-resistant (WP-2 nfr 343) strains.

proved (*20, 21*). This is an example of a compound which was shown to be a carcinogen because it was first discovered to be mutagenic, and again demonstrates the value of the mutagenicity test as the screening method for carcinogens.

Many mutagens and also carcinogens are known to interact in some way with DNA and the resulting modification of DNA is thought to be the primary event in cellular mutation and probably also malignant transformation. Conversion of AF-2 to some metabolite by intact bacteria was actually demonstrated. For this, AF-2 labeled with ^{14}C at carbon 3 of the acrylamide moiety was incubated with intact cells of the wild strain of *E. coli* WP-2 for various times and the radioactivity in its metabolite was assayed by thin-layer chromatography. As shown in Fig. 6

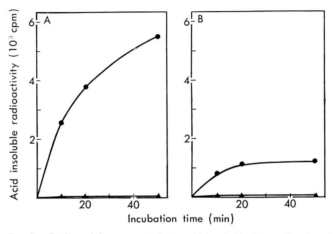

FIG. 7. Radioactivity converted to acid-insoluble form after incubation for various times of [^{14}C]-AF-2 and extracts from *E. coli* cells with and without denatured DNA. WP-2 and WP-2 nfr 343 are wild and nitrofuran-resistant strains, respectively of *E. coli*. A: with acceptor (denatured DNA). B: without acceptor (denatured DNA). ● WP-2; ▲ WP-2 nfr 343.

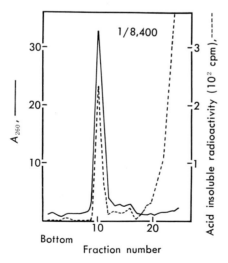

FIG. 8. Cs$_2$SO$_4$ isopycnic centrifugation pattern of denatured DNA incubated with [^{14}C]-AF-2, xanthine oxidase, and NADH.

the radioactivity in the metabolite at the origin increased with time of incubation of [^{14}C]-AF-2 with the bacteria. However, when [^{14}C]-AF-2 was incubated with a nitrofuran-resistant strain of bacteria, WP-2 nfr 343, provided by McCalla (45) no radioactivity was recovered in the metabolite.

When [^{14}C]-AF-2 and denatured calf thymus DNA were incubated with an extract of the wild strain of E. coli, the radioactivity recovered in an acid-insoluble form increased rapidly with the time of incubation, but with an extract of a resistant strain, the radioactivity in the acid-insoluble fraction did not increase appreciably, as shown in Fig. 7. These results suggested that metabolically activated AF-2 interacted with DNA. The failure of AF-2 to bind to DNA in resistant strain cells is explained by their deficiency in nitrofuran reductase (45).

The activation of AF-2 and its binding to DNA were actually demonstrated by incubating [^{14}C]-AF-2 with xanthine oxidase from cow milk, NADH, and denatured calf thymus DNA. Figure 8 shows the Cs_2SO_4 isopycnic centrifugation pattern of denatured DNA after incubation in this mixture. The positions of ^{14}C radioactivity and DNA coincided completely in the gradient, showing the covalent attachment of the metabolite of AF-2 to DNA. Under this condition, one molecule of AF-2 metabolite was calculated to bind per 8,400 bases of DNA. When AF-2 was not activated by xanthine oxidase, no binding of radioactivity to DNA was observed.

Mutagenicity of Cigarette Smoke Condensate and Its Relation to Carcinogenic Activity

The hazardous effect of smoking not only on the human cardiovascular systems but also on the respiratory system with induction of lung cancer has long been discussed and a very high correlation between cigarette smoking and the incidence of lung cancer has been demonstrated epidemiologically (46–48). Thus, if humans cannot stop smoking, an urgent problem in prevention of human cancer is to find the causative agents of cancer in cigarettes and regulate or decrease their levels.

There are many reports of animal experiments demonstrating the carcinogenicity of cigarette smoke (49–57). Attempts have also been made to identify the carcinogens in cigarette smoke condensates and the presence of carcinogenic compounds such as benzo(a)pyrene and nitroso compounds like DMN, DEN and nitrosonornicotine have been demonstrated (49, 50, 58–63). However, fractionation of cigarette smoke condensate (64) and tests on the carcinogenicities of the fractions on animals are time-consuming and laborious. Thus, it seems better to test for mutagenic compounds in cigarette smoke condensates. Some experiments along this line have already been reported (65, 66). Recently we also examined the mutagenicity of a cigarette smoke condensate. The cigarette smoke condensate was trapped on glass fiber paper and about 30 mg of condensate were obtained per cigarette by the standard method (64). This condensate was dissolved in DMSO and its mutagenicity was tested on S. typhimurium TA100 or TA98. In Fig. 9 the mutagenicity of cigarette smoke condensate on S. typhimurium TA100 is compared with that of benzo(a)pyrene, a known carcinogen in the cigarette smoke condensate. The cigarette smoke condensate showed clear dose-dependent mutagenicity when it was

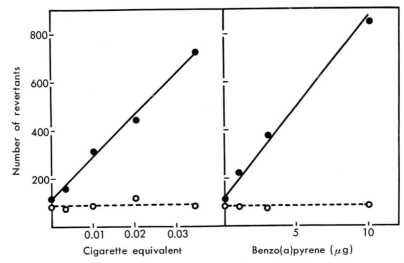

Fig. 9.   Mutagenicities of cigarette smoke condensate and benzo(a)pyrene revealed on *S. typhimurium* TA100. The amount of cigarette smoke condensate is expressed as cigarette equivalent. About 30 mg condensate was obtained from one cigarette by a standard method. ● +S-9 Mix; ○ −S-9 Mix.

activated with liver microsomes, but without S-9 Mix, it showed no mutagenicity. Similar results were obtained with benzo(a)pyrene. One cigarette is reported to contain about 17 ng of benzo(a)pyrene (*49, 67*). However, the mutagenicity of the cigarette smoke condensate was equivalent to 220 μg of benzo(a)pyrene, or more than 10,000-fold its actual benzo(a)pyrene content. This suggests that it contains other mutagenic compounds besides benzo(a)pyrene as also suggested by other workers (*65, 66*). The same is probably true of the carcinogens in cigarettes. The smoke condensate from cigars also showed mutagenicity comparable to that from cigarettes. Attempts have been made to reduce the amounts of nicotine and benzo(a)pyrene in cigarettes but judging from the mutation test described above, this alone will not reduce the amounts of carcinogens in cigarettes very much, and the other more potent mutagen(s) and possibly also carcinogen(s) present must be identified and eliminated. To find these compounds it seems easier to test for compounds which are mutagenic to bacteria, than for those which are carcinogenic to animals.

DISCUSSION AND CONCLUSIONS

There is now known to be a close correlation between carcinogens and mutagens and the mutagenicity test has been shown to be a practically useful method of screening for environmental carcinogens. Once a substance has been found to be mutagenic, great efforts should be made to find out whether it is also carcinogenic, as is evidenced in the case of AF-2. This also seems to be the case with cigarette smoke condensate and other components besides benzo(a)pyrene should be considered as potential carcinogens.

As shown in Figs. 1 and 4, there are still some mutagens which have not been shown to be carcinogenic. One of these is sodium nitrite. However, results suggesting the carcinogenicity of this compound on culture cells have been reported (*68*), and again indicate the necessity for more extensive experiments on its possible carcinogenicity. Conversely, it is also an important and urgent problem to develop more sensitive assay systems to detect the mutagenicities of substances which have so far proved carcinogenic but not mutagenic.

Among the many mutation test systems so far available, that using auxotroph mutants of bacteria is one of the most simple and sensitive and it can be used to test many kinds of substances. This microbial assay system, when used in combination with a drug-activating system from liver microsomes (*7*), has made it possible to demonstrate the mutagenicities of many chemicals, including well-known carcinogens, which did not appear mutagenic using other tests. Furthermore the introduction of the R-factor plasmid into *S. typhimurium* increased its sensitivity to many carcinogens (*24*). Improvements in these systems for detecting mutagens have also facilitated studies on the ultimate or direct forms of metabolites of many carcinogens. Conclusions on the ultimate forms of carcinogens such as azo dyes and dialkylnitrosamines obtained from mutation tests using bacteria and microsomes from rat liver were in good agreement with results on the *in vitro* interactions of these metabolites with intracellular components.

Mutation has long been suggested to be the mechanism of carcinogenesis and the hypothesis that cancer is induced by alteration of the primary structure of DNA seems to be well supported by the correlation of the carcinogenic and mutagenic effects of many compounds. However, it should be mentioned that some of the substances which are both carcinogenic and mutagenic, such as MNNG, N-acetoxy-MAB, and N-benzoyloxy-MAB, interact with proteins as well as DNA. Moreover, many carcinogens and mutagens can interact with RNA as well as DNA. Thus, it is possible that alterations in post-transcriptional events may trigger off the processes of malignant transformation.

The mechanisms of the inductions of cancer and mutation may be different so that carcinogenesis and mutagenesis must be considered separately even though carcinogens have been shown to overlap mutagens. However, it is strongly emphasized that detection of environmental compounds as mutagens is a very useful practical method to screen for carcinogens and thus it contributes greatly to the prevention of cancer.

NOTE ADDED IN PROOF

Extensive study on the correlation between mutagens and carcinogens was made by Ames and his colleagues. Data on mutagenicity and carcinogenicity of various compounds were recently published as a series of papers (J. McCann, E. Choi, E. Yamasaki, and B. N. Ames, Detection of carcinogens as mutagens in the *Salmonella*/microsome test: Assay of 300 chemicals. Proc. Natl. Acad. Sci. U.S., *72*: 5135–5139, 1975; J. McCann and B. N. Ames, Detection of carcinogens as mutagens in the *Salmonella*/microsome test: Assay of 300 chemicals: Discussion. Proc. Natl. Acad. Sci. U.S., *73*: 950–954, 1976).

ACKNOWLEDGMENTS

Authors are indebted to Professor Bruce N. Ames, University of California, Berkeley, and Professor Dennis R. McCalla, McMaster University, Hamilton, Ontario, for providing bacterial strains. This work was supported by grants from the Ministry of Health and Welfare, the Ministry of Education, Science and Culture, Japan, the Society for Promotion of Cancer Research and Nissan Science Foundation.

REFERENCES

1. Wynder, E. L. and Shigematsu, T.   Environmental factors of cancer of the colon and rectum. Cancer, *20*: 1520–1561, 1967.
2. Gregor, O., Toman, R., and Prasova, F.   Gastrointestinal cancer and nutrition. Gut, *10*: 1031–1034, 1969.
3. Drasar, B. S. and Irving, D.   Environmental factors and cancer of the colon and breast. Br. J. Cancer, *27*: 167–172, 1973.
4. Oiso, T.   Incidence of stomach cancer and its relation to dietary habits and nutrition in Japan between 1900 and 1975. Cancer Res., *35*: 3254–3258, 1975.
5. Hirayama, T.   Epidemiology of cancer of the stomach with special reference to its recent decrease in Japan. Cancer Res., *35*: 3460–3463, 1975.
6. Ames, B. N., Lee, F. D., and Durston, W. E. An improved bacterial test system for the detection and classification of mutagens and carcinogens. Proc. Natl. Acad. Sci. U.S., *70*: 782–786, 1973.
7. Ames, B. N., Durston, W. E., Yamasaki, E., and Lee, F. D.   Carcinogens are mutagens: A simple test system combining liver homogenates for activation and bacteria for detection. Proc. Natl. Acad. Sci. U.S., *70*: 2281–2285, 1973.
8. Nakahara, W., Fukuoka, F., and Sugimura, T.   Carcinogenic action of 4-nitroquinoline-N-oxide. Gann, *48*: 129–137, 1957.
9. Pasternak, L.   Mutagene Wirkung von Dimethylnitrosamin bei *Drosophila melanogaster*. Naturwissenschaften, *49*: 381, 1962.
10. Maher, V. M., Miller, E. C., Miller, J. A., and Szybalski, W.   Mutations and decreases in density of transforming DNA produced by derivatives of carcinogens 2-acetylaminofluorene and N-methyl-4-aminoazobenzene. Mol. Pharmacol., *4*: 411–426, 1968.
11. Ames, B. N., Sims, P., and Grover, P. L.   Epoxides of carcinogenic polycyclic hydrocarbons are frameshift mutagens. Science, *176*: 47–49, 1972.
12. Yahagi, T., Degawa, M., Seino, Y., Matsushima, T., Nagao, M., Sugimura, T., and Hashimoto, Y.   Mutagenicities of carcinogenic azo dyes and their derivatives. Cancer Lett., *1*: 91–96, 1975.
13. Druckrey, H., Preussmann, R., Ivankovic, S., Schmidt, C. H., Mennel, H. D., and Stahl, K. W.   Selektive Erzeugung von Blasenkrebs an Ratten durch Dibutyl- und N-Butyl-N-butanol(4)-nitrosamin. Z. Krebsforsh., *66*: 280–290, 1964.
14. Druckrey, H., Preussmann, R., Ivankovic, S., So, B. T., Schmidt, C. H., and Bücheler, J. Zur Erzeugung Subcutaner Sarkome an Ratten. Carcinogen Wirkung von Hydrazodicarbonsäure-bis-methyl-nitrosamid, N-Nitroso-N-*n*-butyl-harnstoff,

N-Methyl-N-nitroso-nitroguanidin und N-Nitroso-imidazolidon. Z. Krebsforsch., *68*: 87–102, 1966.

15. Schoental, R. Carcinogenic activity of N-methyl-N-nitroso-N'-nitroguanidine. Nature, *209*: 726–727, 1966.

16. Sugimura, T., Nagao, M., and Okada, Y. Carcinogenic activity of N-methyl-N'-nitro-N-nitrosoguanidine. Nature, *210*: 962–963, 1966.

17. Mandell, J. D. and Greenberg, J. A new chemical mutagen for bacteria, 1-methyl-3-nitro-1-nitrosoguanidine. Biochem. Biophys. Res. Commun., *3*: 575–577, 1960.

18. Kondo, S. and Ichikawa-Ryo, H. Testing and classification of mutagenicity of furylfuramide in *Escherichia coli*. Japan. J. Genet., *48*: 295–300, 1973.

19. Kada, T. *Escherichia coli* mutagenicity of furylfuramide. Japan. J. Genet., *48*: 301–305, 1973.

20. Ikeda, Y. Chronic toxicity of furylfuramide to mice. Report to Food Sanitary Committee of the Ministry of Health and Welfare, Japan 1974 (in Japanese).

21. Nomura, T. Carcinogenicity of the food additive furylfuramide in foetal and young mice. Nature, *258*: 610–611, 1975.

22. Ames, B. N. The detection of chemical mutagens with enteric bacteria. *In;* A. Hollaender (ed.), Chemical Mutagens. Principles and Methods for Their Detection, vol. 1, pp. 267–282, Plenum Press, New York, 1971.

23. Sugimura, T., Yahagi, T., Nagao, M., Takeuchi, M., Kawachi, T., Hara, K., Yamasaki, E., and Matsushima, T. Validity of mutagenicity tests using microbes as a rapid screening method for environmental carcinogens. *In;* R. Montesano, H. Bartsch, and L. Tomatis (eds.), IARC Scientific Publications No. 12, Lyon, 1976, in press.

24. McCann, J., Spingarn, N. E., Kobori, J., and Ames, B. N. Detection of carcinogens as mutagens: Bacterial tester strains with R factor plasmids. Proc. Natl. Acad. Sci. U.S., *72*: 979–983, 1975.

25. Yoshida, T. Über die Experimentelle Erzeugung von Hepatom durch die Fütterung mit *o*-Aminoazotoluol. Proc. Imp. Acad. Japan, *8*: 464–467, 1932.

26. Druckrey, H., Preussmann, R., Ivankovic, S., and Schmähl, D. Organotrope carcinogene Wirkungen bei 65 verschiedenen N-Nitro-Verbindungen an BD-Ratten. Z. Krebsforsch., *69*: 103–201, 1967.

27. Druckrey, H., Landschutz, Ch., and Preussmann, R. Oesophagus-Carcinome nach Inhalation von Methyl-butyl-nitrosamin (MBNA) an Ratten. Z. Krebsforsh., *71*: 135–139, 1968.

28. Okada, M., Suzuki, E., Aoki, J., Iiyoshi, M., and Hashimoto, Y. Metabolism and carcinogenicity of N-butyl-N-(4-hydroxybutyl)nitrosamine and related compounds, with special reference to induction of urinary bladder tumors. GANN Monogr. Cancer Res., *17*: 161–176, 1975.

29. Lijinsky, W. and Taylor, H. W. Induction of urinary bladder tumors in rats by administration of nitrosomethyldodecylamine. Cancer Res., *35*: 958–961, 1975.

30. Hirao, K., Shimohara, Y., Tsuda, H., Fukushima, S., Takahashi, M., and Ito, N. Carcinogenic activity of quinoline on rat liver. Cancer Res., *36*: 329–335, 1976.

31. Poirier, L. A., Miller, J. A., Miller, E. C., and Sato, K. N-Benzoyloxy-N-methyl-4-aminoazobenzene: Its carcinogenic activity in the rat and its reactions with proteins and nucleic acids and their constituents *in vitro*. Cancer Res., *27*: 1600–1613, 1967.

32. Okada, M., Suzuki, E., Anjo, T., and Mochizuki, M. Mutagenicity of α-acetoxy-

dialkylnitrosamines; model compounds for an ultimate carcinogen. Gann, *66*: 457–458, 1975.

33. Miller, J. A. Carcinogenesis by chemicals: An overview—G. H. A. Clowes memorial lecture. Cancer Res., *30*: 559–576, 1970.

34. Miller, E. C., and Miller, J. A. Studies on the mechanism of activation of aromatic amine and amide carcinogens to ultimate carcinogenic electrophilic reactants. Ann. N.Y. Acad. Sci., *163*: 731–750, 1969.

35. Ames, B. N., Gurney, E. G., Miller, J. A., and Bartsch, H. Carcinogens as frameshift mutagens: Metabolites and derivatives of 2-acetylaminofluorene and other aromatic amine carcinogens. Proc. Natl. Acad. Sci. U.S., *69*: 3128–3132, 1972.

36. Durston, W. E. and Ames, B. N. A simple method for the detection of mutagens in urine; studies with the carcinogen 2-acetylaminofluorene. Proc. Natl. Acad. Sci. U.S., *71*: 737–741, 1974.

37. Hashimoto, Y. and Degawa, M. Synthesis of N-hydroxy-4-(methylamino)azobenzene and its acetate, and their reactivity to amino acids. Gann, *66*: 215–216, 1975.

38. Malaveille, C., Bartsch, H., Grover, P. L., and Sims, P. Mutagenicity of non-K-region diols and diol-epoxides of benz(a)anthracene and benzo(a)pyrene. Biochem. Biophys. Res. Commun., *66*: 693–700, 1975.

39. Wislocki, P. G., Wood, A. W., Chang, R. L., Levin, W., Yagi, H., Hernandez, O., Jerina, D. M., and Conney, A. H. High mutagenicity and toxicity of a diol epoxide derived from benzo[a]pyrene. Biochem. Biophys. Res. Commun., *68*: 1006–1012, 1976.

40. Yahagi, T., Matsushima, T., Nagao, M., Seino, Y., Sugimura, T., and Bryan, G. T. Mutagenicities of nitrofuran derivatives on a bacterial tester strain with an R factor plasmid. Mutat. Res., *40*: 9–14, 1976.

41. Yahagi, T., Nagao, M., Hara, K., Matsushima, T., Sugimura, T., and Bryan, G. T. Relationships between the carcinogenic and mutagenic or DNA-modifying effects of nitrofuran derivatives, including 2-(2-furyl)-3-(5-nitro-2-furyl)acrylamide, a food additive. Cancer Res., *34*: 2266–2273, 1974.

42. Tazima, Y. and Onimaru, K. Results of mutagenicity for some nitrofuran derivatives in a sensitive test system with silkworm oocytes. Mutat. Res., *26*: 440, 1974.

43. Ong, T. and Shahin, M. M. Mutagenic and recombinogenic activities of the food additive furylfuramide in eukaryotes. Science, *184*: 1084–1087, 1974.

44. Wild, D. Mutagenicity of the food additive AF-2, a nitrofuran, in *Escherichia coli* and Chinese hamster cells in culture. Mutat. Res., *31*: 197–199, 1975.

45. McCalla, D. R., Olive, P., Tu, Y., and Fan, M. L. Nitrofurazone-reducing enzymes in *E. coli* and their role in drug activation *in vivo*. Can. J. Microbiol., *21*: 1484–1491, 1975.

46. Ochsner, A. Smoking and Health, Fifth Printing, Julian Messner, Inc., New York, 1962.

47. The Royal College of Physicians of London. Smoking and Health. Pitman Medical Publ. Co., London, 1962.

48. U.S. Public Health Serv. Publ. No. 74-8704. The Health Consequences of Smoking, 1974.

49. Orris, L., Van Duuren, B. L., Kosak, A. I., Nelson, N., and Schmitt, F. L. The carcinogenicity for mouse skin and aromatic hydrocarbon content of cigarette-smoke condensates. J. Natl. Cancer Inst., *21*: 557–561, 1958.

50. Wynder, E. L. and Hoffmann, D.   Experimental Tobacco Carcinogenesis. *In;* A. Haddow and S. Weinhouse (eds.), Adv. Cancer Res., vol. 8, pp. 249–453, Academic Press, New York, 1964.

51. Wynder, E. L. and Hoffmann, D.   Experimental tobacco carcinogenesis. Science, *162*: 862–871, 1968.

52. Van Duuren, B. L.   Tobacco Carcinogenesis. Cancer Res., *28*: 2357–2362, 1968.

53. Bock, F. G., Swain, A. P., and Stedman, R. L.   Bioassay of major fractions of cigarette smoke condensate by an accelarated technic. Cancer Res., *29*: 584–587,1969.

54. Bock, F. G., Swain, A. P., and Stedman, R. L.   Composition studies on tobacco. XLIV. Tumor-promoting activity of subfractions of the weak acid fraction of cigarette smoke condensate. J. Natl. Cancer Inst., *47*: 429–436, 1971.

55. Freeman, A. E., Kelloff, G. J., Gilden, R. V., Lane, W. T., Swain, A .P., and Huebner, R. J.   Activation and isolation of hamster-specific C-type RNA viruses from tumors induced by cell cultures transformed by chemical carcinogens. Proc. Natl. Acad. Sci. U.S., *68*: 2386–2390, 1971.

56. Van Duuren, B. L., Sivak, A., Katz, C., and Melchionne, S.   Cigarette smoke carcinogenesis: Importance of tumor promoters. J. Natl. Cancer Inst., *47*: 235–240, 1971.

57. Rhim, J. S. and Huebner, R. J.   *In vitro* transformation assay of major fractions of cigarette smoke condensate (CSC) in mammalian cell lines. Proc. Soc. Exp. Biol. Bed., *142*: 1003–1007, 1973.

58. Wynder, E. L. and Hoffmann, D.   A study of tobacco carcinogens No. 8. Role of acidic fractions as promoters. Cancer, *14*: 1306–1315, 1961.

59. Serfontein, W. J. and Hurter, P.   Nitrosamines as environmental carcinogens. II. Evidence for the presence of nitrosamines in tobacco smoke condensate. Cancer Res., *26*: 575–579, 1966.

60. Stedman, R. L.   The chemical composition of tobacco and tobacco smoke. Chem. Rev., *68*: 153–207, 1968.

61. Hoffmann, D., Hecht, S. S., Ornaf, R. M., and Wynder, E. L.   N'-Nitrosonornicotine in tobacco. Science, *186*: 265–267, 1974.

62. Hecht, S. S., Ornaf, R. M., and Hoffmann, D.   Chemical studies on tobacco smoke. XXXIII. N'-Nitrosonornicotine in tobacco: Analysis of possible contributing factors and biological implications. J. Natl. Cancer Inst., *54*: 1237–1244, 1974.

63. Hecht, S. S., Thorne, R. L., Maronpot, R. R., and Hoffmann, D.   A study of tobacco carcinogenesis. XIII. Tumor-promoting subfractions of the weakly acidic fraction. J. Natl. Cancer Inst., *55*: 1329–1336, 1976.

64. Swain, A. P., Cooper, J. E., and Stedman, R. L.   Large-scale fractionation of cigarette smoke condensate for chemical and biological investigations. Cancer Res., *29*: 579–583, 1969.

65. Kier, L. D., Yamasaki, E., and Ames, B. N.   Detection of mutagenic activity in cigarette smoke condensates. Proc. Natl. Acad. Sci. U.S., *71*: 4159–4163, 1974.

66. Hutton, J. J. and Hackney, C.   Metabolism of cigarette smoke condensates by human and rat homogenates to form mutagens detectable by *Salmonella typhimurium* TA1538. Cancer Res., *35*: 2461–2468, 1975.

67. Patel, A. R., Hag, M. Z., Innerarity, C. L., Innerarity, L. T., and Weissgraber, K.   Fractionation studies of smoke condensate samples from Kentucky reference cigarettes. Tobacco Sci., *60*: 61–62, 1974.

68. Tsuda, H., Inui, N., and Takayama, S.   *In vitro* transformation of newborn hamster cells by sodium nitrite. Biochem. Biophys. Res. Commun., *55*: 1117–1124. 1973.

Discussion of Paper of Drs. Sugimura et al.

DR. WEISBURGER: How about the problem of the mutagenicity by chemicals like hydroxylamine or 8-hydroxyquinoline which we have tested and found to be non-carcinogenic?

DR. SUGIMURA: Their situation is very close to bromodeoxyuridine (BudR) and NaNO₂. As a first screening test of environmental carcinogens, the mutagenic assay using microbes should include a number of non-carcinogenic but mutagenic compounds. It is necessary to allow a safety margin for the test method itself. In the case of 8-hydroxyquinoline, I feel that more intensive carcinogenesis experiments are required.

DR. WATTENBERG: Does your procedure detect weak carcinogens such as safrole, DDT, and cyclamates?

DR. SUGIMURA: No, I do not think so. Many more modifications and supplementation of the test system are needed to detect weak carcinogens. The use of mouse liver enzymes should also be considered for the activation step.

DR. HIRAYAMA: I should like to ask the chairman to express his comments on Dr. Sugimura's very important and impressive remarks on the mutagenicity of cigarette smoke condensate, especially with regard to the role of benzo(a)pyrene. This is of crucial relevance when one considers production of less harmful cigarettes.

DR. SUGIMURA: Thank you. I would like to emphasize that mutagenicity test using microbes should be introduced more effectively into the technology to develop a so-called "less harmful tobacco product."

DR. GELBOIN: Have you examined the condensates from cigarettes with different tar contents?

DR. SUGIMURA: We have tried many brands of Japanese cigarettes and obtained almost similar mutagenic potentials in their condensates. Condensates from cigars also were very mutagenic.

DR. GELBOIN: (1) Have you examined the effect of the tar on the aryl hydrocarbon hydroxylase (AHH) system? (2) Do the mutagenic effects correlate with the amount of tar in the cigarette?

DR. SUGIMURA: (1) No, I have not tried that. (2) I have no exact data on comparison of mutagenic potentials and total tar content in different cigarettes. However, the specific mutagenic activity per mg tar weight is about same in many specimens.

DR. ANDOH: You listed BudR and $NaNO_2$ as non-carcinogens. BudR induces C-type virus which in turn proved to be carcinogenic. So, this compound might be called a carcinogen. $NaNO_2$ was shown to be carcinogenic in *in vitro* transformation system. What do you think?

DR. SUGIMURA: BudR certainly induces C-type particles. However, I do not think BudR can induce malignant tumors. It is hard to say that BudR is carcinogenic. As Dr. S. Takayama reported, $NaNO_2$ transformed cultured hamster embryonic cells, but no report indicating the carcinogenic action of $NaNO_2$ by itself is available yet. It is reasonable to list BudR and $NaNO_2$ as non-carcinogenic compounds at the present moment.

FUNDAMENTALS IN CANCER PREVENTION, P. N. MAGEE ET AL. (EDS.),
UNIV. OF TOKYO PRESS, TOKYO / UNIV. PARK PRESS, BALTIMORE, PP. 217–228, 1976

Metabolic Activation of 4-Nitroquinoline 1-Oxide and Its Binding to Nucleic Acid

Mitsuhiko TADA and Mariko TADA

Laboratory of Biochemistry, Aichi Cancer Center Research Institute, Nagoya, Japan

Abstract: 4-Hydroxyaminoquinoline 1-oxide (4HAQO), the reduced metabolite
of 4-nitroquinoline 1-oxide (4NQO), was bound to nucleic acid *in vitro via* catalysis
of seryl-tRNA synthetase from yeast. Studies on the mechanism of the enzyme
reaction revealed that 4HAQO was activated through acylation by seryl-AMP
formed on the intermediary complex in the seryl-tRNA synthetase reaction. The
isolated seryl-AMP-enzyme complex or synthetic seryl-AMP can activate 4HAQO.
The reactive metabolite produced in the reaction may be assumed to be an aminoacylated derivative which may attack purine residues in nucleic acid.

Among the aminoacyl-tRNA synthetases in baker's yeast cells, only seryl-
tRNA synthetase had the ability to activate 4HAQO. Seryl- and prolyl-tRNA
synthetases in rat liver and seryl- and phenylalanyl-tRNA synthetases in *Escherichia
coli* may participate in the activation of 4HAQO.

In the *in vitro* enzyme reaction, 4HAQO bound to poly(G) and poly(A) to give
rise to three kinds of adducts (two guanine-adducts and one adenine-adduct) which
were identical with the major products found in the RNA isolated from 4NQO-
treated cells. In DNA isolated from 4NQO-treated cells, an additional adduct was
found other than these three. Chemical structure of adenine adduct was proposed
to be either 3-(N[6]-adenyl)-4-aminoquinoline 1-oxide or 3-(N[1]-adenyl)-4-amino-
quinoline 1-oxide.

Since Nakahara *et al.* found the carcinogenicity of 4-nitroquinoline 1-oxide
(4NQO) (*1*), extensive studies have been carried out on the mechanisms of carcinogenic and mutagenic action of this compound (see Refs. *2–4*). Studies on the
metabolism of 4NQO *in vivo* (*5, 6*) and *in vitro* (*7–9*) revealed that 4NQO was
converted to 4-hydroxyaminoquinoline 1-oxide (4HAQO) and then to noncarcinogenic 4-aminoquinoline 1-oxide (4AQO). In rat liver the reduction is catalysed
by cytosol and microsomal enzymes with the oxidation of NADH or NADPH.
The same metabolic conversion was observed in microbes such as *Escherichia coli*

217

and *Aspergillus niger* in which 4HAQO proved its mutagenic activity (*10, 11*). A good correlation was found between carcinogenic activity and the susceptibility of various 4NQO derivatives to enzymic reduction to give the corresponding 4HAQO derivatives (*8*). From these results, it has been generally believed that the metabolic reduction of 4NQO to 4HAQO is an essential process in the 4NQO carcinogenesis.

When mammalian or microbial cells were treated with 4NQO or 4HAQO, the carcinogen bound covalently to cellular macromolecules including DNA (*12–20*). Although 4HAQO binds to nucleic acid *in vivo*, the binding rarely occurs in buffer solutions. Therefore we presumed a metabolic activation of 4HAQO to be involved in the *in vivo* binding reaction and demonstrated the presence of an activating enzyme in extracts of rat ascites hepatoma cells (*21, 22*) and baker's yeast (*22*). The cytosol fractions of these cells catalysed the binding of 4HAQO to nucleic acid or protein in the presence of ATP and Mg^{2+} (*21*); however, the enzyme, when further purified, required a factor present in the heated extract of the hepatoma cell cytosol fraction other than ATP and Mg^{2+}. The main active substance in the extract was isolated and identified as amino acid L-serine (*22*). The elucidation of the requirement for the enzyme reaction made it possible to achieve further purification of the enzyme (*23*). In this paper we will report our recent findings on the mechanism of 4HAQO activation and the binding of the metabolite to nucleic acid.

Mechanism of 4HAQO Activation by Aminoacyl-tRNA Synthetase

The 4HAQO-activating enzyme was purified from commercial baker's yeast to homogeneity. Studies on the reaction mechanism of 4HAQO activation by this enzyme revealed that the purified enzyme was seryl-tRNA synthetase (*23*). The conclusion was drawn from the following results. (1) The enzyme preparation is essentially homogeneous as judged by polyacrylamide gel electrophoresis and sedimentation analysis. (2) The enzyme requires ATP and L-serine for the 4HAQO activation. In the reaction ATP is converted to AMP and pyrophosphate, while L-serine remains unchanged. (3) The purified enzyme has seryl-tRNA synthesizing activity. (4) The specific activity of seryl-tRNA synthesis in the final preparation is as high as that of the highly purified yeast seryl-tRNA synthetase reported by Heider *et al.* (*24*). (5) Seryl-tRNA synthetase activity is associated with the 4HAQO-activating enzyme throughout the purification steps. (6) These two activities cannot be separated by chromatography on DEAE-cellulose or Sephadex G-200 or by centrifugation on a sucrose density gradient. (7) Both activities show the same stability against heat inactivation.

The reaction of most aminoacyl-tRNA synthetases have been considered to occur in two consecutive steps:

$$\text{Amino acid} + \text{ATP} + \text{Enzyme} \rightleftharpoons \text{Aminoacyl-AMP-enzyme} + \text{PP}_i$$

$$\text{Aminoacyl-AMP-enzyme} + \text{tRNA} \rightleftharpoons \text{Aminoacyl-tRNA} + \text{AMP} + \text{Enzyme}$$

In the first reaction aminoacyl-AMP is made on the enzyme molecule and in the second reaction the intermediary complex transfers amino acid to tRNA. We assume that 4HAQO is acylated by seryl-AMP formed on sreyl-tRNA synthetase and that

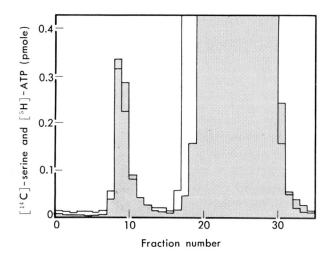

FIG. 1.   Isolation of seryl-AMP-enzyme complex on Sephadex G-75. Seryl-tRNA synthetase from yeast (800 μg) was incubated with 4 μmoles of [¹⁴C]-ʟ-serine (specific activity, 10 μCi/μmole), 0.8 μmole [³H]-ATP (specific activity, 10 μCi/μmole), 4 μmoles of Mg(OAc)₂, 0.8 μmole of dithiothreitol (DTT), and 40 μmoles of sodium borate (pH 8.9) in a final volume of 0.8 ml. After incubation for 5 min at 30°C, the mixture was chromatographed on a Sephadex G-75 column (0.8 × 28 cm), preequilibrated at 4°C with 0.02 ᴍ sodium succinate (pH 6.0) containing 1 mᴍ Mg(OAc)₂, 1 mᴍ EDTA-MgNa₂, and 1 mᴍ DTT ; elution was carried out with the same buffer and 1-ml fractions were collected.   ¹⁴C □ ;   ³H ▨.

TABLE 1.   4HAQO-binding Reaction in Various Activation Systems

	Reaction system		
	(1)[a]	(2)[b]	(3)[c]
	Enzyme ʟ-Serine ATP Mg(OAc)₂ DTT Buffer [³H]-4HAQO RNA	Seryl-AMP-enzyme complex DTT Buffer [³H]-4HAQO RNA	Seryl-AMP DTT Buffer [³H]-4HAQO RNA
Amount of 4HAQO bound to RNA	32.5 (nmole/nmole enzyme/min)	0.53 (nmole/nmole complex)	0.32 (nmole/nmole seryl-AMP)

[a] Reaction mixture (0.1 ml) for the system (1) contained 1 mᴍ [³H]-4HAQO (1.5 μCi/μmole), 3 mᴍ ATP, 10 mᴍ ʟ-serine, 3 mᴍ Mg(OAc)₂, 1 mᴍ DTT, 100 μg/ml bovine serum albumin, 20 mg/ml yeast RNA, 50 mᴍ Bicine-KOH (pH 9.0), and enzyme (1 μg of protein). After incubation at 30°C for 10 min, radioactivity of [³H]-4HAQO converted into acid-insoluble form was determined as described elsewhere (*21*, *23*).   [b] [³H]-4HAQO (1 mᴍ, 30 μCi/μmole) was reacted with yeast RNA (20 mg/ml) in the presence of seryl-AMP-enzyme complex (164 pmoles), 1 mᴍ DTT, and 50 mᴍ Bicine-KOH (pH 8.0) in the final volume of 0.2 ml at 0°C for 10 min.   [c] Reaction mixture contained 0.5 mᴍ seryl-AMP, 1 mᴍ [³H]-4HAQO (1.5 μCi/μmole), 1 mᴍ DTT, 50 mᴍ sodium borate (pH 8.0), and 20 mg/ml yeast RNA. Incubation was carried out at 30°C for 10 min (*23*).

seryl-4HAQO ultimately reacts with nucleic acid. The assumed mechanism of the reaction is as shown below.

$$\text{Serine} + \text{ATP} + \text{Enzyme} \rightleftharpoons \text{Seryl-AMP-enzyme} + \text{PP}_i$$

$$\text{Seryl-AMP-enzyme} + 4\text{HAQO} \longrightarrow \text{Seryl-4HAQO} + \text{AMP} + \text{Enzyme}$$

$$\text{Seryl-4HAQO} + \text{Nucleic acid} \longrightarrow 4\text{HAQO-nucleic acid} + \text{Serine}$$

To prove this assumption, we have isolated the seryl-AMP-enzyme complex and examined its ability to activate 4HAQO. When yeast seryl-tRNA synthetase was incubated with L-serine and ATP in the presence of Mg²⁺, the seryl-AMP-enzyme complex was formed. This was detected by use of radioactive substrate ([¹⁴C]-serine or [³H]-ATP) and gel filtration of the reaction mixture on Sephadex G-75. As can be seen in Fig. 1, fractions eluted just ahead of bulk serine and ATP contained the complex which consists of 1–2 moles of seryl-AMP and 1 mole of enzyme. The isolated complex was able to transfer serine to tRNA and was also able to activate 4HAQO to bind it to nucleic acid in the absence of serine and ATP in the reaction mixture (Table 1). The binding of 4HAQO to nucleic acid occurred even by the addition of synthetic seryl-AMP in the absence of the enzyme (23). This nonenzymic 4HAQO-binding reaction occurred by other kinds of

TABLE 2.   4HAQO Binding to RNA by Aminoacyl-AMP

	[³H]-4HAQO binding (cpm)
Seryl-AMP	7,003
Leucyl-AMP	15,200
Phenylalanyl-AMP	8,706
Prolyl-AMP	3,694

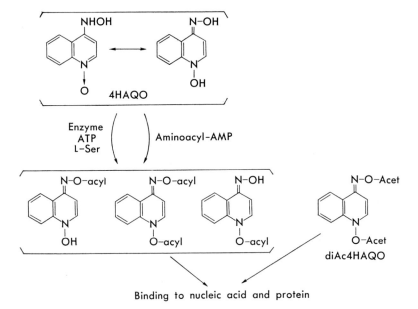

FIG. 2.   A possible mechanism of 4HAQO binding to nucleic acid and protein.

aminoacyl-AMP such as leucyl-AMP (Table 2). These results support our assumption that 4HAQO is activated through acylation by seryl-AMP formed on the intermediary complex in the seryl-tRNA synthetase reaction.

O,O′-Diacetyl-4HAQO which was synthesized by Kawazoe and Araki (*25*) readily reacts with nucleic acid (*26, 27*). From this model reaction, the reactive metabolite of 4HAQO produced in the enzyme system may be assumed to be an aminoacylated derivative which may attack the nucleophilic center of adenine and guanine in nucleic acid as shown in Fig. 2.

Aminoacyl-tRNA Synthetases Capable of 4HAQO Activation

Since many aminoacyl-tRNA synthetases are known to form aminoacyl-AMP-enzyme complexes as their reaction intermediates, it is expected that these amino-

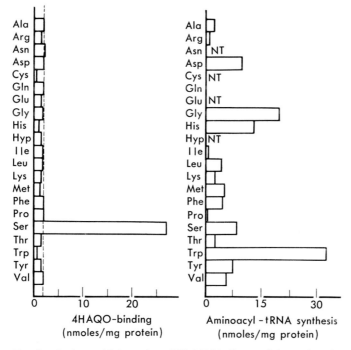

FIG. 3.   Amino acid-dependent 4HAQO-binding activity and aminoacyl-tRNA synthetases in baker's yeast. The disrupted cells from a French press were centrifuged at $105,000 \times g$ and the supernatant was dialysed against 0.02 M potassium phosphate (pH 7.0) containing 1 mM Mg(OAc)$_2$, 1 mM EDTA-MgNa$_2$, 1 mM mercaptoethanol, and 5% glycerol. The reaction mixture (0.1 ml) for the 4HAQO-binding assay contained 1 mM [^{3}H]-4HAQO (1.5 μCi/μmole), 2 mM ATP, 3 mM Mg(OAc)$_2$, 1 mM DTT, 10 mM phosphoenolpyruvate, 40 μg/ml pyruvate kinase, 20 mg/ml yeast RNA, 50 mM Bicine-KOH (pH 8.0), the dialysed $105,000 \times g$ supernatant (100 μg protein), and 10 mM one of amino acids indicated, except that tyrosine was added to yield 0.1 mM as a final concentration. The assay of aminoacyl-tRNA synthetase activity was carried out in 0.05 ml containing 0.1 mM [^{3}H]- or [^{14}C]-amino acid, 2 mM ATP, 10 mM Mg-(OAc)$_2$, 1 mM DTT, 10 mM phosphoenolpyruvate, 40 μg/ml pyruvate kinase, 5 mg/ml yeast tRNA, 50 mM Bicine-KOH (pH 8.0), and dialysed $105,000 \times g$ supernatant (26.5 μg protein). Both reactions were carried out at 37°C for 30 min (*23*). Broken line shows the level of the 4HAQO binding without the addition of amino acids.

acyl-tRNA synthetases are also effective for 4HAQO activation. It has been noted previously, however, that the 4HAQO-binding reaction, including the crude enzyme of baker's yeast, is stimulated only by L-serine (22). The reaction with the dialysed 105,000×g supernatant fraction of baker's yeast was stimulated by L-serine but not by other amino acids, although the fraction contained most kinds of aminoacyl-tRNA synthetases as shown in Fig. 3. This suggests that in yeast cells only seryl-tRNA synthetase has the ability to activate 4HAQO. Examination of the dependency of the 4HAQO-binding reaction with the dialysed 105,000×g supernatant fractions indicated that seryl- and prolyl-tRNA synthetases in rat liver or rat hepatoma cells and seryl- and phenylalanyl-tRNA synthetases in E. coli might participate in the activation of 4HAQO (Fig. 4). Association of the 4HAQO-binding activity with these aminoacyl-tRNA synthetases was demonstrated by DEAE-cellulose chromatography of the rat liver supernatant fraction (Fig. 5). As shown in Table 2 synthetic aminoacyl-AMPs are generally able to activate 4HAQO; however, a few particular aminoacyl-tRNA synthetases are able to activate 4HAQO. Aminoacyl-tRNA synthetases which are capable of 4HAQO activation may have a unique conformation around the aminoacyl-AMP binding site enabling them to aminoacylate the N-hydroxy group of the carcinogen. These aminoacyl-tRNA synthetases may participate *in vivo* in the metabolism not only

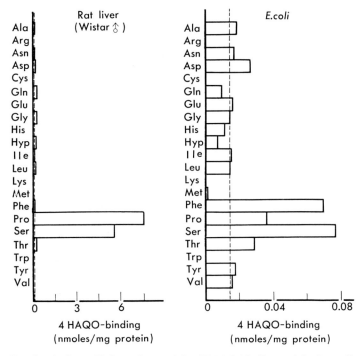

FIG. 4.　Amino acid dependency of the 4HAQO-binding activity in rat liver and *E. coli*. The activities in the dialysed 105,000×g supernatant of rat liver (male Wistar) and *E. coli* B were measured in the presence of amino acid. The reaction was carried out using dialysed 105,000×g supernatant of (A) rat liver (0.6 mg protein) and (B) *E. coli* (1.4 mg protein). Broken lines show the level of the 4HAQO binding without the addition of amino acids.

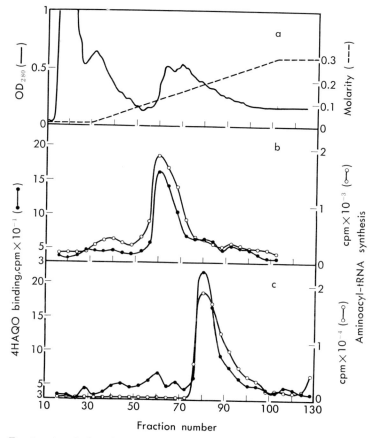

FIG. 5.   Association of the 4HAQO-binding activity with prolyl- and seryl-tRNA synthetases of rat liver. Livers from male Wistar rats were homogenized with 2 volumes of 0.1 M Tris-HCl (pH 7.5) by an Ultra Turrax homogenizer. The dialysed $105,000 \times g$ supernatant of the homogenate (360 mg protein) was applied to a DEAE-cellulose column (2.5×28 cm). Proteins were eluted with a linear gradient from 0.02 to 0.3 M potassium phosphate (pH 7.0) (a) 4HAQO-binding activities were assayed in the presence of either (b) L-proline or (c) L-serine. Prolyl- and seryl-tRNA synthetase activities were measured in the presence of rat liver tRNA.

of 4HAQO but also of some other N-hydroxy compounds through their amino-acylating capacity.

Adducts of 4HAQO with Guanine and Adenine

It has been suggested that the metabolite of 4NQO is bound covalently to the purine residues of nucleic acid *in vivo* (*14, 16*). The adducts derived from the reaction of purine with the carcinogen are detected by paper chromatography in the acid hydrolysate of RNA and DNA isolated from the hepatoma cells exposed to radioactive 4NQO (*14*). The same adducts are formed in RNA and DNA respectively reacted with 4HAQO *in vitro via* catalysis of seryl-tRNA synthetase from yeast or rat hepatoma cells (*21, 28*). In the *in vitro* enzyme system, we have examined the binding of 4HAQO with synthetic homopolyribonucleotides. As shown in Table

TABLE 3. Binding of 4HAQO to Homopolyribonucleotides[a]

Polynucleotide	Extent of 4HAQO binding (mmoles/mole P of nucleotide)
Poly (A)	9.4
Poly (G)	14.1
Poly (U)	1.2
Poly (C)	2.7

[a] Reaction mixture was as described in Table 1 except 10 μmoles P/ml of homopolyribonucleotides were used instead of yeast RNA.

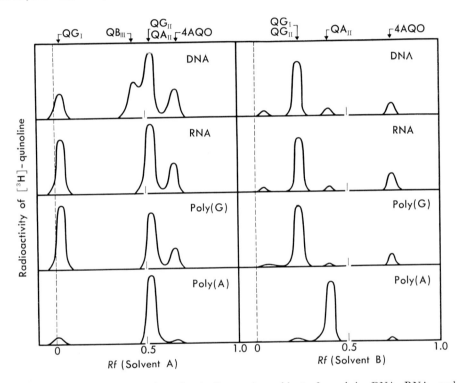

FIG. 6. Radiochromatography of quinoline-purine adducts formed in DNA, RNA, and homopolynucleotides. DNA and RNA were isolated from rat ascites hepatoma cells (AH130) exposed to [^{3}H]-4NQO (14). Poly (G) and poly (A) were reacted with [^{3}H]-4HAQO in the yeast seryl-tRNA synthetase system. DNA, RNA, and homopolynucleotides were hydrolysed by 1 N HCl and the hydrolysates were chromatographed on Whatman No. 1 filter paper either in solvent A (ethanol-water, 4 : 1, v/v) or in solvent B (n-butanol-formic acid-water, 77 : 10 : 13, v/v/v) (14).

3, 4HAQO bound specifically to poly(G) and poly(A), but negligibly to poly(U) and poly(C). Chromatographic analysis of the acid hydrolysates of poly(G) and poly(A) reacted with 4HAQO revealed two guanine adducts (QG$_I$ and QG$_{II}$) and one adenine adduct (QA$_{II}$) (Fig. 6). These three kinds of adducts were identical with the major products found in RNA and DNA isolated from 4NQO-treated cells. As reported previously (14) an additional adduct other than these three was

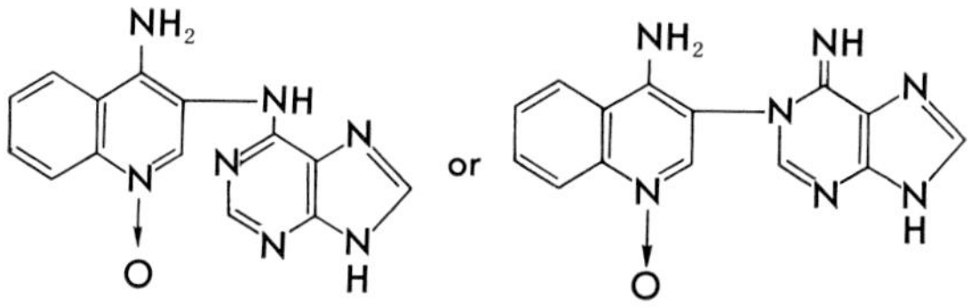

FIG. 7.   Proposed structure of quinoline-adenine adduct (QA$_{II}$).

found in DNA isolated from 4NQO-treated cells. This seemingly DNA-specific adduct (QB$_{III}$) could not be produced by the *in vitro* reaction of 4HAQO with synthetic homopolyribonucleotides.

We have isolated adenine adduct (QA$_{II}$) from poly(A) reacted with 4HAQO in the *in vitro* enzyme system. Working in cooperation with Kawazoe *et al.*, its chemical structure was proposed to be either 3-(N^6-adenyl)-4-aminoquinoline 1-oxide or 3-(N^1-adenyl)-4-aminoquinoline 1-oxide (*29*) (Fig. 7). Determination of the structure of the other adducts is in progress. For the elucidation of the molecular mechanism of carcinogenesis, mutagenesis, and DNA repair, these adducts await complete chemical identification.

ACKNOWLEDGMENTS

We are greatly indebted to Dr. Y. Kawazoe, National Cancer Center Research Institute (Tokyo), for his valuable discussions and gift of [^{3}H]-4HAQO throughout this work. This work was supported in part by Grants-in-Aid for Cancer Research from the Ministry of Education, Science and Culture, Japan.

REFERENCES

1. Nakahara, W., Fukuoka, F., and Sugimura, T.   Carcinogenic action of 4-nitro-quinoline 1-oxide. Gann, *48*: 129–137, 1957.
2. Endo, H., Ono, T., and Sugimura, T. (eds.). Chemistry and Biological Actions of 4-Nitroquinoline 1-Oxide, Springer-Verlag, Berlin, pp. 1–101, 1971.
3. Kawazoe, Y. and Araki, M.   Chemical problems in 4NQO carcinogenesis. *In;* W. Nakahara (ed.), Chemical Tumor Problems, pp. 45–104, Japanese Society for the Promotion of Science, Tokyo, 1970.
4. Nagao, M. and Sugimura, T.   Molecular biology of the carcinogen, 4-nitroquinoline 1-oxide. *In;* G. Klein and G. Weinhouse (ed.), Advances in Cancer Research, vol. 23, pp. 132–169, Academic Press, New York, 1976.
5. Okabayashi, T. and Yoshimoto, A.   Reduction of 4-nitroquinoline 1-oxide by microorganism. Chem. Pharm. Bull. (Tokyo), *10*: 1221–1226, 1962.
6. Sugimura, T., Okabe, K., and Endo, H.   The metabolism of 4-nitroquinoline 1-oxide. I. Conversion of 4-nitroquinoline 1-oxide to 4-aminoquinoline 1-oxide by rat liver enzyme. Gann, *56*: 489–501, 1965.
7. Sugimura, T., Okabe, K., and Nagao, M.   The metabolism of 4-nitroquinoline 1-oxide. III. An enzyme catalyzing the conversion of 4-nitroquinoline 1-oxide to 4-hydroxyaminoquinoline 1-oxide in rat liver and hepatomas. Cancer Res., *26*: 1717–1721, 1966.
8. Kato, R., Takahashi, A., and Oshima, T.   Characteristics of nitro reduction of the carcinogenic agent, 4-nitroquinoline N-oxide. Biochem. Pharm., *19*: 45–55, 1970.

9. Okabayashi, T., Yoshimoto, A., and Ide, M.   Mutagenic activity of 4-hydroxyamino-quinoline 1-oxide. Chem. Pharm. Bull. (Tokyo), *12*: 257–261, 1964.

10. Okabayashi, T., Ide, M., Yoshimoto, A., and Otsubo, M.   Mutagenic activity of 4-nitroquinoline 1-oxide and 4-hydroxyaminoquinoline 1-oxide on bacteria. Chem. Pharm. Bull. (Tokyo), *13*: 610–611, 1965.

11. Morita, T. and Mifuchi, I.   Characterization of respiration deficient mutant of *Saccharomyces cerevisiae* lacking cytochromes *a* and *c*. Biochem. Biophys. Res. Commun., *38*: 191–196, 1970.

12. Tada, M., Tada, M., and Takahashi, T.   Interaction of a carcinogen, 4-hydroxy-aminoquinoline-1-oxide with nucleic acid. Biochem. Biophys. Res. Commun., *29*: 469–477, 1967.

13. Tada, M., Tada, M., and Takahashi, T.   Interactions of chemical carcinogens and cellular macromolecules: 4-Hydroxyaminoquinoline-1-oxide and polynucleotides. *In;* Genetic Concepts and Neoplasia, pp. 214–227, Williams and Wilkins, Baltimore, 1970.

14. Tada, M. and Tada, M.   Interaction of a carcinogen, 4-nitroquinoline 1-oxide, with nucleic acids: Chemical degradation of the adducts. Chem.-Biol. Interact., *3*: 225–229, 1971.

15. Matsushima, T., Kobuna, I., and Sugimura, T.   *In vivo* interaction of 4-nitroquino-line-1-oxide and its derivatives with DNA. Nature, *216*: 508, 1967.

16. Ikegami, S., Nemoto, N., Sato, S., and Sugimura, T.   Binding of ^{14}C-labeled 4-nitroquinoline-1-oxide to DNA *in vivo*. Chem.-Biol. Interact., *1*: 321–330, 1969/70.

17. Andoh, T., Kato, K., Takaoka, T., and Katsuta, H.   Carcinogenesis in tissue culture. XIII. Binding of 4-nitroquinoline 1-oxide-^{3}H to nucleic acids and proteins of L·P3 and JTC-25·P3 cells. Int. J. Cancer, *7*: 455–467, 1971.

18. Kawazoe, Y., Huang, G.-F., Araki, M., and Koga, C.   Chemical binding of carcinogenic 4-nitroquinoline 1-oxide derivatives with DNA *in vivo* and *in vitro*. Gann, *63*: 161–166, 1972.

19. Ikenaga, M., Ishii, Y., Tada, M., Kakunaga, T., Takebe, H., and Kondo, S.   Excision-repair of 4-nitroquinoline 1-oxide damage responsible for killing, mutation and cancer. *In;* P. C. Hanawalt and R. B. Setlow (eds.), Molecular Mechanisms for Repair of DNA, part B, pp. 763–771, Plenum Press, New York, 1975.

20. Ikenaga, M., Ichikawa-Ryo, H., and Kondo, S.   The major cause of inactivation and mutation by 4-nitroquinoline 1-oxide in *Escherichia coli*: Excisable 4NQO-purine adducts. J. Mol. Biol., *92*: 341–356, 1975.

21. Tada, M. and Tada, M.   Enzymatic activation of the carcinogen 4-hydroxyamino-quinoline-1-oxide and its interaction with cellular macromolecules. Biochem. Biophys. Res. Commun., *46*: 1025–1032, 1972.

22. Tada, M. and Tada, M.   Requirement of L-serine for enzymic activation of carcinogen, 4-hydroxyaminoquinoline 1-oxide. Gann, *65*: 281–284, 1974.

23. Tada, M. and Tada, M.   Seryl-tRNA synthetase and activation of the carcinogen 4-nitroquinoline 1-oxide. Nature, *255*: 510–512, 1975.

24. Heider, H., Gottschalk, E., and Cramer, F.   Isolation and characterization of seryl-tRNA synthetase from yeast. Eur. J. Biochem., *20*: 144–152, 1971.

25. Kawazoe, Y. and Araki, M.   Studies on chemical carcinogens. V. *O,O′*-Diacetyl-4-hydroxyaminoquinoline 1-oxide. Gann, *58*: 485–487, 1967.

26. Enomoto, M., Sato, K., Miller, E. C., and Miller, J. A.   Reactivity of the diacetyl derivative of the carcinogen 4-hydroxyaminoquinoline 1-oxide with DNA, RNA, and other nucleophiles. Life Sci., *7*: 1025–1032, 1968.

27. Tada, M., Tada, M., Huang, G.-F., Araki, M., and Kawazoe, Y. Unpublished.
28. Tanooka, H., Tada, M., and Tada, M. Reparable lethal DNA damage produced by enzyme-activated 4-hydroxyaminoquinoline 1-oxide. Chem.-Biol. Interact., *10*: 11–18, 1975.
29. Kawazoe, Y., Araki, M., Huang, G.-F., Okamoto, T., Tada, M., and Tada, M. Chemical structure of QA_{II}, one of the covalently bound adducts of carcinogenic 4-nitroquinoline 1-oxide with nucleic acid bases of cellular nucleic acids. Chem. Pharm. Bull. (Tokyo), *23*: 3041–3043, 1975.

Discussion of Paper of Drs. Tada and Tada

DR. TROLL: Did you find 4-hydroxyaminoquinoline 1-oxide (4HAQO) to be mutagenic in yeast since you find the appropriate activating enzyme in this system?

DR. TADA: The mutagenicity of 4NQO, the parent carcinogen of 4HAQO has been reported by several authors (see Ref. *4*).

DR. SUTHERLAND: (1) What method of hydrolysis did you use on your synthetic polynucleotides? (2) Did you heat the mixtures? (3) Do you think that you might have adducts which are not stable to your hydrolysis procedures?

DR. TADA: (1) Hydrochloric acid. (2) Yes, in boiling water for 1 hr. (3) Yes, guanine adducts are fairly unstable and about 20% decomposed during hydrolysis adopted in the present study.

DR. LIEBERMAN: How have you identified your adenine adducts?

DR. TADA: The work has been done in cooperation with Dr. Kawazoe *et al.* He may be able to give a good explanation.

DR. KAWAZOE: We isolated about 1 mg of QA_{II} adduct from the treated nucleic acid. The structure was proposed on the basis of the data from NMR, mass spectra, and also pKa measurements of the preparation we isolated.

DR. GOLDTHWAIT: Do you have any idea of the structure of the guanine derivatives?

DR. TADA: No, not at the moment.

DR. GELBOIN: Does your rat liver preparation include microsomes?

DR. TADA: No, we used the $105,000 \times g$ supernatant fraction.

FUNDAMENTALS IN CANCER PREVENTION, P. N. MAGEE ET AL. (EDS.),
UNIV. OF TOKYO PRESS, TOKYO / UNIV. PARK PRESS, BALTIMORE ,PP. 229–249, 1976

Damage to DNA by Activated Nitrofurans

D. R. McCalla, P. L. Olive, and Yu Tu

Department of Biochemistry, McMaster University Health Sciences Centre, Hamilton, Ontario, Canada

Abstract: *Escherichia coli* contains three enzymes that reduce nitrofuran derivatives. Of these nitrofuran reductase I is active in air while the others are active only at low oxygen tensions. All catalyse the "activation" of nitrofurans to reactive compounds (identity unknown) which bind to protein, and to DNA. Breakage of DNA is observed when bacteria are incubated with nitrofurans under conditions which permit reduction of the drugs. No breaks or mutations are observed when there is no reduction. The end products of these enzymatic reductions are biologically inactive.

Mutations, like DNA breaks, are induced only when nitrofurans are activated. Strains lacking excision repair (*uvr⁻*) are more sensitive to both the lethal and mutagenic effects of nitrofurans, indicating that nitrofuran-induced lesions are repaired by "cut and patch" mechanisms. In *rec⁻* or *exr⁻* strains no mutations are observed implying that mutations are the consequence of repair *via* the "error prone" repair system.

The nature of the breaks formed in DNA has been probed using *E. coli* minicells which contain λdv DNA in a supercoiled form and nitrofuran reductase I. With this system we have shown that activated nitrofurazone causes both "true breaks" which are detected in neutral sucrose gradients as well as alkali-labile lesions which are converted into breaks in alkali. These two kinds of lesions are found in roughly equal numbers. It seems quite likely that the breaks are the result of nuclease action on nitrofurazone-damaged DNA since additional breaks result when DNA from treated minicells are incubated with extracts of *Micrococcus luteus*. In minicells the breaks and the lesions which are sensitive to *M. luteus* nuclease are repaired but alkali-labile lesions are not.

Mammalian cells contain several enzymes that reduce nitrofurans provided the O_2 tension is low. One or more of these enzymes activates nitrofurans to form compounds which break DNA. Again no breaks are observed when there is no reductive activation.

However, nitrofurans themselves have toxic effects on mammalian cells.

Exposure to the drugs in air results in a decrease in the rate of synthesis of macro-molecules and in lethality. However, as might be expected the lethal effects are much more pronounced under anoxic conditions than in air.

The DNA of mice was labelled by injecting [³H]-thymidine into newborn animals. These were later fed a diet containing 0.1% nitrofurazone. Nitrofurazone appeared to increase the rate of loss of labelled DNA from liver, lung, and brain while the rate of loss from kidney and spleen first increased and then decreased (probably as a consequence of reutilization of [³H]-thymidine released from degraded DNA). No histological changes were observed in the tissue of nitrofurazone-treated animals.

During the early 1940's, research groups in the United States and Germany prepared a number of derivatives of 5-nitro-2-furaldehyde and found that the presence of a nitro group at the 5 position of the furan ring produced a dramatic increase in antibacterial activity (1, 2). Some derivatives were highly effective *in vivo* and rapidly came into wide use in clinical medicine. Figure 1 shows the structures of some nitrofurans. In North America, nitrofurantoin, particularly, has found of considerable use in the treatment of urinary tract infections, nitrofurazone has been used in topical application and ophthalmic preparations and furazolidone is used to treat intestinal infections. In tropical areas yet other nitrofurans have been used as potential antischistosomal agents and against Chagas' disease (3). Nitrofuran derivatives are also added to feed for livestock and poultry as prophylaxis against parasites and bacterial infections and in Japan nitrofurazone and later furylfuramide (AF-2) were added to fish meal sausage, soy curd, and other foods to prevent bacterial spoilage (4).

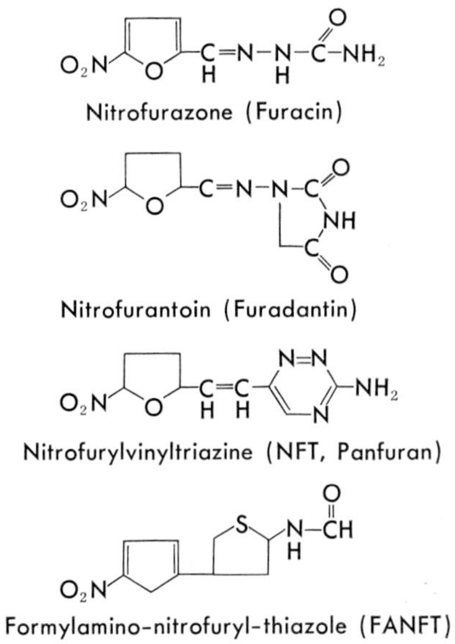

Nitrofurazone (Furacin)

Nitrofurantoin (Furadantin)

Nitrofurylvinyltriazine (NFT, Panfuran)

Formylamino-nitrofuryl-thiazole (FANFT)

FIG. 1.   Structural formulas of some nitrofuran derivatives.

By 1967, some 7,000 papers concerning the synthesis and use of nitrofurans had appeared (3). This vast literature continues to swell; several new derivatives being patented each year.

Although, as we will describe, there were clues in the published literature as far back as 1954 that nitrofurans might do genetic damage, it is only in the past few years that there has been real concern about the continued use of these compounds on humans.

This paper reviews current knowledge of the metabolic activation of nitrofurans, and the reaction of activated compounds with cellular constituents (in particular, DNA) and finally repair of nitrofuran-damaged DNA. We deal first with work on *Escherichia coli* where drug-resistant mutants have provided useful insight and then with work on mammalian cells.

Early studies established that nitrofurans are readily metabolized both by bacteria and animal tissues (5–7). Figure 2 summarizes some of this work. It is important to realize that the putative intermediates between the nitro and amino derivatives are based on indirect evidence and have never been isolated. Knowledge of the rate of buildup of the unstable intermediates which are believed to be the active agents is completely lacking. Other work has documented side-chain modifications of a number of derivatives (*e.g.*, 8–10) but most of these conversions are probably essentially irrelevant to a basic understanding of how nitrofurans exert their effects.

In 1958, a report by Asnis (6) indicated that reduction of nitrofurans produced compounds which were more toxic than the nitrofurans themselves. Normal,

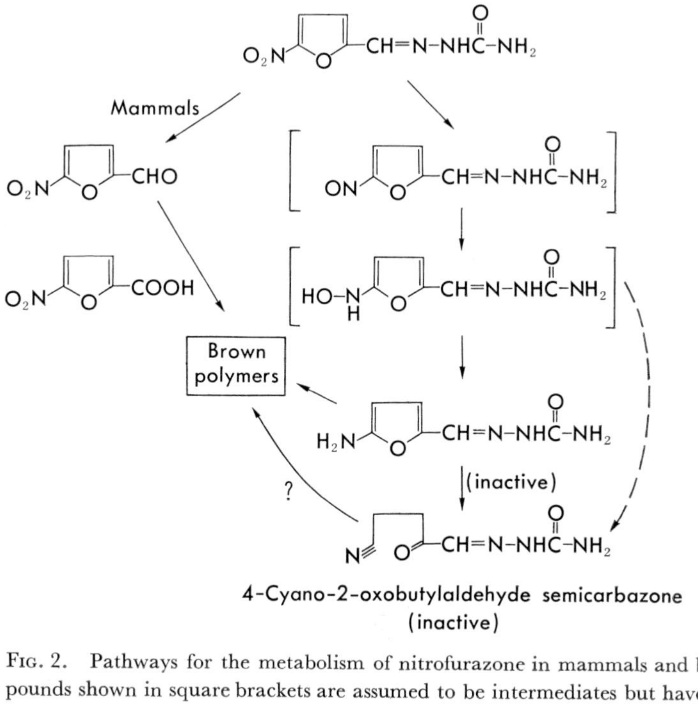

4-Cyano-2-oxobutylaldehyde semicarbazone
(inactive)

FIG. 2. Pathways for the metabolism of nitrofurazone in mammals and bacteria. The compounds shown in square brackets are assumed to be intermediates but have not been isolated.

sensitive bacteria contained a flavoprotein enzyme (reductase I) which reduced nitrofurazone to a compound now known to be 4-cyano-2-oxobutyraldehyde semi-carbazone as the stable end product (7). In contrast, resistant mutants lacked this enzyme. Since the cyano derivative is biologically inactive, Asnis' result implies that some intermediate formed during the course of reduction must be responsible for the killing of the bacteria.

Asnis also recognized that there is other nitrofuran reductase activity (reductase II) still present in drug-resistant bacteria. These enzymes are quite strongly inhibited by oxygen and are maximally active under anaerobic conditions. Asnis observed that his "resistant" mutants became as sensitive as the wild type when incubated with nitrofurazone under anaerobic conditions (11), showing that reductase II as well as reductase I converted nitrofurazone to a more toxic compound.

Early studies which examined the action of nitrofurazone on bacteria and on mammalian tissue established that glucose metabolism was disrupted and that under some conditions, at least, pyruvic dehydrogenase was inhibited (12–14). The possibility that bacterial pyruvate oxidation was the primary target was eliminated by the demonstration that this process was affected equally in sensitive and resistant bacteria (11). A number of other enzymes were found to be inhibited by the drug (15, 16).

As early as 1954 there were indications that nitrofurazone might act on DNA. Szybalski and Nelson (17) found that *E. coli* B/r was more resistant to nitrofurazone than *E. coli* B—a difference which can now be attributed to the greater ability of strain B/r to stop growing until DNA damage is repaired.

Szybalski (18) was also the first to report that some nitrofurans induced reversion of bacteria from streptomycin dependence to streptomycin independence. However, several derivatives which are now known to be mutagenic did not induce mutations with this system. Somewhat later the mutagenicity of nitrofurazone was demonstrated using two different bacterial systems (19, 20). The past two years have seen several additional papers on the mutagenicity of nitro furans in bacteria (21–23), fungi (24), and animal cells (25, 26), and the subject has been thoroughly reviewed by Tazima *et al.* (27). At least 41 different derivatives have now been tested on *E. coli* WP2 or its *uvrA⁻* derivative. Of these, only one, 5-nitro-2-furoic acid, gave negative results—perhaps because it was not taken up by the cells. Furan analogues (*i.e.*, compounds in which the nitro group is replaced by hydrogen) were not mutagenic, indicating that the nitro group plays an important role.

In 1966, Stein *et al.* reported that some nitrofurans are carcinogenic (28). Thereafter followed a rapid succession of papers which clearly established that most nitrofurans are carcinogenic (29 and references in 22 and 23) and that the furan analogues of active carcinogens do not induce tumors (30). Thus, the nitro group appears to be required for carcinogenicity as well as for mutagenicity and strong antibacterial activity.

Work with Bacteria

We began our work with the hypothesis that reduction of nitrofurans produces compounds which damage cellular constituents and set about trying to get more evidence for the involvement of such intermediates and to discover what they do to protein and nucleic acids. Our ultimate objective is to understand the details of the chemical and biochemical processes involved. Initially we used *E. coli*, largely because Asnis' work had shown that useful mutants could be isolated easily and because it seemed worthwhile to obtain more knowledge concerning the antibacterial mode of action of these compounds.

First, we isolated nitrofurazone-resistant (*nfr*) mutants of *E. coli* B/r (*31*). Our mutants are similar to those of Asnis (*6*) in that one of the nitroreductases has been lost and the mutants are about 8- to 10-fold resistant in air. Some properties of *E. coli* nitrofuran reductases are shown in Table 1 (*32*). All these enzymes reduce a wide variety of nitrofuran derivatives at roughly the same rate.

TABLE 1. Properties of *E. coli* Nitrofuran Reductases

	Reductase I	Reductase II	
		a	b
Molecular weight	50,000	120,000	700,000
Cofactor	NADPH or NADH	NADH	NADH
Sensitive to O_2	No	Yes	Yes
Present in *nfr* mutants	No	Yes	Yes

We then exposed the strains to nitrofurazone labelled with [^{14}C] in the semi-carbazone side chain and found that much radioactivity was bound to trichloro-acetic acid (TCA)-insoluble material in *E. coli* B/r but only a little bound in *nfr*-207 (a reductase-I-less) mutant. Fractionation experiments showed that most of the bound radioactivity was associated with protein.

Using cell-free extracts we were able to show that binding of [^{14}C] to protein took place only if the added protein was present during reduction of the nitro-furazone and not if the protein was added after reduction was complete. Addition of cysteine to the reaction mixture reduced the protein binding by 60%—probably by competition of the -SH group for activated nitrofurazone. Lysine also reduced binding, but to a smaller extent. (We have put a good deal of effort into trying to characterize these and similar products but owing to the small amounts available and to the instability of the compounds we have not yet been successful.) The label which becomes bound to protein is stable to cold acid but not to alkali. It resisted dialysis for 16 hr against urea suggesting covalent binding.

A much smaller amount of radioactivity binds to DNA. With the low specific activity nitrofurazone that we have prepared, the counts found in DNA are close to the limits of detectability. Our best estimate is that only 1/1,000 as much [^{14}C] binds to DNA as to protein. Miss Takeuchi in Dr. Sugimura's laboratory has detected binding of activated AF-2 to DNA, polyA, polyG, and polyC.

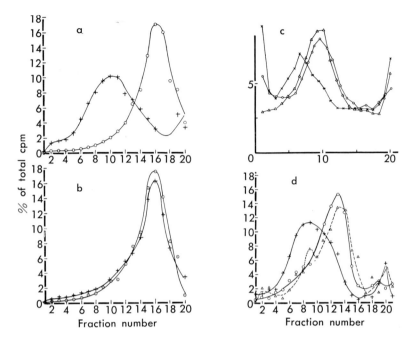

Fig. 3. Alkaline sucrose gradient analysis of DNA from control and nitrofurazone-treated *E. coli.* (a) Strain B/r: ○ control ; + exposed to 50 μg nitrofurazone per ml for 30 min. (b) Strain *nfr*-207 (a mutant of B/r which is resistant to nitrofurazone because it lacks reductase I) : ⊙ control ; + exposed to 50 μg of nitrofurazone per ml for 30 min. (c) *nfr*-207 exposed to 50 μg nitrofurazone per ml in air (△) or nitrogen (×). ○ indicates control values (controls are identical whether incubated in air or under N_2). (d) Strain B/r: ○ control ; + exposed to 25 μg nitrofurazone per ml for 15 min and then reincubated in drug-free medium for 30 min.

Exposure of sensitive bacteria to nitrofurazone causes breaks in their DNA *(33)* (Fig. 3a). There are two especially interesting points to be made about this damage. First, DNA breaks are found only when nitrofurazone has been reduced. Thus, in air, reductase I-containing strains show breaks in their DNA but *nfr* strains which lack this enzyme do not (Fig. 3b). Recall, however, that the *nfr* strains still contain two other nitrofuran reductases which are active only at low oxygen concentrations. When *nfr* strains are exposed to nitrofurazone under N_2, breaks in DNA are observed *(32)* (Fig. 3c). Thus, we can turn at least some of the effects of nitrofurazone and other nitrofurans "on and off" by varying the oxygen content of the gas phase—nitrofurans being activated when the oxygen concentration is low but not when there is a substantial amount of O_2 present. In *nfr*-strains mutagenesis, like breakage of DNA, is dependent on anaerobiosis *(32)*. This is shown in Table 2. The *nfr* derivative of *E. coli* WP2 *uvrA⁻* (*trp⁻*) reverts to *trp⁺* 10 times as frequently under anaerobic as under aerobic conditions.

The second interesting feature is that incubation of the treated bacteria in drug-free medium after exposure to nitrofurans leads to extensive repair as judged by the return of the sedimentation constant of the DNA to the same value as is found with untreated controls (Fig. 3d). We have observed repair after damage of

TABLE 2. Induction of *trp*+ Revertants of *E. coli* Strain *nfr* 343 by 16 μg/ml Nitrofurazone under Aerobic and Anaerobic Conditions

Expt. No.	Oxygen	Induced revertants per 10^8 surviving cells
1	+	50
	−	452
2	+	70
	−	589

DNA by nitrofurazone, FANFT, and nitrofurantoin, although with the latter agent few breaks are obtained. We have no direct evidence as to the molecular details of the repair but we do know that *uvrA*⁻ mutants are more sensitive than are their *uvr*+ counterparts indicating that at least a portion of the damage is repaired by the "cut and patch" system. We also observe that *exrA*⁻ or *recA*⁻ strains are not mutated by nitrofurans, a result which implies that most, if not all, of the nitrofuran-induced mutations arise as a result of mistakes made by the "error prone" repair system (*22*).

In order to try to learn more about the general nature of the damage caused to DNA by activated nitrofurans and in particular to try to determine whether or not the breaks are present before the DNA is treated with alkali, we have used an *E. coli* minicell system which was described by Paterson and Setlow (*34*). This strain of *E. coli* carries λdv CCC (covalently closed circular)-DNA (supercoiled) as a plasmid. This strain also divides unevenly so as to produce minicells which contain the plasmid DNA but not *E. coli* DNA. Minicells are easily isolated and purified by sucrose density gradient centrifugation. Fortunately for our purposes, the minicells also contain nitrofurazone reductase I. Thus, we have a system in which nitrofurans are activated and in which DNA breaks can be detected in neutral as well as alkaline solution since a single break, regardless of the way it is formed, allows unwinding of the supercoiled DNA in neutral solution to yield a relaxed but still double-stranded circle having a substantially reduced sedimentation constant (Fig. 4 (left)). Addition of alkali will denature a relaxed circle to give a linear piece and a single-stranded circle. These single-stranded circles and linear pieces sediment together at a much lower rate than the CCC-DNA. If alkali-labile lesions rather than breaks are present, the DNA will remain supercoiled in neutral solution but will yield single-stranded circles and linear pieces in alkali.

In our initial experiments (*35*) we treated minicells with 75 μg nitrofurazone per ml for 1 hr and then lysed them on either neutral or alkaline gradients. Drug-treated cells contained less supercoiled DNA than did controls when analysed on neutral gradients. This implies that breaks were really present even before the cells were lysed (Fig. 4, left). However, when the DNA is analysed on an alkaline gradient, about twice as many breaks are seen, indicating that there are other lesions in the DNA which react with alkali to produce breaks.

Figure 4 (right) summarizes data from a series of experiments in which minicells were exposed to various concentrations of nitrofurazone for 1 hr—a period which allowed complete reduction of nitrofurazone at the highest concentration

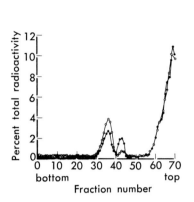
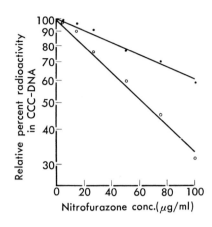

FIG. 4 (left).   Neutral sucrose sedimentation profile of DNA from lysates of nitrofurazone-treated and control minicells. The minicells incubated with nitrofurazone (75 μg/ml) for 1 hr were lysed and subjected to centrifugation on neutral sucrose gradients. The faster-sedimenting component contains supercoiled DNA while the slower component contains relaxed circles having one or more single-strand breaks.   ○ control ; ● drug-treated.

FIG. 4 (right).   Dose response curve for the breakage by nitrofurazone of DNA in intact mini-cells. Minicells were treated with drug for 1 hr, then lysed and the DNA sedimented on neutral or alkaline gradients to determine the percentage of total radioactivity in the supercoiled form. The data were then expressed as a percentage of the total counts found in supercoiled DNA from the treated minicells compared to those in supercoiled DNA from untreated cells.   ○ alkali ; ● neutral.

used. Both types of lesion were formed with first-order kinetics and about one alkali-labile lesion was found for every overt break.

The existence of alkali-labile lesions was confirmed directly by isolating CCC-DNA from drug-treated minicells on a neutral gradient and then examining the sedimentation of samples of this material in either neutral or alkaline gradients. When CCC-DNA prepared from untreated minicells using a neutral gradient was resedimented in alkaline gradients, the recovery of radioactivity in CCC-DNA was 20–25% less than that obtained in neutral gradients. This result, which is similar to that reported by Paterson and Setlow, has been attributed to the presence of alkali-labile lesions in normal λdv DNA. When similar DNA preparations from drug-treated minicells were resedimented in alkali, the recovery of CCC-DNA was much lower than that obtained with untreated minicells. This, together with the *in vivo* results described above, leads us to conclude that nitrofurazone induces alakli-labile lesions in DNA.

We next examined the effect of activated nitrofurazone on CCC-DNA in cell-free extracts. As is shown in Table 3, exposure at CCC-DNA to drug alone did not cause any breaks or alkali-labile lesions. Incubation with preparations containing nitrofurazone reductase caused breaks in about 33% of the circles, presumably as a result of endonuclease present in the preparation. When nitrofurazone as well as the enzyme extract is added, breakage was increased to 54% in neutral solution and 68% in alkali. Thus, in spite of the complications introduced by the nucleases which contaminate reductase preparations, these *in vitro* experiments confirm the results obtained with intact minicells and demonstrate once again that reductive activation is required before nitrofurazone can damage DNA.

Our next series of experiments probed the ability of minicells to repair nitrofuran-damaged DNA. As in our earlier experiments with normal bacteria, minicells were exposed to nitrofurazone for an appropriate period, harvested by centrifuga-

TABLE 3. Breakage of DNA by Activated Nitrofurans *in Vitro*

Conditions		% DNA circles nicked as observed in:	
Nitrofurazone	Reductase preparation	Neutral gradients	Alkaline gradients
—	—	0	0
+	—	0	0
—	+	32	35
+	+	54	68

Reaction mixtures contained 4,000 cpm (spec. act. 4.7×10^5 cpm/μg) of supercoiled-DNA isolated from [^{3}H]-labelled minicells, 20 μg NADPH, 0.24 mg glucose 6-phosphate and 0.2 units of glucose 6-phosphate dehydrogenase. Where indicated, 15 μg nitrofurazone and/or 0.5 μl of *E. coli* enzyme preparation were also added. The final volume was 200 μl. After incubation for 30 min at 37°C, the DNA was analysed on gradients.

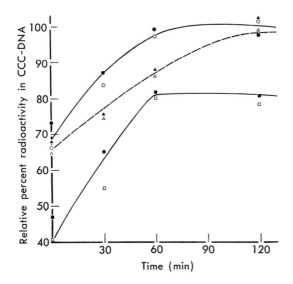

FIG. 5. Time course for the repair of DNA in *E. coli* minicells after exposure to 75 μg/ml nitrofurazone for 1 hr. The times indicated represent the period of reincubation in drug-free medium. The upper curve labelled "breaks on neutral gradient" represents data from minicells lysed and analysed on neutral gradients: ● Expt. 1; ○ Expt. 2. The lower curve labelled "breaks on alkaline gradient" represents data from the same minicell preparations lysed and analysed on neutral gradients: ■ Expt. 1; □ Expt. 2. The dashed line represents the percentages of the total of control radioactivity found in supercoiled DNA after isolated supercoiled DNA from drug-treated minicells on neutral gradients was exposed to *Micrococcal* endonuclease and then analysed on alkaline gradients relative to that found in a parallel supercoiled DNA sample which was not exposed to the extract: ▲ Expt. 1; △ Expt. 2.

tion and resuspended in drug-free medium. At intervals, samples were taken and the DNA analysed by neutral alkaline sucrose-gradient centrifugation. Figure 5 shows that at the end of one hour's exposure to drug, 68% of the DNA was super-coiled on a neutral gradient but only 44% was supercoiled after exposure to alkali. Thus, we conclude that about 32% of the DNA molecules had overt breaks and an additional 34% had alkali-labile lesions. Upon reincubation in drug-free medium, the breaks observed on neutral gradients were completely repaired in 60 min. However, analysis in alkali showed that over 20% of the molecules contained alkali-labile lesions even after two hours' reincubation, suggesting that if alkali-labile lesions are repaired in minicells, their repair is very slow.

It would be of interest to know whether or not the breaks which are found in DNA after nitrofurazone treatment are due to direct chemical reactions with the DNA which lead to strand scission or whether the initial reaction products leave the DNA intact but render it susceptible to nucleases (perhaps repair nucleases). Our information at present is too limited to permit a clear distinction between these two possibilities. We do know, however, that CCC-DNA isolated from treated minicells contains lesions which are converted to breaks upon treatment with a partially purified *Micrococcus luteus* extract containing repair nuclease. Figure 6 shows, in fact, that approximately 32% of the molecules contained *Micrococcal* endonuclease-sensitive lesions immediately after one hour's treatment with drug. Upon reincubation of the cells, these nuclease-sensitive lesions disappeared from the DNA. We believe that the overt breaks which are seen on neutral gradients may

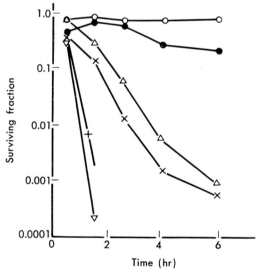

FIG. 6.   Survival curves for L cells in buffer under various conditions. Cells were harvested and resuspended in phosphate-buffered saline (PBS) containing glucose and exposed to the appropriate gas mixture for 1 hr before addition of nitrofurazone to a final concentration of 500 μM. ○ control cells in 21% O_2 (air) ; ● control cells in N_2 ; △ nitrofurazone treated in air ; × nitrofurazone treated in 5% O_2 in N_2 ; △ nitrofurazone treated in 2% O_2 in N_2 ; ▽ nitrofurazone treated in N_2.

well reflect lesions that have been hydrolysed by repair endonucleases to yield gaps which have not yet been completely patched. The fact that essentially all of the lesions which are sensitive to *Micrococcal* endonuclease have disappeared from the DNA of minicells at the time breaks have disappeared is consistent with this possibility. So is the observation that when reductase I preparations obtained from a *uvrA⁻*, *exrA⁻* strain which lacks a "repair endonuclease" (*15*) (and is much more sensitive to nitrofurazone than its wild-type counterpart (*4*)) were used to activate nitrofurazone *in vitro*, less of the CCC-DNA was converted to the relaxed form than when a *uvrA⁺*, *exrA⁺* strain served as the source of enzyme (unpublished results). Critical examination of whether or not endonuclease is required before any breaks are formed will require purification of nitrofurazone-reductase free of endonuclease.

It is of interest that repair of γ-ray-induced breaks occurs much faster in minicells than does repair of nitrofurazone-induced damage. It is also of interest that the alkali-labile lesions induced by radiation are not repaired in *E. coli* minicells (*34*) although they appear to be repaired by intact, repair competent, bacteria.

In the foregoing we have concentrated on effects upon DNA. It must be emphasized, however, that activated nitrofurans do affect other processes including glucose metabolism and ATP synthesis. Work by ourselves and others has also shown that different nitrofuran derivatives have widely different potencies as mutagens, carcinogens, and in breaking DNA. At one end of the spectrum are compounds like AF-2 and FANFT which damage DNA at low concentrations; at the other is nitrofurantoin which has much weaker mutagenic and carcinogenic activity. Nitrofurazone is intermediate in potency. The most potent agents appear to be specific inhibitors of bacterial DNA synthesis—probably because at low concentrations they damage the DNA template without having other significant effects. Higher concentrations of the weaker agents are required to cause the same amount of DNA damage. These higher concentrations have a multitude of effects on cellular processes. Glucose metabolism is impaired with a resulting lowering of the ATP concentration (Tu, McCalla, and Fan, unpublished) (a change which may affect the repair capacity of the bacteria as well as rates of RNA and protein synthesis). Ribosomes are damaged so that they show a much reduced rate of poly U-directed polyphenylalanine synthesis.

Work on Mammalian Cells and Tissues

A good deal of work by several groups can be summarized by saying that at least three mammalian enzymes reduce a wide variety of nitroheterocyclic compounds including nitrofuran derivatives. These are: xanthine oxidase (*11*, *36*, *37*), microsomal NADPH cytochrome-P450 reductase (*37*, *38*), and aldehyde oxidase (*39*). All of these are flavoproteins and all are relatively inactive in reducing nitrofurans in air. The activities of these enzymes toward nitrofurans are assayed by measuring the disappearance of the absorption maximum of the nitro compound.

We have found that all of the permanent mammalian cell lines tested reduced

TABLE 4. Reduction of Nitrofurazone by Mammalian Cells and by Mouse Liver Homogenate

Intact cells	% O_2	Rate[a]
L-929	0	2.1
KB	0	1.3
BHK-21	0	0.4
HeLa	0	1.0
Ehrlich ascites	0	0.5
Rat liver	0	18.7
Mouse liver homogenate[b]	0	8.2
Mouse liver homogenate	2	4.5
Mouse liver homogenate	5	1.7
Mouse liver homogenate	21	0

[a] μmoles/hr/10^8 cells or μmoles/hr/g liver.   [b] Mouse liver homogenate (1 ml of $9,000 \times g$ supernatant) was incubated with nitrofurazone (1 ml of 250 μM) at 37°C under 0, 2, 5, or 21% oxygen in nitrogen.

nitrofurazone under N_2 at a low but significant rate. Primary liver cultures were 10- to 20-fold more active (Table 4). Neither intact cells nor liver homogenates reduced nitrofurazone in air. However, a concentration of 2% O_2 in N_2 gave about half maximal rates of reduction. Since 2% O_2 in N_2 is equivalent to an oxygen tension of about 15 mmHg and corresponds roughly to the p_{O_2} values which are found in liver, kidney, and spleen (40), we conclude that the "nitrofuran reductases" of mammalian tissues can be expected to be active in intact animals.

Drawing on our knowledge of the action of nitrofurans on bacteria, we next asked questions about the binding of [^{14}C] from labelled nitrofurazone to TCA-insoluble material in organ slices and cell-free extracts. Not surprisingly we found much more extensive binding in tissues such as liver, kidney, and testes which rapidly metabolize nitrofurans than in spleen which does not (41).

In cell-free extracts of liver we have found that both xanthine oxidase and a microsomal enzyme, presumably NADPH: cytochrome c reductase activate nitrofurazone to yield compounds which bind tightly and probably covalently to protein. Wang et al. (42) have obtained similar results with N-[4-(5-nitro-2-furyl)-2-thiazolyl]acetamide. Tatsumi et al. (43) have reported reduction of nitrofurans by xanthine oxidase preparations from intestinal mucosa and suggested that nitrofurans may be reductively activated as they are absorbed from the gut (43).

Indirect evidence suggests that the 5-hydroxylaminofuryl derivatives may be produced by xanthine oxidase (35) and that the same compound may be formed when NADPH: cytochrome c reductase catalyses the reduction of nitrofurans (38). The hydroxylamine of niridazole (a nitrothiazolyl derivative) has been isolated from reaction mixtures containing NADPH: cytochrome c reductase and characterized by means of mass spectroscopy (44).

These results and the well-known fact that hydroxylamines (or esters of hydroxylamines) formed from many aromatic amines are known to be the active form of amine carcinogens have led some authors to assume that hydroxylaminofurans are the proximal or ultimate carcinogens and mutagens of nitrofurans. While this may well prove to be the case, it seems best at present to retain an open mind. Mason and Holtzman have recently found that micromolar concentrations of the

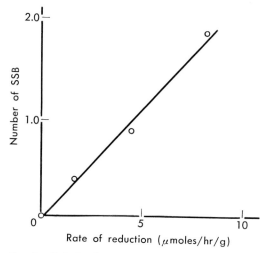

FIG. 7. Relation between the number of single-strand breaks (SSB) in DNA and the rate of reduction of nitrofurazone by intact L cells. The different rates of reduction were obtained using 21, 5, 2, and 0% O_2 in N_2. The number of breaks per cell was calculated from sedimentation data using the equation of Bergi and Hershey (51).

nitrofuryl radical anion are formed during reduction of nitrofurazone and FANFT by a liver microsomal "nitroreductase" preparation (45) and suggested that such compounds might be the proximal activated forms of nitroheterocyclic mutagens and carcinogens (46).

Survival curves obtained in our laboratory and by Mohindra and Rauth in Toronto (private communication) show that nitrofurans are more toxic to mammalian cells in N_2 than in air (Fig. 6). However, both groups find that cells are killed when exposed to nitrofurans in air. While we do not really know how nitrofurans kill cells in air, we do know that ATP levels are reduced and macromolecule synthesis inhibited (Olive and McCalla, unpublished).

When the DNA of cultured mammalian cells is examined for single-strand breaks after treatment with nitrofurans, a familiar pattern is seen: the lower the oxygen tension, the greater the amount of drug reduced and the greater the number of breaks (Fig. 7) (47). Under a given set of conditions the amount of damage increases with the amount of nitrofuran used and with time of exposure at least for the first hour.

When L cells were partially synchronized by treatment with hydroxyurea for 12 hr followed by colcemid for 15 hr before being washed and resuspended in fresh medium, the results shown in Fig. 8 were obtained. With both agents tested there was considerable breakage of DNA at all stages of the cell cycle but G_1–early S cells were most sensitive.

Our data on the repair of nitrofuran-induced damage by mammalian cells is rudimentary. However, we know that reincubation of treated cells in drug-free medium results in disappearance of breaks (47). Damage induced in L cells by 500 μM nifuroxime for 2 hr was repaired within 4 hr but the greater amount of damage

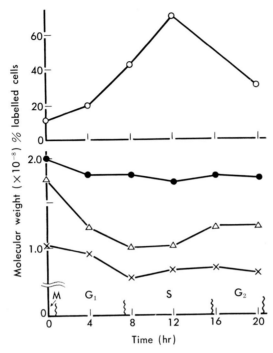

Fig. 8.   Effect of nitrofurans on the DNA of partially synchronized L cells at various stages of the cell cycle. Top panel shows the frequency of cells synthesizing DNA as determined by autoradiography after a 15-min pulse of [³H]-thymidine at various stages of the cell cycle. The lower panel shows average molecular weights of DNA (measured in alkaline sucrose gradients) after exposure of the cells to 430 μM nitrofurantoin or 630 μM nifuroxime for 2 hr in PBS containing glucose. ● control ; △ nifuroxime ; × nitrofurantoin.

caused by the same concentration of nitrofurantoin did not appear to be completely rejoined even after 16 hr. Experiments with Ehrlich ascites cells in mice suggests that cells *in vivo* repair nitrofuran-induced damage more rapidly.

To try to get some insight into whether DNA is degraded and repaired in intact animals we have attempted to use prelabelled mice to examine DNA turnover—a technique similar to that used by Goodman and Potter (48). Two labelling procedures were used. In the first, [³H]-thymidine was injected into partially hepatectomized mice while liver regeneration took place. In the second, we injected labelled thymidine into newborn mice, thus labelling a wide variety of tissues. After several weeks, the labelled animals were divided into various groups which were then fed either control or nitrofuran-containing diets. The activity and specific activity of the DNA was determined at intervals.

The first experiment indicated that 0.1% nitrofurazone in the diet caused progressive loss of label from the DNA but that 0.05% FANFT in the diet did not significantly reduce the activity in the DNA. With nitrofurazone there was a slight enlargement of the liver. No abnormalities were seen by microscopic examination of sections of the livers from treated mice.

A more elaborate experiment was then carried out using mice that had been

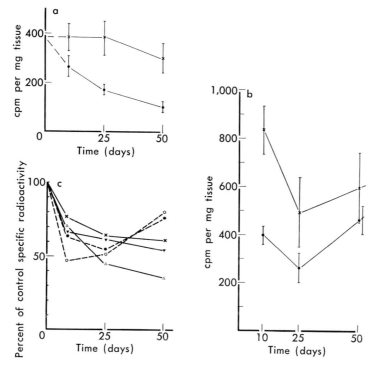

FIG. 9. Effect of nitrofurazone as 0.1% of the diet on the turnover of radioactivity from mice prelabelled with [³H]-thymidine shortly after birth. (a) Radioactivity in the liver : × control ; ● nitrofurazone. (b) Radioactivity in the spleen (bars represent standard errors of the means) × control ; ● nitrofrazone. (c) Summary of the effects seen in various organs : ○ spleen ; ● kidney ; × brain ; ▲ lung ; △ liver.

labelled as newborns and which were later fed 0.1% nitrofurazone in the diet. Results of this experiment can be summarized by saying that there seems to be significant nitrofurazone-induced loss of radioactivity in liver (Fig. 9a), lung, and brain. Spleen (Fig. 9b) and kidney showed considerable initial loss of counts upon nitrofurazone feeding but at later times actually showed an increase in the amount of label per g tissue. The results expressed as percent of control values for all of these tissues are shown in Fig. 9c. The same general picture emerges if the data are expressed as cpm per organ rather than cpm per mg tissue. We believe that the increase in radioactivity in kidney and spleen seen at 50 days is the result of scavenging of the [³H] which is produced by turnover of DNA. Autoradiography showed that in the kidney areas of high grain counts were associated with the blood vessels and proximal convoluted tubules.

The nitrofuran-induced reduction in the specific activity of DNA could be due to: (1) an increase in the mass and DNA content of the tissue, (2) death, lysis, and replacement of some cells in the tissue, or (3) to increased turnover of DNA within the cells. Alternative (1) appears to be eliminated by direct measurement of organ weights. It is, however, not possible to distinguish between loss of some cells and increased turnover within cells even though no marked histological changes are observed. It should also be noted that while liver is known to be damaged by high doses of nitrofurazone (49), it is not a site of tumor development at least in nitro-furazone-fed rats (50).

CONCLUDING REMARKS

In conclusion, work carried out over the past 6 years by ourselves and others has shown that nitrofurans have many features in common with other aromatic carcinogens. They are activated *in vivo* to form electrophilic compounds that react with cellular nucleophiles including DNA. It is interesting that bacteria as well as mammalian tissues have the enzymes required for activation of nitrofurans. Much of the damage to DNA is repaired by enzymatic repair systems, but through mistakes made during repair, or because of residual unrepaired damage mutations are induced. While we cannot at this point exclude reactions of activated nitrofurans with other cellular constituents as having a role in the carcinogenic process, it does seem reasonable to postulate that it is damage to DNA produced by nitrofurans that ultimately leads to tumor formation.

While one can derive some satisfaction from the progress that has been made, many important details are still unclear. The exact chemical nature of the ultimate carcinogens and mutagens, the structure of the derivatives formed when these compounds react with cellular constituents and the reasons for the wide differences both in potency and target specificity of various nitrofuran derivatives remain problems for the future.

ACKNOWLEDGMENTS

Rebecca Berry, Christel Kaiser, Antoon Reuvers, and Donna Voutsinos also contributed to the work from our laboratory. Our work has been supported by the National Cancer Institute of Canada and the National Research Council of Canada.

REFERENCES

1. Dodd, M. C. and Stillman, W. B.   The *in vitro* bacteriostatic action of some simple furan derivatives. J. Pharmacol. Exp. Ther., *82*: 11–18, 1944.
2. Dan, O. and Möller, E. F.   Bacteriostatic effects of nitrocompounds of thiophene and furan. Chem. Ber., *80*: 23–36, 1947.
3. Greenberg, E. and Titsworth, E. H.   Chemotherapeutic properties of heterocyclic compounds: Monocyclic compounds with five-membered rings. Annu. Rev. Microbiol., *27*: 317–346, 1973.
4. Matsuda, T.   Review on recent nitrofuran derivatives used as food preservatives. Hakko Kogaku Zasshi, *44*: 495–508, 1966.
5. Paul, H. E., Austin, F. L., Paul, M. E., and Ells, V. R. Metabolism of the nitrofurans. Ultraviolet absorption studies of urinary end-products after oral administration. J. Biol. Chem., *180*: 345–363, 1949.
6. Asnis, R. E.   The reduction of furacin by cell-free extracts of furacin-resistant and parent-susceptible strains of *Escherichia coli*. Arch. Biochem. Biophys., *66*: 208–216, 1957.
7. Gavin, J. J., Ebetino, F. F., Freedman, R., and Waterbury, W. E.   The aerobic

degradation of 1-(5-nitrofurfurylideneamino)-2-imidazolidinone (NF-246) by *Escherichia coli*. Arch. Biochem. Biophys., *113*: 399–404, 1966.

8. Pugh, D. L., Olivard, J., Snyder, H. R., Jr., and Heotis, J. P. Metabolism of 1-[(5-nitrofurfurylidene)amino]-2-imidazolidinone. J. Med. Chem., *15*: 270–273, 1972.

9. Craine, E. M. and Ray, W. H. Metabolites of furazolidone in urine of chickens. J. Pharm. Sci., *61*: 1495–1497, 1972.

10. Wang, C. Y. and Bryan, G. T. Deacylation of carcinogenic 5-nitrofuran derivatives by mammalian tissues. Chem.-Biol. Interact., *9*: 423–428, 1974.

11. Asnis, R. E., Cohen, F. B., and Gots, J. S. Studies on bacterial resistance to furacin. Antibiot. Chemother., *2*: 123–129, 1952.

12. Green, M. N. The effect of furacin (5-nitro-2-furaldehyde semicarbazone) on the metabolism of bacteria. Arch. Biochem., *19*: 397–406, 1948.

13. Paul, M. F., Bryson, M. J., and Harrington, C. Effect of furacin on pyruvate metabolism. J. Biol. Chem., *219*: 463–471, 1956.

14. Asnis, R. E., Glick, M. C., and Fritz, M. Effect of furacin on the dissimilation of pyruvate and formate by cell-free extracts of bacteria. J. Biol. Chem., *227*: 863–869, 1957.

15. Green, M. N., Heath, E. C., and Yall, I. Effect of furacin (5-nitro-2-furaldehyde semicarbazone) on various sulfhydryl and non-sulfhydryl enzymes. Proc. Soc. Exp. Biol. Med., *76*: 152–155, 1951.

16. Buzard, J. A., Kopko, F., and Paul, M. F. Inhibition of glutathione reductase by nitrofurantoin. J. Lab. Clin. Med., *56*: 884–890, 1960.

17. Szybalski, W. and Nelson, T. C. Genetics of bacterial resistance to nitrofurans and radiation. Bacteriol. Proc., 51–52, 1954.

18. Szybalski, W. Special microbiol systems. II. Observations on chemical mutagenesis. Ann. N. Y. Acad. Sci., *76*: 475–489, 1958.

19. Zampieri, A. and Greenberg, J. Nitrofurazone as a mutagen in *Escherichia coli*. Biochem. Biophys. Res. Commun., *14*: 172–176, 1964.

20. Cook, T. M., Goss, W. A., and Deitz, W. H. Mechanism of action of nalidixic acid on *Escherichia coli*. V. Possible mutagenic effect. J. Bacteriol., *91*: 780–783, 1966.

21. Kada, C. *Escherichia coli* mutagenicity of furylfuramide. Japan. J. Genet., *48*: 301–305, 1973.

22. McCalla, D. R. and Voutsinos, D. On the mutagenicity of nitrofurans. Mutat. Res., *26*: 3–16, 1974.

23. Yahagi, T., Nagao, M., Hara, K., Matsushima, T., Sugimura, T., and Bryan, G. T. Relationships between the carcinogenic and mutagenic or DNA-modifying effects of nitrofuran derivatives, including 2-(2-furyl)-3-(5-nitro-2-furyl)acrylamide, a food additive. Cancer Res., *34*: 2266–2273, 1974.

24. Ong, T. and Shahim, M. M. Mutagenic and recombinogenic activities of the food additive furylfuramide in eukaryotes. Science, *184*: 1086–1087, 1974.

25. Tonomura, A. and Sasaki, M. S. Chromosome aberration and DNA repair synthesis in cultured human cells exposed to nitrofurans. Japan. J. Genet., *48*: 291–294, 1973.

26. Sugiyama, T., Goto, K., Uenaka, U., and Nishio, K. Acute cytogenetic effect of 2-(2-furyl)-3-(5-nitro-2-furyl)acrylamide (AF-2), a food preservative on rat bone marrow cells *in vivo*. Mutat. Res., *31*: 241–246, 1975.

27. Tazima, Y., Kada, T., and Murakami, A. Mutagenicity of nitrofuran derivatives, including furylfuramide, a good preservative. Mutat. Res., *32*: 55–80, 1975.

28. Stein, R. J., Yost, O., Petroliunas, F., and von Esch, A. Carcinogenic activity of nitrofurans: A histologic evaluation. Fed. Proc., *25*: 291, 1966.

29. Morris, J. E., Price, J. M., Lalich, J. J., and Stein, R. J. The carcinogenic activity of some 5-nitrofuran derivatives in the rat. Cancer Res., *29*: 2145–2156, 1969.

30. Ertürk, E., Morris, J. E., Cohen, S. M., Von Esch, A. M., Crovetti, A. J., and Bryan, G. T. Comparative carcinogenicity of formic acid 2-[4-(5-nitro-2-furyl)-2-thiazolyl]-hydrazide and related chemicals in the rat. J. Natl. Cancer Inst., *47*: 437–445, 1971.

31. McCalla, D. R., Reuvers, A., and Kaiser, C. Mode of action of nitrofurazone. J. Bacteriol., *104*: 1126–1134, 1970.

32. McCalla, D. R., Olive, P., Tu, Y., and Fan, M. L. Nitrofurazone-reducing enzymes in *E. coli* and their role in drug activation *in vivo*. Can. J. Microbiol., *21*: 1484–1491, 1975.

33. McCalla, D. R., Reuvers, A., and Kaiser, C. Breakage of bacterial DNA by nitrofuran derivatives. Cancer Res., *31*: 2184–2188, 1971.

34. Paterson, M. C. and Setlow, R. B. Endonucleolytic activity from *Micrococcus luteus* that acts on γ-ray-induced damage in plasmid DNA of *Escherichia coli* minicells. Proc. Natl. Acad. Sci. U.S., *69*: 2927–2931, 1972.

35. Tu, Y. and McCalla, D. R. Effect of activated nitrofurans on DNA. Biochim. Biophys. Acta, *402*: 142–149, 1975.

36. Taylor, J. D., Paul, H. D., and Paul, F. M. Metabolism of nitrofurans. III. Studies with xanthine oxidase *in vitro*. J. Biol. Chem., *191*: 223–231, 1951.

37. Feller, D. R., Morita, M., and Gillette, J. R. Reduction of heterocyclic nitro compounds in the rat liver. Proc. Soc. Exp. Biol. Med., *137*: 433–437, 1971.

38. Wang, C.-Y., Chiu, C.-W., Kaiman, B., and Bryan, G. T. Identification of 2-methyl-4-(5-amino-2-furyl)thiazole as the reduced metabolite of 2-methyl-4-(5-nitro-2-furyl)thiazole. Biochem. Pharmacol., *24*: 291–293, 1975.

39. Wolpert, M. K., Althaus, J. R., and Johns, D. G. Nitroreductase activity of mammalian liver aldehyde oxidase. J. Pharm. Exp. Ther., *185*: 202–213, 1973.

40. Jamieson, D. and von den Brenk, H. A. S. Effect of electrode dimensions on tissue pO_2 measurement *in vivo*. Nature, *201*: 1227–1228, 1964.

41. McCalla, D. R., Reuvers, A., and Kaiser, C. "Activation" of nitrofurazone in animal tissues. Biochem. Pharmacol., *20*: 3532–3537, 1971.

42. Wang, C. Y., Behrens, B. C., Ichikawa, M., and Bryan, G. T. Nitroreduction of 5-nitrofuran derivatives by rat liver xanthine oxidase and reduced nicotinamide adenine dinucleotide phosphate-cytochrome *c* reductase. Biochem. Pharmacol., *23*: 3395–3404, 1974.

43. Tatsumi, K., Ou, T., Yamaguchi, T., and Yashimura, H. The metabolic fate of nitrofuran derivatives. II. Degradation by small intestinal mucosa and absorption from gastrointestinal tract. Chem. Pharm. Bull., *21*: 191–201, 1973.

44. Feller, D. R., Morita, M., and Gillette, J. R. Enzymatic reduction of niridazole by rat liver microsomes. Biochem. Pharmacol., *20*: 203–226, 1971.

45. Mason, R. P. and Holtzman, J. L. ESR spectra of free radicals formed from nitroaromatic drugs by microsomal nitroreductase. Pharmacologist, *16*: 496, 1974.

46. Mason, R. P. and Holtzman, J. L. The mechanism of microsomal and mitochondrial nitroreductase. Electron spin resonance evidence for nitroaromatic free radical intermediates. Biochemistry, *14*: 1626–1632, 1975.

47. Olive, P. L. and McCalla, D. R. Damage to mammalian cell DNA by nitrofurans. Cancer Res., *35*: 781–784, 1975.

48. Goodman, J. I. and Potter, V. R.   Evidence for DNA repair synthesis and turnover in rat liver following ingestion of 3'-methyl-4-dimethylaminoazobenzene. Cancer Res., *32*: 766–775, 1972.

49. Dodd, M. C.   The chemotherapeutic properties of 5-nitro-2-furaldehyde semicarbazone (Furacin). J. Pharm. Exp. Ther., *86*: 311–323, 1946.

50. Morris, J. E., Price, J. M., Lalich, J. J., and Stein, R. J.   The carcinogenic activity of some 5-nitrofuran derivatives in the rat. Cancer Res., *29*: 2145–2156, 1969.

51. Bergi, E. and Hershey, A. D. Sedimentation rate as a measure of molecular weight of DNA. Biophys. J., *3*: 309–321, 1963.

Discussion of Paper of Drs. McCalla et al.

DR. SATO: (1) What kind of protein did you use as the acceptor in the experiment of binding of nitrofurazone? (2) What is the radioactive material at the top of neutral sucrose density gradient?

DR. McCALLA: (1) In crude extracts, label from activated nitrofurazone is bound to bacterial proteins and no increase is observed with added protein. When 50-fold purified enzyme is used to activate nitrofurazone, an increase in binding of ^{14}C has been observed with bovine serum albumin, bovine serum globulin, cytochrome *c* and histone. (2) This radioactivity at the top of the gradient is always seen. We do not know what it represents.

DR. KONDO: (1) According to your summarizing diagram, you indicated there are (a) an alkaline-labile sensitive lesion, and (b) an endonuclease-sensitive lesion. Did you not get any excisable lesion? (2) If excision repair takes place, we expect that the molecular weight of DNA decreases with increase in postincubation time. (3) I understand minicells usually contain less activity of repair enzyme than the intact bacterial cell.

DR. McCALLA: (1) The endonuclease-sensitive lesions are excisable. (2) The molecular weight of the DNA will decrease at first as the endonuclease acts and then increase again as the final stages of repair take place. (3) That is correct. Repair of breaks is much slower in minicells than in wild-type bacteria.

DR. CRADDOCK: What happens to the alkali-labile lesions in DNA in the cell? Are they never repaired?

DR. McCALLA: In minicells it appears that they are not repaired. However, in wild-type bacteria the molecular weight of the DNA in alkaline gradients returns to the control value, implying that the alkali-labile lesions are repaired by these cells.

DR. TAKEBE: Am I correct to understand that you did not identify the strand breaks in alkaline gradient to determine whether they were caused by the direct defect of the chemical or caused during the course of excision repair by comparing the wild-type and *uvrA⁻* mutants?

Dr. McCalla: That is correct. We have not used minicells derived from *uvrA⁻* bacteria.

Dr. Maher: Did I understand correctly that in mammalian cells there is no reduction if they are treated in air (high O_2 tension) and correspondingly, no breaks are found under such conditions? I wonder then if you find cytotoxic effects of nitrofurans in cells treated under the regular tissue culture conditions.

In this regard, I will show, tomorrow, differential survival curves in normally repairing and excision repair-deficient human cells treated with furylfuramide.

Dr. McCalla: We are unable to detect activation (reduction) or DNA breaks by mammalian cells in air. However, we do see cell killing in air. The extent of killing is progressively increased as the oxygen tension is reduced.

Dr. Kada: Do you think that there is only one type of reductase required for activation of the nitrofuran in *E. coli*?

Dr. McCalla: We really do not know how many enzymes are involved in the activation of nitrofurans. There certainly may be a need for more than one enzyme. However, we are only able to assay the disappearance of nitrofurans, *i.e.*, the first step in activation and have only been able to obtain mutants which lack reductase I.

Dr. Weisburger: We need to consider that mutational events are detected by reverse mutations. However, carcinogenic events very likely involve a forward event.

FUNDAMENTALS IN CANCER PREVENTION, P. N. MAGEE ET AL. (EDS.),
UNIV. OF TOKYO PRESS, TOKYO / UNIV. PARK PRESS, BALTIMORE, PP. 251–266, 1976

Metabolic Aspects in Organotropic Carcinogenesis by Dialkylnitrosamines

Masashi OKADA

Tokyo Biochemical Research Institute, Tokyo, Japan

Abstract: Metabolic fate of N-butyl-N-(4-hydroxybutyl)nitrosamine (BBN) and
N,N-dibutylnitrosamine (DBN) in the rat was investigated in order to elucidate a
possible relationship between metabolism and organotropic carcinogenicity to the
urinary bladder of these N-nitrosamines. The principal urinary metabolite of
BBN as well as of DBN was identified as N-butyl-N-(3-carboxypropyl)nitrosamine
(BCPN), which was demonstrated to be the common active metabolite (proximate
or ultimate form) of these compounds as bladder carcinogen.

In vivo metabolism, carcinogenicity and target organs in rats of a number of
BBN analogs having 4-hydroxybutyl, 3-hydroxypropyl, or 2-hydroxyethyl groups
were investigated. Their principal urinary metabolite was found usually to be the
corresponding carboxylic acid formed by the oxidation of the primary alcoholic
hydroxyl group leaving the other one intact, *i.e.*, N-alkyl-N-(3-carboxypropyl)-,
N-alkyl-N-(2-carboxyethyl)- or N-alkyl-N-(carboxymethyl)nitrosamine, respectively. It was revealed that the dibutyl structure was not an essential requirement for
inducing bladder cancer as presumed and the presence of a 4-hydroxybutyl chain
in BBN analogs was essential but not sufficient enough for the selective induction of
bladder cancer, whereby the principal urinary metabolite possessing the 3-carboxy-
propyl chain was responsible for the organospecific effect.

BBN analogs which had a 3-hydroxypropyl group was not carcinogenic, while
those having a 2-hydroxyethyl group induced hepatoma as well as papilloma in the
esophagus, but not bladder cancer. A possible correlation of structure and metabolism with organotropic carcinogenicity of N,N-dialkylnitrosamines is discussed,
with special reference to selective induction of bladder cancer.

The mutagenic action on microorganism was demonstrated with N-alkyl-N-α-
acetoxyalkylnitrosamines, model compounds of an ultimate form of N,N-dialkyl-
nitrosamines, without using any metabolic activation system.

One of the most intriguing findings reported by Druckrey *et al.* (*1*) in their

TABLE 1.   Carcinogenic Effects of N,N-Dialkylnitrosamines in Rats (p.o.)

Compound	Target organs	Compound	Target organs
$ON\text{–}N(CH_3)(CH_3)$	L	$ON\text{–}N(CH_3)(CH_2CH_2CH_2CH_3)$	E (inhalation)
$ON\text{–}N(CH_2CH_3)(CH_2CH_3)$	L, E	$ON\text{–}N(CH_2CH_3)(CH_2CH_2CH_2CH_3)$	E, L
$ON\text{–}N(CH_2CH_2CH_3)(CH_2CH_2CH_3)$	L, E	$ON\text{–}N(CH_2CH_2CH_3)(CH_2CH_2CH_2CH_3)$	L, E
$ON\text{–}N(CH_2CH_2CH_2CH_3)(CH_2CH_2CH_2CH_3)$	L, E, B B (s.c.)	$ON\text{–}N(CH_2CH_2CH_2CH_3)(CH_2CH_2CH_2CH_2OH)$	B
$ON\text{–}N(CH_2CH_2CH_2CH_2CH_3)(CH_2CH_2CH_2CH_2CH_3)$	L	$ON\text{–}N(CH_2CH_2CH_2CH_3)(CH_2CH_2CH_2CH_2CH_3)$	L (s.c.)

L, liver;   E, esophagus;   B, urinary bladder;   p.o., per os;   s.c., subcutaneous.

comprehensive study on the carcinogenicity and target organs of numerous N-nitroso compounds in rats was that of all the compounds investigated, only two, namely N,N-dibutylnitrosamine (DBN) and its ω-hydroxylated derivative, N-butyl-N-(4-hydroxybutyl)nitrosamine (N-butyl-N-butanol-(4)-nitrosamine) (BBN), induced tumors of the urinary bladder. Especially, it is worth notice that BBN has a potent and selective action on the urinary bladder by the oral administration.

In Table 1 are listed symmetric N,N-dialkylnitrosamines and asymmetric N,N-dialkylnitrosamines having a butyl group and their target organs in rats in the carcinogenicity test. They are taken from the work of Druckrey et al. (1) except N-propyl-N-butylnitrosamine, the carcinogenic effect of which has been examined in our laboratory (2). Only asymmetric N,N-dialkylnitrosamines having a butyl group are given in the table, since the presence of this group is supposed to be essentially important for the induction of bladder tumors. Based on their observations indicated in the table, Druckrey et al. (3) assumed that the dibutyl structure was responsible for the induction of bladder tumors because neither symmetric N,N-dialkylnitrosamines other than DBN nor asymmetric N,N-dialkylnitrosamines having a butyl grcup such as N-ethyl-N-butylnitrosamine induced bladder tumors. In order to elucidate a possible relationship between the metabolism and the organotropic effect on the urinary bladder of BBN or DBN, the metabolic fate of these nitrosamines in the rat was investigated.

Metabolic Fate of BBN and DBN in the Rat

After oral administration of BBN (II) or DBN (I) to rats, urinary metabolites which retained the nitrosamino moiety were separated and characterized as reported previously (2). Based on the urinary metabolites characterized, the metabolic pathway of BBN in the rat was revealed by us as indicated in Chart 1 (4, 5). The main urinary metabolite obtained in more than 40% of the dose was identified as N-butyl-N-(3-carboxypropyl)nitrosamine (BCPN) (VI). Besides BCPN, several N-nitroso compounds were characterized as minor metabolites; glucuronic acid conjugates of BBN and BCPN (III and VII); subsequent transformation products of BCPN by β-oxidation according to the Knoop mechanism, i.e., N-butyl-N-(2-hydroxy-3-carboxypropyl)nitrosamine (BHCPN) (X), N-butyl-N-(carboxymethyl)-nitrosamine (BCMN) (XI), and N-butyl-N-(2-oxopropyl)nitrosamine (BOPN) (XII). No BBN could be detected in the urine.

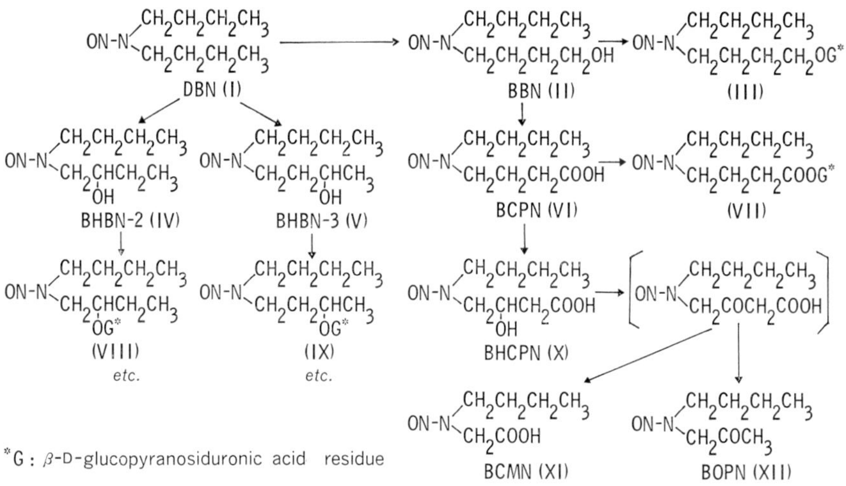

CHART 1.   Metabolic fate of BBN and DBN.

The metabolic fate of DBN in the rat was similarly elucidated by us and by Blattmann et al. (5–9), as indicated in the same chart. Thus, DBN underwent metabolic transformation in at least three ways. First it was metabolized via BBN, whereby it underwent ω-oxidation of the one butyl group, giving also BCPN as the principal metabolite which was estimated to be about 10% of the dose. Secondly, DBN underwent (ω-1)-oxidation of the one butyl group, and thirdly, (ω-2)-oxidation of the one alkyl chain. The monohydroxylated metabolites, N-butyl-N-(3-hydroxybutyl)nitrosamine (BHBN-3) (V) and N-butyl-N-(2-hydroxybutyl)ni-trosamine (BHBN-2) (IV), were in turn conjugated with glucuronic acid to form the glucuronides (IX and VIII) or they underwent further oxidative metabolic transformation through the corresponding oxo compounds, N-butyl-N-(3-oxobutyl)-nitrosamine (BOBN-3) and N-butyl-N-(2-oxobutyl)nitrosamine (BOBN-2), as described below in connection with the multiple carcinogenic effects of DBN on different organs.

Carcinogenic Effect of BBN, DBN, and Their Metabolites

The carcinogenic effect of BBN, DBN, and their metabolites was investigated

TABLE 2.   Induction of Tumors in Rats by DBN, BBN, and Their Metabolites

Compound	Period for drinking water (weeks)		Effective No. of rats	Target organs, incidence, and histology of tumors		
	With compound	Without compound		Urinary bladder Cancer No. (%)	Liver Hepatoma No. (%)	Esophagus Papilloma No. (%)
DBN (Druckrey *et al.*)			40	14 (35)	23 (58)	18 (45)
DBN	20	0–2	9	0[a]	5 (56)	0
BBN	20	10	7	7 (100)	0	0
BCPN	20	10	5	5 (100)	0	0
BCMN	20	10	7	0	0	0
BOPN	10–17	10	5	0	3 (60)	0
BOBN-2	20	0–3	9	0	9 (100)	0
BOBN-3	20	0–4	10	0	2 (20)[b]	0
BHBN-3	20	10	7	0	0	0

[a] Hyperplasia: 5 (56).   [b] Hyperplasia: 10 (100).

in rats as described previously (*2*) and the results are summarized in Table 2 (*10*–*13*). Selective induction of bladder cancer by BBN was observed as reported by other investigators (*3, 14*), while DBN induced no bladder cancer but only hepatomas in our experimental conditions. BCMN was found to be noncarcinogenic, being more than 60% of the dose recovered unchanged from urine. Hepatomas were induced by treatment with BOPN, but esophageal tumors were not found. BHBN-3 induced no tumors in our experimental conditions, although degenerative changes in the liver were observed histologically in a few rats treated. BOBN-3 as well as BOBN-2, on the other hand, induced hepatomas as did BOPN. The carcinogenic effect of BHCPN has not yet been examined.

In view of the finding that the principal urinary metabolite of BBN as well as of DBN was BCPN, and more than 40% of the dose was recovered unchanged from the urine of rats given BCPN, the carcinogenic effect of BCPN itself was examined. It was proved definitely that BCPN is a selective and potent bladder carcinogen by the oral administration as BBN in rats (*10*). Moreover, direct carcinogenic action of BCPN on the bladder epithelium was demonstrated by inducing bladder tumors in female rats through intravesicular instillation of BCPN (*15*). Finally, *in vitro* neoplastic transformation of epithelial cells of rat bladder by BCPN was elaborated by Hashimoto *et al.* (*16*) in our laboratory. It seems quite reasonable therefore to conclude that the induction of bladder cancer by BBN or DBN is ascribable to their common major urinary metabolite, BCPN. Previous observations concerning species variations in response to BBN or DBN might be explained on the basis of the different urinary excretion rates of BCPN in various animal species (*2*).

Metabolic Fate of BBN Analogs in the Rat

In order to elucidate a possible relationship among chemical structure, *in vivo* metabolism, and organotropic specificity of BBN, a number of N-alkyl-N-(ω-

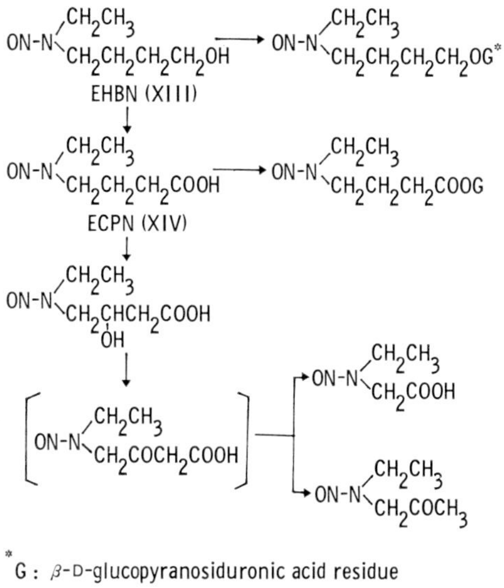

$$
\begin{array}{ccc}
\text{ON-N} \begin{smallmatrix} \text{CH}_2\text{CH}_3 \\ \text{CH}_2\text{CH}_2\text{CH}_2\text{CH}_2\text{OH} \end{smallmatrix} & \longrightarrow & \text{ON-N} \begin{smallmatrix} \text{CH}_2\text{CH}_3 \\ \text{CH}_2\text{CH}_2\text{CH}_2\text{CH}_2\text{OG}^* \end{smallmatrix}
\end{array}
$$

EHBN (XIII)

$$
\begin{array}{ccc}
\text{ON-N} \begin{smallmatrix} \text{CH}_2\text{CH}_3 \\ \text{CH}_2\text{CH}_2\text{CH}_2\text{COOH} \end{smallmatrix} & \longrightarrow & \text{ON-N} \begin{smallmatrix} \text{CH}_2\text{CH}_3 \\ \text{CH}_2\text{CH}_2\text{CH}_2\text{COOG} \end{smallmatrix}
\end{array}
$$

ECPN (XIV)

$$
\text{ON-N} \begin{smallmatrix} \text{CH}_2\text{CH}_3 \\ \text{CH}_2\text{CHCH}_2\text{COOH} \\ \text{OH} \end{smallmatrix}
$$

$$
\left[\text{ON-N} \begin{smallmatrix} \text{CH}_2\text{CH}_3 \\ \text{CH}_2\text{COCH}_2\text{COOH} \end{smallmatrix} \right]
$$

$$
\text{ON-N} \begin{smallmatrix} \text{CH}_2\text{CH}_3 \\ \text{CH}_2\text{COOH} \end{smallmatrix}
$$

$$
\text{ON-N} \begin{smallmatrix} \text{CH}_2\text{CH}_3 \\ \text{CH}_2\text{COCH}_3 \end{smallmatrix}
$$

* G : β-D-glucopyranosiduronic acid residue

CHART 2. Metabolic fate of EHBN in the rat.

hydroxyalkyl)nitrosamines related to BBN were synthesized, and their metabolic fate and carcinogenicity in rats were investigated.

The metabolic fate of N-ethyl-N-(4-hydroxybutyl)nitrosamine (EHBN) (XIII) is given in Chart 2 (17) as an example of BBN homologs which have the 4-hydroxy-butyl group. The principal urinary metabolite of EHBN was identified as N-ethyl-N-(3-carboxypropyl)nitrosamine (ECPN) (XIV), and the urinary excretion was estimated to be about 50% of the dose. Other minor metabolites indicated in the chart were formed according to the same way as shown with BBN (Chart 1). Essentially similar metabolic pattern was demonstrated with other BBN homologs having the 4-hydroxybutyl chain, e.g., N-methyl-N-(4-hydroxybutyl)nitrosamine (MHBN) (17), N-propyl-N-(4-hydroxybutyl)nitrosamine (PHBN) (18), N-tert-butyl-N-(4-hydroxybutyl)nitrosamine (t-BBN) (19). Thus the principal urinary metabolite of these compounds was the corresponding 3-carboxypropyl compound, i.e., N-methyl-N-(3-carboxypropyl)nitrosamine (MCPN), N-propyl-N-(3-carboxy-propyl)nitrosamine (PCPN), and N-tert-butyl-N-(3-carboxypropyl)nitrosamine (t-BCPN), respectively. On the other hand, the metabolic fate of N-amyl-N-(4-hydroxybutyl)nitrosamine (AHBN) which is also a BBN homolog having the 4-hydroxybutyl group was found to be somewhat different from that of other homologs described above. No less than 9 urinary metabolites were characterized, however, the principal one was not the corresponding 3-carboxypropyl compound, i.e., N-amyl-N-(3-carboxypropyl)nitrosamine (ACPN), but the carboxymethyl compound N-amyl-N-(carboxymethyl)nitrosamine, a further degradation product formed by metabolic β-oxidation from the former (2, 17).

The metabolic fate of N-butyl-N-(3-hydroxypropyl)nitrosamine (BHPN) (XV), a BBN analog having a 3-hydroxypropyl group, was disclosed by us as indicated in Chart 3 (18). The main urinary metabolite was N-butyl-N-(2-carboxyethyl)nitro-

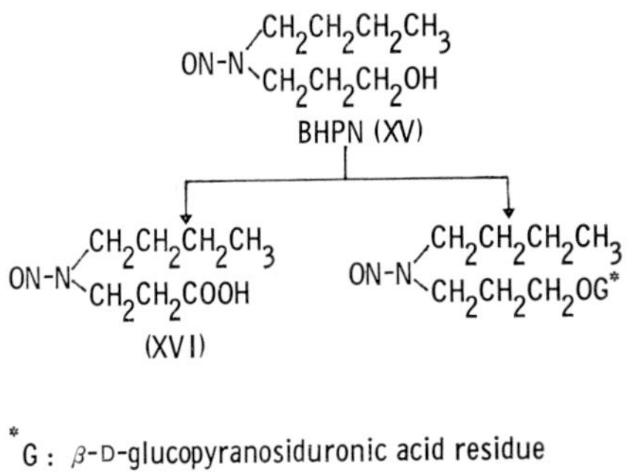

CH₂CH₂CH₂CH₃
ON-N
CH₂CH₂CH₂OH
BHPN (XV)

CH₂CH₂CH₂CH₃
ON-N
CH₂CH₂COOH
(XVI)

CH₂CH₂CH₂CH₃
ON-N
CH₂CH₂CH₂OG*

* G : β-D-glucopyranosiduronic acid residue

CHART 3.   Metabolic fate of BHPN in the rat.

samine (XVI) and the urinary excretion amounted to approximately 70% of the dose. Substantially similar metabolic pattern was demonstrated with the ethyl homolog, N-ethyl-N-(3-hydroxypropyl)nitrosamine (EHPN) (20).

In Chart 4 is given the metabolic fate of N-butyl-N-(2-hydroxyethyl)nitrosamine (BHEN) (XVII), a BBN analog having a 2-hydroxyethyl group (18). The principal urinary metabolite of BHEN was identified as BCMN (XI), a minor metabolite of BBN or DBN as described previously (Chart 1). The urinary excretion was estimated to be about 40% of the dose. Essentially similar metabolic pattern was demonstrated with the ethyl homolog, N-ethyl-N-(2-hydroxyethyl)-nitrosamine (EHEN) (20).

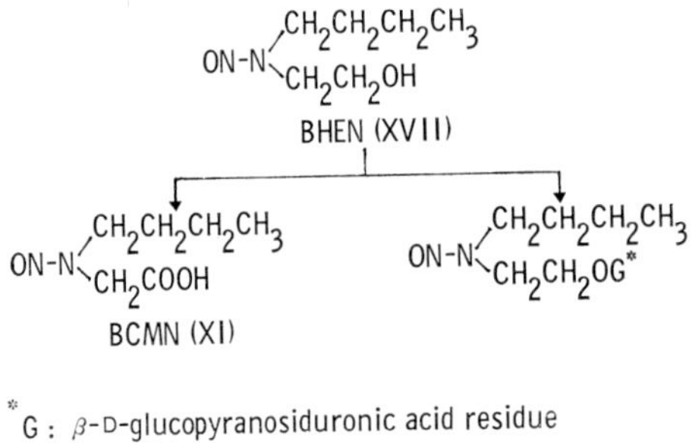

CH₂CH₂CH₂CH₃
ON-N
CH₂CH₂OH
BHEN (XVII)

CH₂CH₂CH₂CH₃
ON-N
CH₂COOH
BCMN (XI)

CH₂CH₂CH₂CH₃
ON-N
CH₂CH₂OG*

* G : β-D-glucopyranosiduronic acid residue

CHART 4.   Metabolic fate of BHEN in the rat.

Furthermore, the metabolic fate of N,N-di-(ω-hydroxyalkyl)nitrosamines which have the 4-hydroxybutyl chain was investigated. They were N-(2-hydroxyethyl)-N-(4-hydroxybutyl)nitrosamine (HEHBN) (XVIII), N-(3-hydroxypropyl)-N-(4-hydroxybutyl)nitrosamine (HPHBN)* (XIX), and N,N-di-(4-hydroxybutyl)nitrosamine (DHBN) (XX). Based on the urinary metabolites characterized, their metabolic fate in the rat is indicated in Chart 5 (20). The principal metabolite of HEHBN as well as HPHBN was identified as the corresponding 3-carboxypropyl derivative, and the urinary excretion was estimated to be about 60% and 30% of the dose, respectively. The main metabolite of DHBN, on the other hand, was

* HPHBN was obtained as a principal product when spermidine was treated with nitrite under acidic conditions (21).

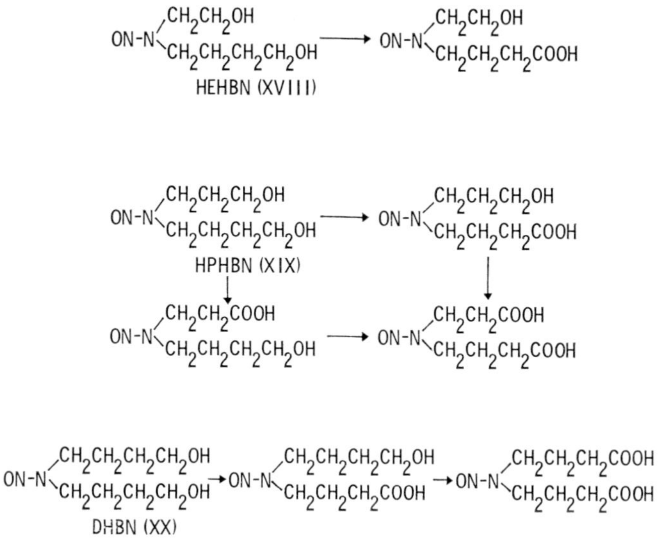

ON-N$\big\langle$ CH$_2$CH$_2$OH / CH$_2$CH$_2$CH$_2$CH$_2$OH $\longrightarrow$ ON-N$\big\langle$ CH$_2$CH$_2$OH / CH$_2$CH$_2$CH$_2$COOH

HEHBN (XVIII)

ON-N$\big\langle$ CH$_2$CH$_2$CH$_2$OH / CH$_2$CH$_2$CH$_2$CH$_2$OH $\longrightarrow$ ON-N$\big\langle$ CH$_2$CH$_2$CH$_2$OH / CH$_2$CH$_2$CH$_2$COOH

HPHBN (XIX)

ON-N$\big\langle$ CH$_2$CH$_2$COOH / CH$_2$CH$_2$CH$_2$CH$_2$OH $\longrightarrow$ ON-N$\big\langle$ CH$_2$CH$_2$COOH / CH$_2$CH$_2$CH$_2$COOH

ON-N$\big\langle$ CH$_2$CH$_2$CH$_2$CH$_2$OH / CH$_2$CH$_2$CH$_2$CH$_2$OH $\rightarrow$ ON-N$\big\langle$ CH$_2$CH$_2$CH$_2$CH$_2$OH / CH$_2$CH$_2$CH$_2$COOH $\rightarrow$ ON-N$\big\langle$ CH$_2$CH$_2$CH$_2$COOH / CH$_2$CH$_2$CH$_2$COOH

DHBN (XX)

CHART 5. Metabolic fate of N-(ω-hydroxyalkyl)-N-(4-hydroxybutyl)nitrosamines (HEHBN, HPHBN, and DHBN) in the rat.

the di-3-carboxypropyl compound and the urinary excretion was about 35% of the dose. The preferential metabolic oxidation of the 4-hydroxybutyl chain to the 3-carboxypropyl group in N-alkyl-N-(ω-hydroxyalkyl)nitrosamines had been observed previously in *in vitro* experiments using slices or homogenates prepared from rat liver (22).

Carcinogenic Effect of BBN Analogs

The results of the carcinogenicity test carried out in our laboratory with the above BBN analogs are summarized in Table 3 (10–13, 23). Selective induction of bladder cancer was demonstrated not only with BBN but also with its several homologs, MHBN, EHBN, and PHBN. No bladder cancer was induced, however, by AHBN and t-BBN which are also BBN homologs in our experimental conditions, although induction of papilloma in the bladder was observed in a few rats treated with AHBN. ECPN, the principal urinary metabolite of EHBN (Chart 2), did also selectively induce bladder cancer as effectively as the original compound (23), so that ECPN is responsible for the organospecific carcinogenicity of EHBN to the urinary bladder as in the case with BCPN and BBN described above.

BHPN as well as EHPN which have a 3-hydroxypropyl chain induced neither bladder tumors nor any tumors in other organs in our experimental conditions. No induction of any tumor was demonstrated even after one year of treatment with BHPN. On the other hand, BHEN which has a 2-hydroxyethyl group induced hepatoma as well as papilloma in the esophagus as reported by Druckrey et al. (1) on EHEN.

All the three N,N-di-(ω-hydroxyalkyl)nitrosamines (HEHBN, HPHBN, and

TABLE 3.   Induction of Tumors in Rats by BBN Analogs

Compound	Period for drinking water (weeks)		Effective No. of rats	Target organs, incidence, and histology of tumors		
	With compound	Without compound		Urinary bladder Cancer No. (%)	Liver Hepatoma No. (%)	Esophagus Papilloma No. (%)
BBN	20	10	7	7 (100)	0	0
MHBN	20	10	6	6 (100)	0	0
EHBN	20	0	10	10 (100)	0	0
PHBN	20	10	7	7 (100)	0	0
AHBN	20	10	7	0[a]	0	0
t-BBN	20	10	7	0	0	0
ECPN	20	0	9	9 (100)	0	0
BCPN	20	10	5	5 (100)	0	0
BHEN	20	0	9	0	8 (90)	9 (100)
EHEN (Druckrey et al.)			40	0	40 (100)	3 (8)
BHPN	20[b]	10	7	0	0	0
EHPN	20	10	7	0	0	0

[a] Papilloma: 3 (43).   [b] No tumors on 52 weeks.

DHBN) having the 4-hydroxybutyl chain induced neither bladder tumor nor any tumor in other organs (20, 21).

Correlation of Structure and Metabolism with Organotropic Carcinogenesis

The results concerning the principal urinary metabolite and the urinary excretion rate of N-alkyl-N-(4-hydroxybutyl)nitrosamines (BBN homologs) are summarized in Table 4, together with their carcinogenic effect and target organs in rats. The carcinogenic activity of the BBN homologs so far investigated are arranged in the following order: EHBN > BBN = MHBN > PHBN > AHBN > t-BBN, the last being inactive. The carcinogenic effect of the 3-carboxypropyl compounds, MCPN and PCPN, which were the major metabolites of MHBN and PHBN has not yet been examined, however, it seems quite reasonable to suppose that they should be selectively carcinogenic to rat urinary bladder by analogy of the relationship demonstrated between BBN and BCPN as well as between EHBN and ECPN, while the carcinogenic effect of the 3-carboxypropyl compound t-BCPN, the principal metabolite of t-BBN, should not be expected. The carcinogenic effect of the 3-carboxypropyl compound ACPN which was identified as a minor urinary metabolite of AHBN, has also not been tested, since it was found that only about 2% of the dose was recovered unchanged from the urine of rats given ACPN.

In Table 5, the results regarding the principal metabolite and the urinary excretion rate of BBN analogs having the 3-hydroxypropyl or the 2-hydroxyethyl group are summarized, together with their carcinogenicity and target organs. It is very surprising as well as interesting that N-alkyl-N-(3-hydroxypropyl)nitrosamines which excreted a very large amount of the 2-carboxyethyl metabolites into urine did not induce any tumors in any organs of rats in our experimental

TABLE 4. Principal Urinary Metabolite, Carcinogenicity, and Target Organs of N-Alkyl-N-(4-hydroxybutyl)nitrosamines (BBN Homologs)

Compound	Principal urinary metabolite (% of dose)		Carcinogenicity and target organs
ON–N(CH$_2$CH$_2$CH$_2$CH$_3$ / CH$_2$CH$_2$CH$_2$CH$_2$OH)	ON–N(CH$_2$CH$_2$CH$_2$CH$_3$ / CH$_2$CH$_2$CH$_2$COOH)	(43)	+ B
ON–N(CH$_3$ / CH$_2$CH$_2$CH$_2$CH$_2$OH)	ON–N(CH$_3$ / CH$_2$CH$_2$CH$_2$COOH)	(42)	+ B
ON–N(CH$_2$CH$_3$ / CH$_2$CH$_2$CH$_2$CH$_2$OH)	ON–N(CH$_2$CH$_3$ / CH$_2$CH$_2$CH$_2$COOH)	(48)	+ B
ON–N(CH$_2$CH$_2$CH$_3$ / CH$_2$CH$_2$CH$_2$CH$_2$OH)	ON–N(CH$_2$CH$_2$CH$_3$ / CH$_2$CH$_2$CH$_2$COOH)	(40)	+ B
ON–N(CH$_2$CH$_2$CH$_2$CH$_2$CH$_3$ / CH$_2$CH$_2$CH$_2$CH$_2$OH)	ON–N(CH$_2$CH$_2$CH$_2$CH$_2$CH$_3$ / CH$_2$COOH)	(7)	− (B: papilloma)
ON–N(C(CH$_3$)$_3$ / CH$_2$CH$_2$CH$_2$CH$_2$OH)	ON–N(C(CH$_3$)$_3$ / CH$_2$CH$_2$CH$_2$COOH)	(75)	−

TABLE 5. Principal Urinary Metabolite, Carcinogenicity, and Target Organs of N-Alkyl-N-(3-hydroxypropyl)- and N-Alkyl-N-(2-hydroxyethyl)nitrosamines

Compound	Principal urinary metabolite (% of dose)		Carcinogenicity and target organs
ON–N(CH$_2$CH$_2$CH$_2$CH$_3$ / CH$_2$CH$_2$CH$_2$OH)	ON–N(CH$_2$CH$_2$CH$_2$CH$_3$ / CH$_2$CH$_2$COOH)	(70)	−
ON–N(CH$_2$CH$_3$ / CH$_2$CH$_2$CH$_2$OH)	ON–N(CH$_2$CH$_3$ / CH$_2$CH$_2$COOH)	(62)	−
ON–N(CH$_2$CH$_2$CH$_2$CH$_3$ / CH$_2$CH$_2$OH)	ON–N(CH$_2$CH$_2$CH$_2$CH$_3$ / CH$_2$COOH)	(40)	+ L, E
ON–N(CH$_2$CH$_3$ / CH$_2$CH$_2$OH)	ON–N(CH$_2$CH$_3$ / CH$_2$COOH)	(67)	+ L, E

conditions. N-Alkyl-N-(2-hydroxyethyl)nitrosamines, on the other hand, induced hepatoma as well as papilloma in the esophagus, but did not induce any bladder tumors in spite of excreting a large quantity of the carboxymethyl metabolites into urine. In view of these findings it could be mentioned that N-alkyl-N-(2-carboxyethyl)- as well as N-alkyl-N-(carboxymethyl)nitrosamines should not be involved in the induction of bladder tumors in rats.

It is quite evident from the above results that the dibutyl structure in N,N-dialkylnitrosamines is not an indispensable requirement for inducing bladder cancer as presumed by Druckrey *et al.* (*3*). It might be mentioned further that the essential structural requirement in N,N-dialkylnitrosamines for the selective induction of bladder cancer is to possess a 4-hydroxybutyl chain which undergoes metabolic transformation to a 3-carboxypropyl group, resulting in a considerable excretion of a metabolite having this group into urine. The presence of a 4-hydroxybutyl chain, however, is essential but not sufficient enough for the selective induction of bladder cancer, as illustrated with AHBN, *t*-BBN, and N-(ω-hydroxyalkyl)-N-(4-hydroxybutyl)nitrosamines (HEHBN, HPHBN, and DHBN). So far the highest urinary excretion of the 3-carboxypropyl metabolite (*t*-BCPN) was demonstrated with *t*-BBN, which was found to be noncarcinogenic. In this connection, N,N-dialkylnitrosamines having a *tert*-butyl group were reported to be noncarcinogenic (*1, 24*). It may be worthy of note further that N,N-di-(2-hydroxyethyl)nitrosamine induced hepatoma as did N,N-diethylnitrosamine and EHEN (*1*), while of the three compounds (DBN, BBN, and DHBN) investigated, which possessed the dibutyl structure, DHBN induced neither bladder tumors nor any tumors in other organs.

Quite recently, Lijinsky *et al.* (*25*) reported that oral treatment of rats with N-methyl-N-dodecylnitrosamine (MDN) (XXI) for 50 weeks gave rise to 100% incidence of urinary bladder tumors. We have investigated the metabolic fate of this N,N-dialkylnitrosamine having a long alkyl chain in the rat. The metabolic pathway of MDN has been disclosed in our laboratory as indicated in Chart 6 (*20*). The principal urinary metabolite was not MCPN (XXII) as expected but N-nitrososarcosine (XXIII), and the urinary excretion was estimated to be about 3% and 15%, respectively. Taking the fairly long-term treatment with MDN into consideration, however, it seems reasonable to suppose that the induction of bladder tumors by MDN is due to its urinary metabolite MCPN. In this connection, considering the metabolic shortening of the alkyl chain by β-oxidation according to the Knoop mechanism, it may be mentioned on the whole that N,N-dialkylnitrosamines having a long alkyl chain could induce bladder tumors only when the number of carbon atoms of the chain is even, as illustrated with MDN.

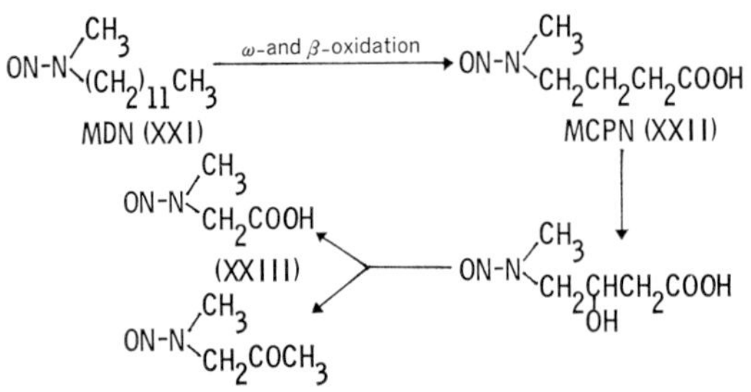

CHART 6.   Metabolic fate of MDN in the rat.

Among a number of N,N-dialkylnitrosamines only DBN induced bladder cancer as well as tumors of the liver and the esophagus by oral administration. Other N,N-dialkylnitrosamines so far examined induced tumors principally in the liver or the esophagus (*1*). From the metabolic point of view, it seems quite reasonable to assume that ω-oxidation of DBN is responsible for the induction of bladder cancer, while (ω-1)-, (ω-2)-, or (ω-3) ($=\alpha$)-oxidation may be responsible for inducing tumors of the liver and the esophagus. The former part of this assumption was clearly demonstrated with BBN, the ω-hydroxy-DBN, which selectively induced bladder cancer. In order to substanciate the latter part of the assumption, the carcinogenic effect of the (ω-1)-hydroxylated DBN metabolite, BHBN-3 (V) (Chart 1), was first examined in rats. It did not induce any tumors in our experimental conditions as described (Table 2). The principal urinary metabolite of BHBN-3 as well as of BHBN-2 (IV), the (ω-2)-hydroxylated DBN metabolite (Chart 1), on the other hand, was found to be the glucuronide (*7*). Moreover, other metabolites characterized of these hydroxylated derivatives of DBN were proved to have a 3-oxobutyl or a 2-oxobutyl group and/or to be further transformation products of the oxobutyl derivatives (*7, 26*). Thus, in the light of the potent carcinogenic effect on rat liver of BOPN (*11*) and N-propyl-N-(2-oxopropyl)nitrosamine, a presumed metabolite of N,N-dipropylnitrosamine (*27, 28*), the carcinogenic effect of N-butyl-N-(3-oxobutyl)nitrosamine (BOBN-3) (XXIV) and N-butyl-N-(2-oxobutyl)nitrosamine (BOBN-2) (XXV) was investigated. Both oxo compounds induced hepatomas (Table 2).

We have investigated, on the other hand, the metabolic fate of BOBN-3 and BOBN-2 in the rat and the result is given in Chart 7 and 8, respectively (*7, 19*). It should be noticed that the principal metabolite of both oxo compounds was BCMN, the main metabolite of BHEN which had a potent carcinogenic effect on the liver (Table 3). Actually, BHEN itself as well as its glucuronide were characterized as metabolite of BOBN-3 (Chart 7).

Based on the above observations concerning the metabolic fate and the organotropic effect of DBN and its metabolites, it could be stated that there are two,

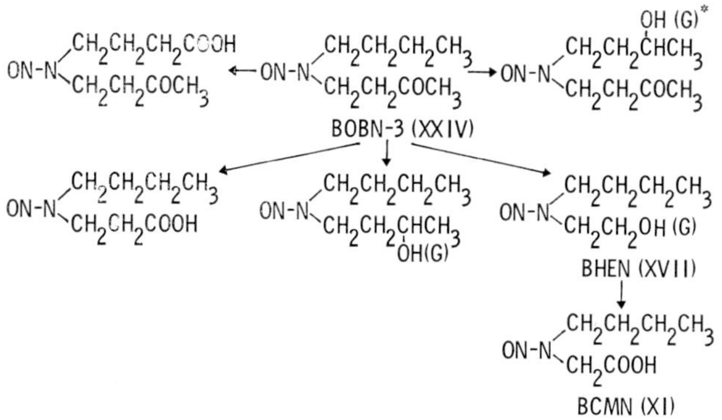

(G)* : the glucuronide was characterized together with the free compound.

CHART 7.   Metabolic fate of BOBN-3 in the rat.

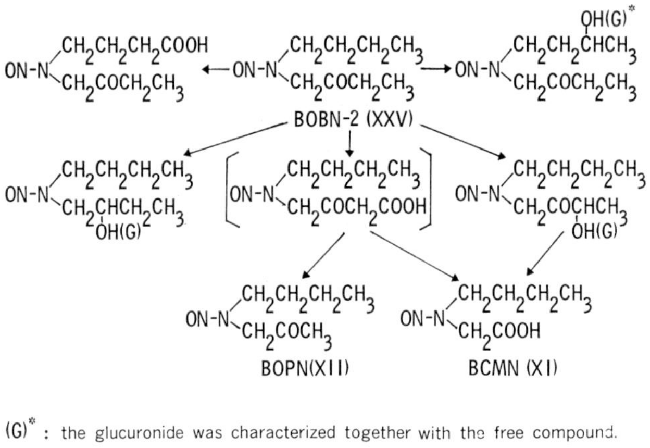

$$ON-N\begin{cases}CH_2CH_2CH_2COOH\\CH_2COCH_2CH_3\end{cases} \longleftarrow ON-N\begin{cases}CH_2CH_2CH_2CH_3\\CH_2COCH_2CH_3\end{cases} \longrightarrow ON-N\begin{cases}CH_2CH_2\overset{OH(G)^*}{C}HCH_3\\CH_2COCH_2CH_3\end{cases}$$

BOBN-2 (XXV)

$$ON-N\begin{cases}CH_2CH_2CH_2CH_3\\CH_2\underset{OH(G)}{C}HCH_2CH_3\end{cases} \qquad \left[ON-N\begin{cases}CH_2CH_2CH_2CH_3\\CH_2COCH_2COOH\end{cases}\right] \qquad ON-N\begin{cases}CH_2CH_2CH_2CH_3\\CH_2CO\underset{OH(G)}{C}HCH_3\end{cases}$$

$$ON-N\begin{cases}CH_2CH_2CH_2CH_3\\CH_2COCH_3\end{cases} \qquad ON-N\begin{cases}CH_2CH_2CH_2CH_3\\CH_2COOH\end{cases}$$

BOPN(XII)   BCMN (XI)

(G)* : the glucuronide was characterized together with the free compound.

CHART 8. Metabolic fate of BOBN-2 in the rat.

three or more different "proximate" forms of DBN according to their organotropic action, while the "ultimate" form(s) of DBN derivable from the "proximate" forms may be identical or may not be identical. Accordingly, at present it should be correctly mentioned with DBN as follows: BBN is the "proximate" and BCPN is the "more proximate" (or "ultimate") form of DBN as urinary bladder carcinogen, while BHBN-3 as well as BHBN-2 are the "proximate" and BOBN-3 as well as BOBN-2 are the "more proximate" forms of DBN as hepatocarcinogen. Multiple effect on different organs of an "indirect" carcinogen may be due to the diversity in its metabolic activation.

N-Alkyl-N-α-acetoxyalkylnitrosamines: Model Compounds of an Ultimate Form of N,N-Dialkylnitrosamines

In view of the α-hydroxylation hypothesis (*29*) concerning the metabolic activation of N,N-dialkylnitrosamines leading to the ultimate alkylating species probably being a carbonium ion, we have synthesized several N-alkyl-N-α-acetoxyalkylnitrosamines and examined their mutagenic effects by means of rapid microbial assay methods (*30*). The compounds are N-butyl-N-(1-acetoxybutyl)nitrosamine (**XXVI**), N-butyl-N-(acetoxymethyl)nitrosamine (**XXVII**), N-*sec*-butyl-N-(acetoxymethyl)nitrosamine (**XXVIII**), and N-*tert*-butyl-N-(acetoxymethyl)nitrosamine (**XXIX**) indicated in Chart 9. So far as we know, owing to its instability the synthesis of the N-alkyl-N-α-hydroxyalkylnitrosamine has never been successful, although the synthesis of N-alkyl-N-α-acetoxyalkylnitrosamines has been elaborated recently in several laboratories (*30–35*). In our extensive studies on the *in vivo* metabolism of N,N-dialkylnitrosamines (*2*), a metabolite hydroxylated at α-carbon atom has not yet been detected. It was demonstrated that N-alkyl-N-α-acetoxyalkylnitrosamines (**XXVI, XXVII,** and **XXVIII**) except the *tert*-butyl derivative (**XXIX**) had the mutagenic action on a microorganism (*Salmonella typhimurium* strain TA 1535) without using any metabolic activation system. Furthermore, the structure of the butyl chain in these compounds profoundly affected the activity in the

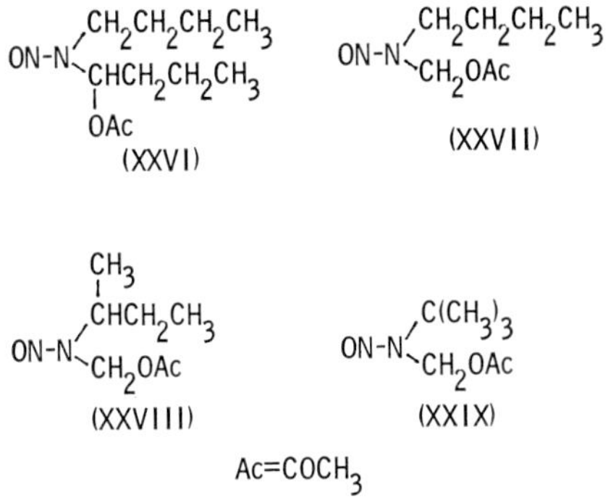

ON-N⟨CH₂CH₂CH₂CH₃ / CHCH₂CH₂CH₃ | OAc   (XXVI)

ON-N⟨CH₂CH₂CH₂CH₃ / CH₂OAc   (XXVII)

ON-N⟨CHCH₂CH₃ (CH₃) / CH₂OAc   (XXVIII)

ON-N⟨C(CH₃)₃ / CH₂OAc   (XXIX)

Ac=COCH₃

CHART 9.   N-Alkyl-N-α-acetoxyalkylnitrosamines.

order of *n*-butyl (XXVII) > *sec*-butyl (XXVIII) > *tert*-butyl (XXIX), the last being inactive. These results on the mutagenicity of N-alkyl-N-α-acetoxyalkylnitrosamines may anyhow strongly support the α-hydroxylation hypothesis concerning the metabolic activation of N,N-dialkylnitrosamines.

ACKNOWLEDGMENTS

This presentation represents in part a summarization of work carried out in numerous collaborations. The author would like to mention the names of the collaborators, E. Suzuki, J. Aoki, Y. Hashimoto, K. Suzuki, C. Kurashima, M. Iiyoshi, Y. Takeda, M. Mochizuki, and T. Anjo. He is grateful to S. Odashima, and his colleagues, National Institute of Hygienic Sciences, Tokyo, for histological examinations. Works reported in this presentation were supported in part by Grants-in-Aid for Cancer Research from the Ministry of Education, Science and Culture, Japan.

REFERENCES

1. Druckrey, H., Preussmann, R., Ivankovic, S., and Schmähl, D.   Organotrope carcinogene Wirkungen bei 65 verschiedenen N-Nitroso-Verbindungen an BD-Ratten. Z. Krebsforsch., *69*: 103–201, 1967.
2. Okada, M., Suzuki, E., Aoki, J., Iiyoshi, M., and Hashimoto, Y.   Metabolism and carcinogenicity of N-butyl-N-(4-hydroxybutyl)nitrosamine and related compounds, with special reference to induction of urinary bladder tumors. GANN Monogr. Cancer Res., *17*: 161–176, 1975.
3. Druckrey, H., Preussmann, R., Ivankovic, S., Schmidt, C. H., Mennel, H. D., and Stahl, K. W.   Selektive Erzeugung von Blasenkrebs an Ratten durch Dibutyl- und N-Butyl-N-butanol-(4)-nitrosamin. Z. Krebsforsch., *66*: 280–290, 1964.
4. Okada, M. and Suzuki, E.   Metabolism of butyl(4-hydroxybutyl)nitrosamine in rats. Gann, *63*: 391–392, 1972.
5. Suzuki, E., Aoki, J., and Okada, M.   Metabolism of butyl(4-hydroxybutyl)nitrosamine (BBN) and dibutylnitrosamine (DBN). Proc. Japan. Cancer Assoc., 31st Annu. Meet., p. 9, 1972 (in Japanese).
6. Okada, M., Suzuki, E., Iiyoshi, M., Suzuki, K., and Hashimoto, Y.   Studies on the correlation of structure and metabolism with organotropic carcinogenicity of N-nitrosodialkylamines, with special reference to induction of urinary bladder

tumors. Proc. 6th Symp. on Drug Metabolism and Action, pp. 50–53, 1974 (in Japanese).

7. Suzuki, E., Iiyoshi, M., and Okada, M.   *In vivo* metabolism and target organs of dibutylnitrosamine. Abstr. 95th Annu. Meet., Pharm. Soc. Japan, III, p. 230, 1975 (in Japanese).

8. Blattmann, L. and Preussmann, R.   Struktur von Metaboliten carcinogener Dialkylnitrosamine im Rattenurin. Z. Krebsforsch., *79*: 3–5, 1973.

9. Blattmann, L. and Preussmann, R.   Biotransformation von carcinogenen Dialkylnitrosaminen. Weitere Urinmetaboliten von Di-*n*-butyl- und Di-*n*-pentylnitrosamin. Z. Krebsforsch., *81*: 75–78, 1974.

10. Hashimoto, Y., Suzuki, E., and Okada, M.   Induction of urinary bladder tumors in ACI/N rats by butyl(3-carboxypropyl)nitrosamine, a major urinary metabolite of butyl(4-hydroxybutyl)nitrosamine. Gann, *63*: 637–638, 1972.

11. Okada, M. and Hashimoto, Y.   Carcinogenic effect of N-nitrosamines related to butyl(4-hydroxybutyl)nitrosamine in ACI/N rats, with special reference to induction of urinary bladder tumors. Gann, *65*: 13–19, 1974.

12. Hashimoto, Y., Suzuki, K., Odashima, S., and Okada, M.   Studies on carcinogenicity of butyl(4-hydroxybutyl)nitrosamine analogs in ACI rats, with special reference to carcinogenesis in urinary bladder (II). Proc. Japan. Cancer Assoc., 33rd Annu. Meet., p. 58, 1974 (in Japanese).

13. Hashimoto, Y., Okada, M., and Odashima, S.   Studies on carcinogenicity of butyl-(4-hydroxybutyl)nitrosamine analogs in ACI rats, with special reference to carcinogenesis in urinary bladder (III). Proc. Japan. Cancer Assoc., 34th Annu. Meet., p. 22, 1975 (in Japanese).

14. Ito, N., Hiasa, Y., Tamai, A., Okajima, E., and Kitamura, H.   Histogenesis of urinary bladder tumors induced by N-butyl-N-(4-hydroxybutyl)nitrosamine in rats. Gann, *60*: 401–410, 1969.

15. Hashimoto, Y., Suzuki, K., and Okada, M.   Induction of urinary bladder tumors by intravesicular instillation of butyl(4-hydroxybutyl)nitrosamine and its principal urinary metabolite, butyl(3-carboxypropyl)nitrosamine in rats. Gann, *65*: 69–73, 1974.

16. Hashimoto, Y. and Kitagawa, H. S.   *In vitro* neoplastic transformation of epithelial cells of rat urinary bladder by nitrosamines. Nature, *252*: 497–499, 1974.

17. Iiyoshi, M. and Okada, M.   Metabolism of N-methyl-N-(4-hydroxybutyl)nitrosamine, N-ethyl-N-(4-hydroxybutyl)nitrosamine, and N-amyl-N-(4-hydroxybutyl)-nitrosamine in the rat. Abstr. 94th Annu. Meet., Pharm. Soc. Japan, III, p. 20, 1974 (in Japanese).

18. Okada, M., Suzuki, E., and Aoki, J.   Metabolism and carcinogenicity of N-nitrosamines related to butyl(4-hydroxybutyl)nitrosamine in the rat. Proc. Japan. Cancer Assoc., 32nd Annu. Meet., p. 136, 1973 (in Japanese).

19. Suzuki, E., Iiyoshi, M., and Okada, M.   Correlation of structure and metabolism with organotropic carcinogenicity of N-nitrosamines related to DBN and BBN. Proc. Japan. Cancer Assoc., 34th Annu. Meet., p. 41, 1975 (in Japanese).

20. Unpublished results.

21. Takeda, Y., Hashimoto, Y., and Okada, M.   Structure and carcinogenic effect of an N-nitroso compound obtained by the reaction of spermidine with nitrite. Abstr. 95th Annu. Meet., Pharm. Soc. Japan, III, p. 151, 1975 (in Japanese).

22. Hashimoto, Y., Kurashima, C., and Okada, M.   Metabolic transformation of a

urinary bladder carcinogen butyl(4-hydroxybutyl)nitrosamine and its analogs *in vitro*. Proc. Japan. Cancer Assoc., 32nd Annu. Meet., p. 171, 1973 (in Japanese).

23. Hashimoto, Y., Iiyoshi, M., and Okada, M.   Rapid and selective induction of urinary bladder cancer in rats with N-ethyl-N-(4-hydroxybutyl)nitrosamine and by its principal urinary metabolite. Gann, *65*: 565–566, 1974.

24. Heath, D. F.   The decomposition and toxicity of dialkylnitrosamines in rats. Biochem. J., *85*: 72–91, 1962.

25. Lijinsky, W. and Taylor, H. W.   Induction of urinary bladder tumors in rats by administration of nitrosomethyldodecylamine. Cancer Res., *35*: 958–961, 1975.

26. Blattmann, L. and Preussmann, R.   Metaboliten von (2-Hydroxybutyl)-*n*-butylnitrosamine im Rattenurin. Z. Krebsforsch., *83*: 125–127, 1975.

27. Althoff, J., Krüger, F. W., Hilfrich, J., Schmähl, D., and Mohr, U.   Carcinogenicity of β-hydroxylated dipropylnitrosamine. Naturwissenschaften, *60*: 55, 1973.

28. Althoff, J., Hilfrich, J., Krüger, F. W., and Bertram, B.   The carcinogenic effect of 2-oxo-propyl-propylnitrosamine in Sprague-Dawley rats. Z. Krebsforsch., *81*: 23–28, 1974.

29. Druckrey, H.   Chemical carcinogenesis on N-nitroso derivatives. GANN Monogr. Cancer Res., *17*: 107–132, 1975.

30. Okada, M., Suzuki, E., Anjo, T., and Mochizuki, M.   Mutagenicity of α-acetoxy-dialkylnitrosamines: Model compounds for an ultimate carcinogen. Gann, *66*: 457–458, 1975.

31. Eiter, K., Hebenbrock, K.-H., and Kabbe, H.-J.   Neue offenkettige und cyclische α-Nitrosaminoalkyl-äther. Liebigs Ann. Chem., *765*: 55–77, 1972.

32. Wiessler, M.   Synthese α-funktioneller Nitrosamine. Angew. Chem., *86*: 817–818, 1974.

33. Wiessler, M.   Chemie der Nitrosamine II. Synthese α-funktioneller Dimethylnitrosamine. Tetrahedron Lett., 2575–2578, 1975.

34. Roller, P. P., Shimp, D. R., and Keefer, L. K.   Synthesis and solvolysis of methyl-(acetoxymethyl)nitrosamine. Solution chemistry of the presumed carcinogenic metabolite of dimethylnitrosamine. Tetrahedron Lett., 2065–2068, 1975.

35. Rice, J. M., Joshi, S. R., Roller, P. P., and Wenk, M. L.   Methyl(acetoxymethyl)-nitrosamine: A new carcinogen highly specific for colon and small intestine. Proc. Am. Assoc. Cancer Res., *16*: 32, 1975.

Discussion of Paper of Dr. Okada

DR. MAGEE: Does N-butyl-N-(3-carboxypropyl)nitrosamine (BCPN) react directly with DNA or other cellular micromolecules *in vitro*?

DR. OKADA: We have not done any experiments yet but we hope to do so. Quite
recently, Dr. Sugimura *et al.* have demonstrated definitely a mutagenic effect of
BCPN on microorganism without any metabolic activation system. Therefore,
BCPN is a relatively stable compound as an "ultimate" carcinogen, or it might
be a pre-ultimate carcinogen.

FUNDAMENTALS IN CANCER PREVENTION, P. N. MAGEE ET AL. (EDS.),
UNIV. OF TOKYO PRESS, TOKYO / UNIV. PARK PRESS, BALTIMORE, PP. 267–280, 1976

In Vivo and *In Vitro* Aspects of Carcinogenesis of the Urinary Bladder by Nitrosamines

Yoshiyuki Hashimoto,[*1] Hisayo S. Kitagawa,[*2] and Kunihiro Ogura[*3]

Faculty of Pharmaceutical Sciences, Tohoku University, Sendai, Japan,[*1] *Tokyo Biochemical Research Institute, Tokyo, Japan,*[*1,*2] *and Department of Urology, School of Medicine, University of Tokushima, Tokushima, Japan*[*3]

Abstract: Experiments on the *in vivo* and *in vitro* effects of a potent and selective urinary bladder carcinogen, N-butyl- or N-ethyl-N-(4-hydroxybutyl) nitrosamine (BBN or EHBN), to epithelial cells of the urinary bladder of ACI/N rats are described.

In vivo experiments by direct instillations of BBN or its major urinary metabolite, N-butyl-N-(3-carboxypropyl) nitrosamine (BCPN), and by administration of EHBN to rats who have received cutaneocystostomy suggest that bladder cancers can be induced by direct effect of BCPN or N-ethyl-N-(3-carboxypropyl) nitrosamine (ECPN), a major urinary metabolite of EHBN, and that the urinary metabolite must be retained for a certain period in the urinary bladder in order to induce cancer.

Normal epithelial cells of the urinary bladder transformed into neoplastic cells by *in vitro* culture in the presence of BBN or BCPN and urea. Squamous cell carcinomas developed by transplantation of cells of established cell lines into syngeneic adult animals. Other carcinogenic and noncarcinogenic nitrosamines such as EHBN, ECPN, N-butyl-N-(3-hydroxypropyl) nitrosamine, and N-butyl-N-(2-carboxyethyl) nitrosamine also transformed normal epithelial cells of the bladder into neoplastic cells in the coexistence of urea. Cytological characters of transforming and transformed epithelial cells are demonstrated.

N-Butyl-N-(4-hydroxybutyl)nitrosamine (BBN) showed a potent and selective carcinogenic effect to epithelium of the urinary bladder in rats, mice, and dogs (*1, 2, 9, 15*). Metabolic fate of this compound in rats was thoroughly investigated by Okada *et al.* (*13, 14*). They found that BBN given orally was excreted into the urine mainly as its carboxy derivative, N-butyl-N-(3-carboxypropyl)nitrosamine (BCPN). It was shown by *in vitro* and *in vivo* experiments that conversion of BBN to BCPN was mainly conducted by liver enzymes (*6*). Carcinogenic test of BCPN in rats revealed that BCPN was also a potent and selective carcinogen for the urinary bladder like BBN (*7*). These findings suggest that selective carcinogenicity of BBN to the urinary bladder can be attributable to rapid conversion of BBN to BCPN in the liver, and prompt excretion of BCPN into urine, and to the direct carcinogenic effect of BCPN to epithelium of the urinary bladder. In order to ascertain these assumptions further *in vivo* experiments were carried out by direct instillation of BCPN or BBN into a lumen of the urinary bladder and by oral administration of nitrosamine to rats who had received cutaneocystostomy. *In vitro* culture system will be also useful for obtaining further information on the mechanism of carcinogenesis of the urinary bladder. We have succeeded in culturing epithelial cells of the urinary bladder in the presence of nitrosamine, and observed the fate of the cells in the culture and tumorigenicity of the transformed cells in the syngeneic animals (*4*).

The present article summarizes the data of these experiments and discusses the mechanism of carcinogenesis in the urinary bladder of rats by nitrosamines. All animals used in the present experiments were ACI/N rats of a highly inbred strain.

Intravesicular Instillation of Nitrosamine

A rat was anesthetized with ether and a polyethylene tube was inserted into the cavity of the urethra of the rat until the top of the tube reached the bladder lumen. Then 0.2 ml each of nitrosamine solution or distilled water was injected through the tube. All the rats received the injection 3 times a week for 20 weeks and they received once a week an injection of kanamycin solution to prevent infection.

Urinary bladder tumors were not induced in rats who received distilled water alone, whereas 4 out of 7 and 3 out of 8 rats developed bladder cancers when they received BBN and BCPN, respectively (*8*). Most of the rats who developed papillomas and/or cancers held calculi in the bladder but two rats who received BBN developed tumors without calculus formation. Because of the calculus formation it would be irrelevant to conclude from the result that tumor induction was due to the direct action of nitrosamine to the bladder epithelium, however, it was likely that BCPN promoted the induction of tumors, since some control rats had calculi but no tumors. Direct carcinogenic effect of BBN could be also attributable to BCPN, because BBN was found to be easily converted to BCPN by incubation with bladder mucosa (*6*).

Effect of Cutaneocystostomy

We have tested the carcinogenic activity of several nitrosamines whose structure were analogous to BBN and found that N-ethyl-N-(4-hydroxybutyl)nitrosamine (EHBN) was a more potent carcinogen to the urinary bladder than BBN (*3*). The metabolic pattern of EHBN in the rat was quite similar to BBN (*14*) and the principal urinary metabolite, N-ethyl-N-(3-carboxypropyl)nitrosamine (ECPN) showed also potent and selective carcinogenic activity to the urinary bladder. Thus application of EHBN to carcinogenesis of the urinary bladder will be relevant

TABLE 1. Effect of EHBN on Rats That Received Cutaneocystostomy

Sex of rat	Operation[a]	Period of EHBN administration[b] in weeks	No. of rats with urinary bladder tumors/No. of test
M	+	0	0/1
F	+	0	0/4
M	+	8	0/1
M	+	20	0/2
F	+	20	0/4
M	−	20	5/5
F	−	20	5/5

[a] Operation was carried out 3 weeks previous to the start of EHBN administration.   [b] 0.04% EHBN in the drinking water, daily 20 ml, was given to a rat.

to shorten the period for carcinogenesis, whereas the mechanism of the carcinogenesis may be similar to BBN carcinogenesis.

In order to know whether stagnation of urine, containing active metabolite of nitrosamine, in the urinary bladder is required for the carcinogenesis of the bladder, carcinogenic effect of EHBN on rats who had undergone cutaneocystostomy was examined. The urinary bladder of a rat was separated from the urethra and transplanted through the abdominal skin. Rats who received this operation excreted the urine without stagnation in the urinary bladder.

As shown in Table 1, all rats who had not received the operation developed bladder cancers through oral administration of EHBN for 20 weeks, whereas none developed tumors when they had undergone cutaneocystostomy previously.

Tissue Culture Experiment

1. Effect of BCPN and BBN

Trypsin digested cells from the epithelium of the urinary bladder of adult ACI/N rats were inoculated into tissue culture flasks and cultured in Eagle's minimum essential medium (MEM) containing 10% fetal bovine serum for 3 to 4 days. Then the medium was changed to one of the following media, which was refreshed every 7 to 10 days: medium A, Eagle's MEM containing 10% fetal bovine serum (plain medium); B, plain medium plus urea; C, plain medium plus BCPN; D, plain medium plus urea and BCPN; E, plain medium plus BBN; and F, plain medium plus urea and BBN. Concentration of urea in each medium was 0.05% and that of nitrosamine was usually 0.03%.

Fate of epithelial cells in each medium. As illustrated in Fig. 1, the fate of epithelial cells in cultures were divided into 3 stages. Stage 1 was represented by gradual degeneration of inoculated cells which was characterized by formation of polynuclei, abundant cytoplasmic granules and vacuoles, and by rounding up of the cells. Fate of cells cultured in plain medium or in medium containing urea alone or nitrosamine alone usually were terminated in this stage and few epithelial cells were detectable 5 to 6 weeks after inoculation, whereas cells cultured in the medium

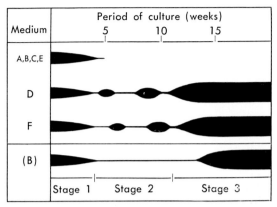

FIG. 1.   Apparent growth patterns of epithelial cells from 39-week-old rats in various media. Medium A, plain medium ; B, plain medium plus urea ; C, plain medium plus BCPN ; D, plain medium plus urea and BCPN ; E, plain medium plus BBN ; F, plain medium plus urea and BBN. (B), proliferation of cells in medium B, which took place in only one flask.

containing both urea and nitrosamine survived in a small number at Stage 1, and they started to proliferate after 4 to 6 weeks. The proliferated cells formed a small colony whose number in a flask was usually 1 or 2. When the cells grew to form a focal monolayer, many cells degenerated in 1 or 2 weeks (Fig. 2). This phenom-

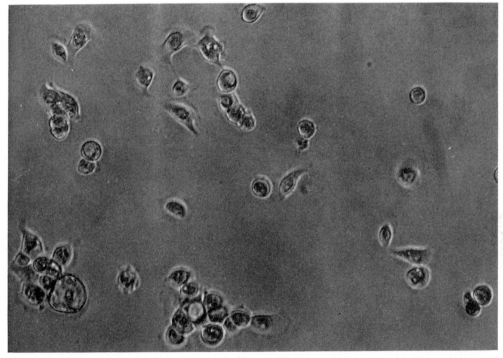

FIG. 2.   Degenerated epithelial cells by contact death phenomenon. Cells in a focal colony developed by culture in medium containing urea and BCPN (44 days after inoculation). Phase contrast.   ×100.

TABLE 2.   Culture of Epithelial Cells of Urinary Bladder in Various Media

Age of donor rats (weeks)	No. of flasks developed cell strains/No. of tested flasks with medium[b] of:					
	A	B	C	D	E	F
12, 15[a]	0/6		0/4		0/4	
8	0/1	0/1	0/1	2/2	0/1	1/1
9	0/1	0/1	0/1	1/2		
12	0/1	0/1	0/1	2/2	0/1	2/2
37	0/2			7/7		
39	0/1	1/2	0/1	3/3	0/1	2/2
Total	0/12	1/5	0/8	15/16	0/7	5/5

[a] Accumulated results of preliminary experiments.   [b] A, plain medium; B, plain medium plus urea; C, plain medium plus BCPN; D, plain medium plus urea and BCPN; E, plain medium plus BBN; F, plain medium plus urea and BBN.

enon was called contact death (4). Contact death was not due to a nutritional factor of the medium, because at this stage of culture the total number of cells was very small and contact death took place even in a fresh medium. Moreover, when two colonies were present in the appart position of a flask, cells in one colony were degenerating but cells in another colony of lower cell density showed active proliferation. Surviving cells after contact death divided again and formed a new

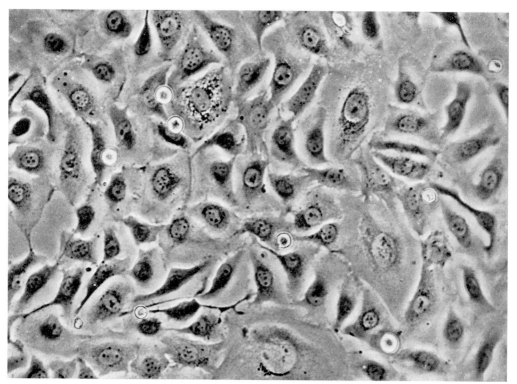

FIG. 3.   An established cell strain, BES3P-16 cells. Phase contrast.   ×100.

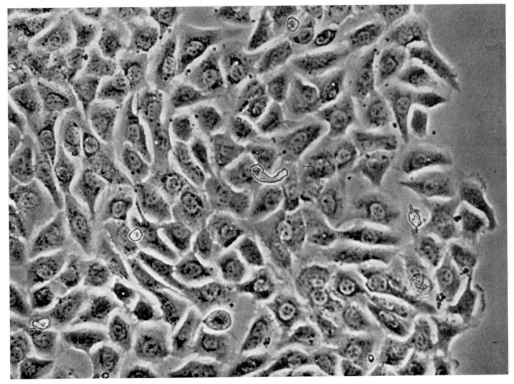

FIG. 4.   BES3B-2 cells. Phase contrast.   × 100.

colony. This process was repeated 2 to 3 times (Stage 2). Contact death tendency in these epithelial cells decreased gradually and finally cells grew without contact death to form a confluent monolayer (Stage 3). It took usually 13 to 15 weeks until cells attained Stage 3. Confluent cells were trypsinized and passed to other new flasks, thus cell strains amenable to serial passages were obtained; they were named as indicated in the footnote of Table 3.

As shown in Table 2, repeated experiments using bladder epithelial cells obtained from 8- to 39-week-old rats gave similar results as above. However, only cells from 39-week-old rats continued to grow without showing the contact death phenomenon in the medium containing urea alone and formed a confluent monolayer, although the start of growth was delayed in the cells cultured in the medium containing both urea and nitrosamine (Fig. 1).

In all cultures fibroblast-like cells were contaminated in the early stage of culture, however, they did not show progressive growth even in the medium where epithelial cells grew, and they gradually disappeared from the culture. Therefore established cell strains consisted of pure epithelial cells (Figs. 3 and 4).

Morphology. Cells of inductive phase and of established strains appeared to be composed of essentially similar epithelial cells to normal ones which were rhombic or fusiform with oval or round nucleus surrounded by spreading cytoplasm. However there was a difference between normal cells and established strains in number of nucleoli. The former cells had one or 2 relatively large nucleoli per nucleus but the latter had more than 2 such nucleoli (Figs. 3 and 4). Piling up of cells in a monolayer was rarely seen in any of the strains. In all cultures, during or after inductive phase, some cornified cells were formed on a cell layer which appeared as relatively large and thin dark flakes under a phase contrast microscope, and after fixation they were stained orangish by Papanicolou stain.

TABLE 3. Chromosome Constitution of Established Cell Strains

Cell strain[a] and the generation	No. of cells observed	Modal No. of chromosome (%)	Constitution[b]
BES3P-8	81	42 (59.0)	19 t+ 9 s+14 m
BES3B-12	124	81 (15.3)	34 t+24 s+23 m
BES3B-T2[c]	104	74 (22.0)	36 t+17 s+22 m
BES6P-9	66	64 (28.8)	32 t+11 s+21 m
BES8P-8	112	75 (13.4)	35 t+10 s+30 m
		79 (12.5)	36 t+18 s+25 m
BES8B-5	63	71 (22.0)	33 t+20 s+19 m
BES8U-9	87	64 (15.0)	30 t+16 s+18 m
		77 (18.4)	39 t+14 s+24 m

[a] Cell strains are named as follows: BE means they derived from bladder epithelial cells; S number denotes the experimental series number, and the last character shows the drug added in the medium, *i.e.*, P, BCPN plus urea; B, BBN plus urea; U, urea alone. [b] t, telocentric; s, subtelocentric; m, metacentric chromosomes. [c] Passage 2 cells which were backcultured from tumor.

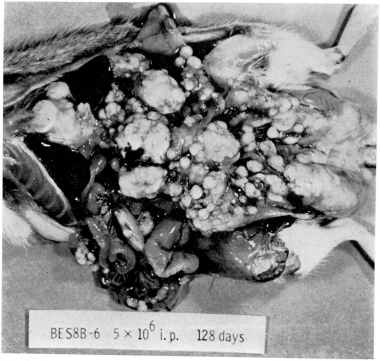

FIG. 5. Tumors developed by intraperitoneal injection of BES8B-6 cells.

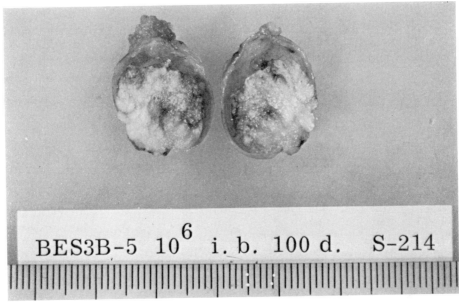

Fig. 6.   Tumor developed by intrabladder wall injection of BES3B-5 cells.

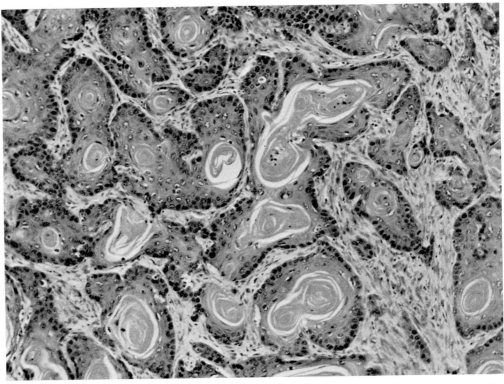

Fig. 7.   Histology of tumor developed from BES3B cells. Hematoxylin and Eosin stain.
×100.

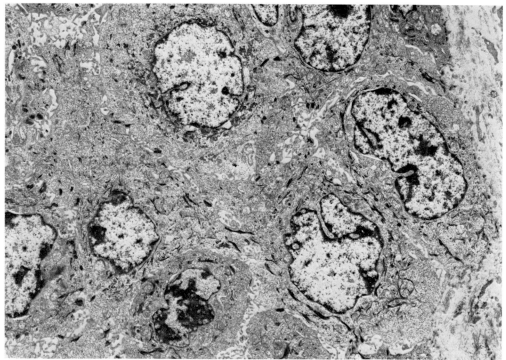

FIG. 8. Electron microscopic pattern of the tumor in Fig. 7.   ×3,600.

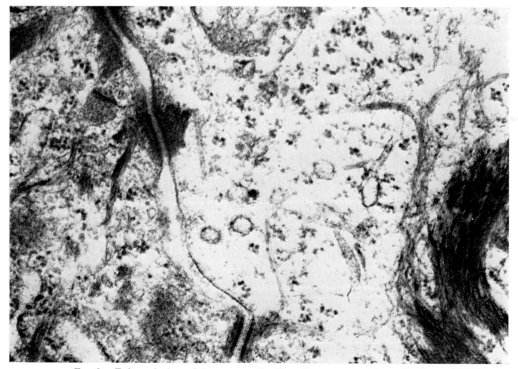

FIG. 9. Enlarged view of the tumor cells. Note desmosomes and tonofibrils.   ×54,000.

Chromosome distributions. Chromosome features of the established cell strains were shown in Table 3. Majority of the cell strains held hypotetraploid complement except one strain, BES3P, whose modal chromosome was ranged in diploid. Cells back-cultured from the tumor of BES3B cells showed a karyogram similar to the original strain. All cell strains had individual marker chromosomes in each strain and they were not common.

Tumorigenicity. Cells of all the established strains developed tumors by intraperitoneal, subcutaneous, or intrabladder wall injection into X-irradiated or unconditioned adult ACI/N rats (*4*). In all cases the growth rate of tumors was slower than that of tumors developed by the transplantation of *in vivo* induced bladder cancer cells (*12*). When the cells were injected subcutaneously or intraperitoneally, tumors became palpable after 1 to 2 months. By intraperitoneal injection many tumor nodules were formed in the peritoneal region (Fig. 5). Tumors located mainly in the omentum, peritoneum, and diaphragm but there was no metastasis in the other organs. By leaving the animals with a tumor for longer than 6 months they died due to the tumor. When $1-2 \times 10^6$ cells were injected into the bladder wall of a rat, all cell strains developed a tumor at the injection site (Fig. 6).

Tumors developed from transformed cells were serially transplantable to adult ACI/N rats by a trocar inoculation of minced tumor fragments.

Morphology of tumor. Tumors developed from the cells of any of the strains showed similar histological patterns and were diagnosed as squamous cell carcinoma (Fig. 7).

Cells of the tumors showed similar ultrastructure in all the cell strains (Figs. 8 and 9). Cells were irregularly spherical, forming cytoplasmic projections and a moderate number of microvilli. Cells were connected with many desmosomes (Fig. 9). Tonofibrils were abundant, especially in cells of an advanced degree of differentiation (cornification). These ultrastructures were quite similar to those of the cells derived from *in vivo* induced bladder cancer (*9*).

2. *Effect of other nitrosamines*

In order to know whether the transforming effect of nitrosamine to normal epithelial cells of the urinary bladder is related to its carcinogenic effect in animals, several nitrosamines whose carcinogenic activities were already known (*3, 14*) were

TABLE 4. Effect of Various Nitrosamines on Cultures of Epithelial Cells of Urinary Bladder

Compound[a] (+urea)	*In vivo* carcino- genicity to bladder	No. of established strains/No. of test[b]	Tumorigenicity of cell strain[c]
EHBN	+	1/2	−
ECPN	+	2/2	+
BHPN	−	1/4	+
BCEN	−	2/4	+

[a] For abbreviation of chemical names see the text.   [b] Normal epithelial cells of the urinary bladder were cultured in the medium containing 0.03% nitrosamine and 0.05% urea.   [c] 10^6 cells were injected intraperitoneally, subcutaneously, or into the bladder wall and the tumor formation was observed until days after the injection.

tested by *in vitro* culture. Normal epithelial cells of the urinary bladder were cultured in a method similar to that described above. As shown in Table 4, not only carcinogenic nitrosamines such as EHBN and its major urinary metabolite, ECPN, but also noncarcinogenic compounds such as N-butyl-N-(3-hydroxypropyl)nitrosamine (BHPN) and its metabolite, N-butyl-N-(2-carboxyethyl)nitrosamine (BCEN), induced proliferation of epithelial cells and gave permanently growing cell strains which formed squamous cell carcinomas by injection into ACI/N rats. In this experiment cells from rather old rats (30-week-old) were employed, so that in order to confirm the present result we will need to perform the experiment using cells from younger animals.

DISCUSSION

Ito *et al.* (*9*) observed that hyperplastic change took place in the epithelium of the urinary bladder when BBN in drinking water was administered to rats for several weeks, and by continuation of the administration of the carcinogen papillomas and cancers were successively induced. However, if the administration was discontinued the hyperplastic change in the early stage returned to normal. This finding suggests that persistent stimulation of the epithelium by active metabolite(s) of the carcinogen may be an important factor in the development of the bladder tumors. The stimulant for the epithelium could be attributable, in the case of BBN carcinogenesis, to a principal urinary metabolite, BCPN (*13*) which showed a potent and selective carcinogenic effect on the urinary bladder by oral administration to rats (*7*). The direct carcinogenic effect of BBN as well as its urinary metabolite, BCPN, was demonstrated by repeating instillations of the compound into the bladder lumen of a rat (*8*).

A question arises as to why transitional epithelium of the renal pelvis and ureter of a rat who is given BBN are little affected by the active metabolite, BCPN, inspite of the continuous exposure to the metabolite. Ito *et al.* (*10*) found that tumors were induced in these tissues if the ureter had been ligated loosely, and they assumed that stagnation of urine, containing an active metabolite, was important in the induction of tumors of the transitional epithelium. This assumption was confirmed by the present experiment using rats who had undergone cutaneocystostomy previous to nitrosamine administration.

Utilization of the tissue culture method will be advantageous for the study on the etiology of nitrosamine carcinogenesis in the urinary bladder. Although cells of urinary bladder tumors were successfully cultured *in vitro* (*11, 16*), establishment of culture cell strains from normal epithelial cells of the rat or mouse urinary bladder have been unsuccessful until our recent report (*4*). As shown in the previous and the present reports, epithelial cells of the urinary bladder of adult ACI/N rats did not grow in the regular tissue culture medium, but they grew in the medium containing BBN or BCPN or their analogues and urea to give cell strains which were amenable sereal passages. Since nitrosamine alone did not induce proliferation of epithelial cells, urea could be an important factor for the establishment of epithelial cell strains. Thus, in *in vivo* too, urea in urine would play some role in the induction of bladder tumors in cooperation with an active urinary metabolite derived from nitrosamine. Cells of all the strains induced by *in vitro* culture held neoplastic character and by injection into adult syngeneic animals, squamous cell carcinomas were developed in the injection site (*4, 5*).

It was observed that in the course from normal to neoplastic cells, epithelial cells of the urinary bladder showed a characteristic growth pattern; a few surviving cells from the initial degeneration process started to grow to form a small focal colony and when the cells contacted each other many cells died leaving a small number of living cells which showed regrowth later. When this character was lost and they were able to grow as a confluent monolayer, they had already acquired a neoplastic character. It is interesting that the period required for the induction of the intermediate cell-colony quite matches that required for the formation of focal hyperplasia of the urinary bladder in the animal experiment with BBN (*9*).

As far as carcinogenesis by BBN or BCPN is concerned, *in vitro* results reflected well the *in vivo* findings, thus the present *in vitro* culture system will be useful for study on the mechanism of carcinogenesis of the urinary bladder by nitrosamine, and may provide information for the research of a preventive method for urinary bladder cancer.

ACKNOWLEDGMENTS

The authors wish to thank Drs. S. Odashima, A. Maekawa, and M. Ishidate, Jr. of the National Institute for Hygienic Sciences, Tokyo, for performing histological and karyological observations, and Dr. M. Okada of the Tokyo Biochemical Research Institute, Tokyo, for supplying the chemicals.

This work was supported in part by a Grant-in-Aid for Cancer Research from the Ministry of Education, Science and Culture, Japan.

REFERENCES

1. Bertram, J. S. and Craig, A. W. Specific induction of bladder cancer in mice by butyl-(4-hydroxybutyl)nitrosamine and the effect of hormonal modifications on the sex difference in response. Eur. J. Cancer, *8*: 587–594, 1972.

2. Druckrey, H., Preussmann, R., Ivankovic, S., and Schmidt, C. H. Selektive Erzeugung von Blasenkrebs an Ratten durch Dibutyl- und N-butyl-N-butanol(4)nitrosamine. Z. Krebsforsch., *66*: 280–290, 1964.

3. Hashimoto, Y., Iiyoshi, M., and Okada, M. Rapid and selective induction of urinary bladder cancer in rats with N-ethyl-N-(4-hydroxybutyl)nitrosoamine and by its principal urinary metabolite. Gann, *65*: 565–566, 1974.

4. Hashimoto, Y. and Kitagawa, S. H. *In vitro* neoplastic transformation of epithelial cells of rat urinary bladder by nitrosamines. Nature, *252*: 497–499, 1974.

5. Hashimoto, Y., Kitagawa, S. H., Ishidate, M., Jr., and Maekawa, A. *In vitro* neoplastic transformation of epithelial cells of rat urinary bladder by nitrosamine and urea—Cytological and histological observations. Submitted to J. Natl. Cancer Inst., 1975.

6. Hashimoto, Y., Kurashima, C., and Okada, M. Metabolic change of an urinary bladder carcinogen, N-butyl-N-(4-hydroxybutyl)nitrosamine, and its analogues *in vitro*. Proc. Japan. Cancer Assoc., 32nd Annu. Meet., p. 171, 1973.

7. Hashimoto, Y., Suzuki, E., and Okada, M.   Induction of urinary bladder tumors in ACI/N rats by N-butyl-N-(3-carboxypropyl)nitrosoamine, a major urinary metabolite of N-butyl-N-(4-hydroxybutyl)nitrosoamine. Gann, *63*: 637–638, 1972.

8. Hashimoto, Y., Suzuki, K., and Okada, M.   Induction of urinary bladder tumors by intravesicular instillation of butyl-(4-hydroxybutyl)nitrosoamine and its principal urinary metabolite, butyl-(3-carboxypropyl)nitrosoamine in rats. Gann, *65*: 69–73, 1974.

9. Ito, N., Hiasa, Y., Tamai, A., Okajima, E., and Kitamura, H. Histogenesis of urinary bladder tumors induced by N-butyl-N-(4-hydroxybutyl)nitrosoamine in rats. Gann, *60*: 401–410, 1969.

10. Ito, N., Makiura, S., Yokota, Y., Kamamoto, Y., Hiasa, Y., and Sugihara, S. Effect of unilateral ureter ligation on development of tumors in the urinary system of rats treated with N-butyl-N-(4-hydroxybutyl)nitrosamine. Gann, *62*: 359–365, 1971.

11. Lavin, P. and Koss, L. G. Studies of experimental bladder carcinoma in Fischer 344 female rats. II. Characterization of 3 cell lines derived from induced urinary bladder carcinomas. J. Natl. Cancer Inst., *46*: 597–614, 1971.

12. Noda, M. and Hashimoto, Y. Transplantability of urinary bladder cancers induced in ACI/N rats by oral administration of butyl-(4-hydroxybutyl)nitrosamine and its acetate. Japan. J. Urol., *64*: 397–401, 1973.

13. Okada, M. and Suzuki, E. Metabolism of butyl-(4-hydroxybutyl)nitrosoamine in rats. Gann, *63*: 391–392, 1972.

14. Okada, M., Suzuki, E., Aoki, J., Iiyoshi, M., and Hashimoto, Y. Metabolism and carcinogenicity of N-*n*-butyl-N-(4-hydroxybutyl)nitrosamine and related compounds, with special references to induction of urinary bladder tumors. GANN Monogr. Cancer Res., *17*: 161–176, 1975.

15. Okajima, E., Motomiya, Y., Ijuin, M., Matsushima, S., Hirao, Y., Yamada, K., Ohara, S., Shiomi, T., Oishi, H., and Hosoki, Y.   Development of urinary bladder tumors in dogs induced by N-butyl-N-(4-hydroxybutyl)nitrosamine (BBN). Proc. Japan. Cancer Assoc., 34th Annu. Meet., p. 22, 1975.

16. Toyoshima, K., Ito, N., Hiasa, Y., Makiura, S., and Kamamoto, Y.   Tissue culture of urinary bladder tumor induced in a rat by N-butyl-N-(4-hydroxybutyl)nitrosamine: Establishment of cell line, Nara bladder tumor II. J. Natl. Cancer Inst., *47*: 979–985, 1971.

Discussion of Paper of Drs. Hashimoto et al.

DR. RAJEWSKY: During the process of neoplastic transformation in culture, have you observed any phenotypic or functional changes in the bladder epithelia (such as, *e.g.*, colony formation in semisolid agar medium) preceding the first demonstrability of tumorigenicity upon reimplantation *in vivo*?

DR. HASHIMOTO: Transformed cells showed 3 dimensional growth on sponge-matrix culture, but because of the shortage of the number of intermediate cells, we have not tested yet the properties of these cells.

DR. KURODA: (1) You can maintain cells continuously in the presence of nitros-amine and urea. Have you obtained similar transformed cells after treatment with chemicals for a limited time? (2) Have you detected any difference in the sensitivity to nitrosamine between the original cells and the transformed cells?

DR. HASHIMOTO: (1) In some experiments, we have observed that if nitrosamine and urea were removed from the culture medium, epithelial cells in an intermediate stage died after 1 or 2 weeks, and further growth did not take palce. In this sense, the presence of nitrosamine and urea may be required until the cell strain is established. (2) The nitrosamine used did not show any cytotoxic effect to either normal or transformed cells even in rather high concentration (*i.e.*, 0.06%).

FUNDAMENTALS IN CANCER PREVENTION, P. N. MAGEE ET AL. (EDS.),
UNIV. OF TOKYO PRESS, TOKYO / UNIV. PARK PRESS, BALTIMORE, PP. 281–292, 1976

Possible Repair of Carcinogenesis by Nitroso Compounds

P. N. Magee, P. F. Swann, U. Mohr,* G. Resnik,* and U. Green*

*Courtauld Institute of Biochemistry, Middlesex Hospital Medical School, London, U.K. and Abteilung für Experimentelle Pathologie, Medizinische Hochschule Hannover, Hannover, West Germany**

Abstract: The data discussed in this paper indicates that there are defensive repair mechanisms in the body against carcinogenesis by nitroso compounds and suggest possible molecular mechanisms by which they may act.

If alkylation of DNA is causally related to the induction of cancer by N-nitroso compounds, recent findings on the differential rates of removal of alkylated bases from the DNA of different organs may clarify hitherto unexplained organotropic actions of these carcinogens.

Several N-nitroso compounds are known to alkylate cellular components *in vivo*, the nitrosamines requiring activation by enzymes whereas the nitrosamides require no such metabolic activation (*1–3*). The role of alkylation in the biological actions of the nitroso compounds, including carcinogenesis, has been extensively investigated and discussed without conclusive results. Most investigations have been concerned with the alkylation of nucleic acids and relatively little has been published on reactions with proteins and other cellular macromolecules. An important reason for this concentration of effort on the nucleic acids is the well-known relationship between the carcinogenic and mutagenic activities of chemicals (*4*) and the belief, held by some workers, that cancer results from a mutation in a somatic cell.

Alkylation of nucleic acids by nitroso compounds and its possible role in carcinogenesis were discussed at the Second International Symposium of The Princess Takamatsu Cancer Research Fund in 1971 (*5, 6*), and again more recently (*2, 3, 7*).

The main site of alkylation of DNA and RNA by a variety of alkylating agents, *in vitro* and *in vivo*, is the 7-position of guanine. For this reason, the earlier quantitative work on methylation and ethylation of nucleic acids in the whole animal (*8, 9*) was confined to measurements of reaction on this position. Although there were some correlations between the degree of alkylation in different organs and the sites of tumour induction there were many discrepancies which led to serious objections to the hypothesis that alkylation of nucleic acids might be causally related to tumour production (*10, 11*).

A major objection to alkylation of DNA as a cause of cancer arose from the findings that methyl and ethyl methanesulphonate were equally or more effective in reacting with guanine on the 7-position in rats *in vivo* but were much less potent as carcinogens than the corresponding methyl and ethyl nitrosamines or nitros-amides. This failure of correlation was particularly marked with methyl methane-sulphonate, which failed to induce kidney tumours after administration to rats in single doses which gave rise to similar degrees of methylation on the 7-position of guanine to those found after treatment with dimethylnitrosamine (*8*). The latter compound, under appropriate dietary conditions, can give rise to tumour induction in every exposed animal (*12*). It is of interest, however, that a small number of brain tumours were induced in rats given methyl methanesulphonate as young adults (*13*) or by the transplacental route (*14*). The situation became more clear in 1969 when Loveless (*15*) reported alkylation of phage DNA on the O^6-position of guanine by nitrosamides, which were powerfully mutagenic to the phage, but with methyl methanesulphonate, which was not mutagenic in the phage, no detectable alkylation of the O^6-position was found. (Methyl methanesulphonate was sub-sequently shown to produce a very small degree of methylation of the O^6-position of guanine in DNA *in vitro* (*16*).) The finding that O^6-alkylguanines in DNA were promutagenic (*17*) whereas 7-methylguanine was not (*18*), gave further support for the idea that O^6-alkylation was particularly important biologically whereas N^7-alkylation was of relatively much less significance.

Although these ideas went some way towards the reestablishment of alkylation as the mechanism of nitrosamine carcinogenesis, they did not explain the various failures of correlation between the extent of reaction and the sites of tumour induc-tion, and led to the putting forward of various alternatives to the hypothesis that nucleic acid alkylation was the crucial event in the induction of cancer by this class of compounds.

Schoental (*19*) suggested that the proximate carcinogens derived from di-alkylnitrosamines are oxidation products retaining the alkylnitrosamine moiety but having acquired a carbonyl function. Such metabolites would probably be multifunctional and might bind with reactive centres of chromatin to form a bridge between, for example, an amino group of a nucleic acid base and a thiol group of protein. There is no direct evidence for such a cross-linking of proteins and nucleic acids but Fahmy and Fahmy (*20*), based on their extensive experimental studies of mutagenesis by nitroso compounds in *Drosophila*, have concluded that their results are not entirely explicable on the simple alkylation of nucleic acids and suggest that they might be better explained by the cross-linking mechanism.

Since however, the cross-linking hypothesis of Schoental requires metabolic activation of the dialkylnitrosamines, it does not provide any better explanation for the organotropic actions of these compounds than nucleic acid alkylation.

Possible Role of DNA Repair in the Organotropic Actions of Nitroso Carcinogens

It now appears that some of the organ specificity in the carcinogenic actions of nitroso compounds can be explained by consideration first, of the distribution of the activating enzyme systems which transform those chemically stable N-nitrosamines into chemically reactive carcinogenic species, and second, the different capacities of different organs to repair lesions in their DNA caused by alkylation of bases.

The different capacities of different organs to metabolise dialkyl and other nitrosamines have been demonstrated (*8, 9, 21–23*) and will not be discussed further. The variable persistence of alkylated bases in DNA of different organs has only recently been recognised and its significance appreciated. This major advance in the understanding of nitrosamine carcinogenesis was made by Goth and Rajewsky (*24, 25*) who compared the persistence of 7-ethylguanine and O^6-ethylguanine in the DNA of brain and liver from young rats given a single pulse dose of N-ethylnitrosourea. An essential feature of this experiment is that, under these conditions, tumours are induced selectively in the brain and other parts of the nervous system, with none or very few in other organs. Since N-ethylnitrosourea has only a very brief existence (a few minutes) after injection, it requires no metabolic activation, and penetrates and alkylates throughout the body, the remarkable organotropic effect was very difficult to explain. Very briefly, Goth and Rajewsky (*24, 25*) found similar initial degrees of ethylation in the DNA of brain and liver in terms of the molar fractions of O^6-ethylguanine, 7-ethylguanine, and 3-ethyladenine but the elimination rate of O^6-ethylguanine over a 240-hr observation period was much slower in brain than in liver, and also much slower than the elimination rates from brain DNA of 7-ethylguanine and 3-ethyladenine. These findings clearly indicate that repair of the O^6-ethylguanine lesion in the brain DNA is much slower than in the liver and suggest a possible explanation for the hitherto inexplicable organ specificity of N-ethylnitrosourea for the brain.

Similar results have been obtained by Kleihues and Margison (*26, 27*) using N-methylnitrosourea. Like the ethyl derivative, this compound can also have a highly selective carcinogenic action on the brain, in this case by repeated intravenous administration to young rats at weekly intervals. After five such weekly injections, O^6-methylguanine accumulated in rat brain DNA to an extent which greatly exceeded that in the kidney, spleen, or intestine. In the liver, the final level of O^6-ethylguanine was less than 1% of that in the brain. The authors concluded that there is no major cell fraction in the brain which can excise chemically methylated bases from DNA and that this repair deficiency could be a determining factor in the selective induction of nervous-system tumours by N-methylnitrosourea and other compounds which induce tumours in this organ.

Recent work at the Courtauld Institute of Biochemistry, Middlesex Hospital Medical School, London, England, using dimethylnitrosamine (*28*) confirms the probable importance of DNA repair processes in determining the sites of tumour induction by this compound which, in contrast to the two alkylnitrosoureas, does require metabolic activation.

Dimethylnitrosamine induces tumours of the liver in rats after continued administration in the food (or in the drinking water) at levels around 50 ppm. Under these conditions, no kidney tumours are induced, but if the rats are given a single large dose of dimethylnitrosamine, kidney tumours but no liver tumours are induced. If large single doses of dimethylnitrosamine (30 mg/kg body wt.), approaching the lethal level, are given, about 20% of the surviving animals develop renal tumours (*29*) and the incidence can be increased to 100% by prior feeding of a protein-deficient diet (*12*) which markedly increases the proportion of the dose metabolised in the kidney (*30*). Under these conditions of high single dosage of dimethylnitrosamine, the extent of methylation of the liver DNA is higher than that of kidney by a factor of 5 to 10, but tumours appear only in the kidney. These findings were again difficult to reconcile with a causative role for DNA alkylation in carcinogenesis, but again, consideration of differential rates of removal of O^6-methylguanine and 7-methylguanine from the two organs provides a reasonable explanation for these apparent discrepancies.

The persistence of O^6-methylguanine and 7-methylguanine in the DNA of rat liver and kidney was studied after a larger dose of dimethylnitrosamine (20 mg/kg body wt.), which would induce some kidney tumours, and a smaller dose (2.5 mg/kg body wt.) which would not. After the larger dose, the 7-methylguanine in both the liver and kidney DNA was lost at a rate corresponding to a half-life of about 60 hr and a similar rate was found in the kidneys of rats treated with the smaller dose, the rate of loss in the liver being slightly slower after this dose. Thus the rate of loss of 7-methylguanine from DNA *in vivo* was only slightly faster than that expected from chemical depurination at neutral pH (*31, 32*). In both organs, the amount of O^6-methylguanine formed in the DNA was only about 10% of that of 7-methylguanine. The rate of loss of O^6-methylguanine, which is chemically stable in DNA at neutral pH, was about the same from the liver after either dose, with a half-life of about 20 hr. This rate is much faster than the loss of 7-methylguanine from the liver and indicates that an enzyme must be involved in the excision of this methylated base. The O^6-methylguanine was lost from the kidney DNA at about the same rate as from the liver after the smaller dose of dimethylnitrosamine. After the larger dose however, there was a striking difference in rate of loss of O^6-methylguanine. After an initial fall of about 30% between 6 and 15 hr after giving the carcinogen, there was almost no loss for the next 35 hr followed by a relatively slow fall after this period. These findings are illustrated graphically in Fig. 1, and show that the potentially mutagenic O^6-methylguanine persists much longer in the kidney after the larger dose which does induce kidney tumours, than after the smaller dose of dimethylnitrosamine, which does not. The much more rapid loss of the O^6-methylguanine from the liver after both doses may explain why liver tumours are not produced under the conditions of the experiment. The enzyme responsible for the excision of the O^6-alkylated guanines from the DNA has not been characterised. It is interesting however, that the enzyme endonuclease II has recently been shown to be capable of excision of O^6-methylguanine and 3-methyladenine from the DNA of *E. coli* previously reacted with N-methylnitrosourea (*33*). It is possible that a similar enzyme may be present, in different amounts, in different mammalian tissues.

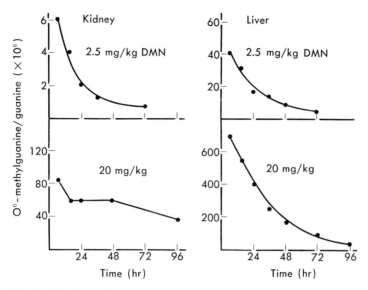

FIG. 1.   The loss of dimethylnitrosamine-produced O⁶-methylguanine from rat liver DNA and
from rat kidney DNA. The rats were given either a large single dose of dimethylnitrosamine
(20 mg/kg body wt.) which would produce a small incidence of kidney tumours but no liver
tumours, or a small dose (2.5 mg/kg body wt.) which would induce neither liver nor kidney
tumours.

From the evidence so far discussed, it is clear that there are mechanisms in
animal cells which are capable of excising O⁶-methylguanine and 3-methyladenine
from their DNA and that there is some correlation between the distribution of these
mechanisms and the development of tumours in different organs. In no sense however, has a causal relationship been established. In what follows, experiments will
be described that were designed to reveal the existence of repair processes from
carcinogenesis by dimethylnitrosamine in terms of actual tumour yield without
reference to any postulated molecular mechanism of cancer induction.

*Induction of Kidney Tumours in Rats by Two Doses of Dimethylnitrosamine Separated by
Increasing Intervals of Time*

The experimental model used was the induction of kidney tumours in rats by
two consecutive doses of dimethylnitrosamine, the second dose being given at increasing time intervals after the first. Since an initial dose of dimethylnitrosamine
affects the metabolism of a second dose, the second dose has to be adjusted so that
the dose produces the same increment of carcinogenic injury to the kidney as is
obtained when the single dose is increased from 16 to 32 mg/kg body wt. This
"notional dose" was determined by measurement of the alkylation of the kidney
DNA. The second dose (the notional dose) was adjusted so that the total amount
of alkylation produced by the two doses (the first of 16 mg/kg, the second the
notional dose) was the same as that produced by a single dose of 32 mg/kg body
wt. The rats were CFN (Carworth Farms New City, N.Y., U.S.A.) males (now

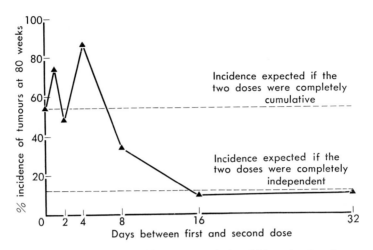

FIG. 2. The incidence of kidney tumours induced 80 weeks after the start of the experiment by a single intraperitoneal injection of dimethylnitrosamine (32 mg/kg body wt.) (100 rats), a single dose of 16 mg/kg (140 rats), or by two doses, the first of 16 mg/kg body wt., the second a nominal 16 mg/kg 1, 2, 4, 8, 16, or 32 days later. (50, 50, 60, 50, 100, and 100 rats in each group). Male CFN rats weighing about 180 g were transferred to a protein-free diet 7 days before the first injection of dimethylnitrosamine. They were maintained on this diet for 5 days after the first injection of dimethylnitrosamine and were then returned to a normal rat diet (MRC 41B, Christopher Hill, Ltd., Poole, Dorset). The second dose was in every case adjusted, as described in the text, so that the total amount of dimethylnitrosamine metabolised to the active intermediate in the kidney when two doses were given, was the same as that resulting from a single dose of 32 mg/kg. This adjustment meant that the actual dose given 1 day after the first was 12 mg/kg ; 2 days 13 mg/kg ; 4 days 12.5 mg/kg ; 8 days 26 mg/kg ; 16 days 24 mg/kg ; and 32 days 25 mg/kg. Tumours have been found in 243 of the 617 rats surviving more than 4 weeks. The upper broken line shows the incidence produced by a single dose of 32 mg/DMN/kg body wt. If the doses were completely cumulative, one would expect the two doses of 16 mg/kg to give this incidence of tumours. If the doses were not cumulative and each dose of 16 mg/kg acted independently of the other, one would expect to get twice the incidence produced by a single dose of 16 mg/kg, i.e., 12% marked by the lower broken line.

available from Charles River, Inc.) weighing 180 g at the start of the experiment. The numbers of animals in the experimental groups varied from 50 to 140.

The dose-response curve for induction of kidney tumours in rats by a single dose of dimethylnitrosamine is very steep. In this strain, the predicted incidence following 16 mg/kg body wt. was 6% of the rats at 80 weeks rising to 10% at 2 years. A single dose of 32 mg/kg dimethylnitrosamine induced an incidence of 55% at 80 weeks and 80% at 2 years. In the experiment now in progress at the Medizinische Hochschule in Hannover, the dietary conditioned rats have received a single dose of 16 mg dimethylnitrosamine/kg body wt. followed at increasing time intervals from 1 to 32 days by a second notional dose calculated as described above, of 16 mg/kg body wt. The experiment, which will last for 2 years, had been going on for 80 weeks when the results shown in Fig. 2 were obtained.

If there is no repair from the carcinogenic damage caused by the first dose of dimethylnitrosamine, the number of tumours arising from the second dose should be the same as from a single dose of 32 mg/kg body wt., *i.e.*, 55% at 80 weeks. If, however, there is some form of defensive repair a less than additive effect should be found, and if the effects of the initial dose were completely repaired, the tumour incidence should be that induced by each dose separately, *i.e.*, 12% (6% plus 6%) at 80 weeks. As shown in Fig. 2, the tumour incidences resulting from the second doses given at 16 or 32 days after the first are both about 12%, indicating that repair of the initial dose had, in fact, taken place. However, doses separated by an interval of 4 days or less, are at least cumulative in their effect. The complex pattern of response when the second dose was given 1, 2, and 4 days after the first, is probably valid because it is based on at least 50 animals per group. The explanation may be related to the effects of prior treatment with the nitrosamine on the excision of O^6-methylguanine resulting from methylation of the kidney DNA by the second dose. If the above interpretation of the results shown in Fig. 2 is valid, it seems necessary to conclude that repair from carcinogenesis by dimethylnitrosamine can occur.

REFERENCES

1. Magee, P. N. and Barnes, J. M. Carcinogenic nitroso compounds. Adv. Cancer Res., *10*: 163–246, 1967.
2. Magee, P. N., Pegg, A. E., and Swann, P. F. Molecular mechanisms of chemical carcinogenesis. *In;* E. Grundmann (ed.), Handbuch der Allgemeinen Pathologie, vol. VI, 5-6, Tumours II, pp. 329–419, Springer-Verlag, Berlin-Heidelberg-New York, 1975.
3. Magee, P. N., Montesano, R., and Preussmann, R. N-Nitroso compounds and related carcinogens. *In;* C. E. Searle (ed.), Chemical Carcinogens, American Chemical Society, New York, in press.
4. Ames, B. N., Durston, W. E., Yamasaki, E., and Lee, F. D. Carcinogens are mutagens: A simple test system combining liver homogenates for activation and bacteria for detection. Proc. Natl. Acad. Sci. U.S., *70*: 2281–2285, 1973.
5. Lawley, P. D. The action of alkylating mutagens and carcinogens on nucleic acids: N-Methyl-N-nitroso compounds as methylating agents. *In;* W. Nakahara, S. Takayama, T. Sugimura, and S. Odashima (eds.), Topics in Chemical Carcinogenesis, pp. 237–256, University of Tokyo Press, Tokyo and University Park Press, Baltimore, 1972
6. Magee, P. N. Possible mechanisms of carcinogenesis and mutagenesis by nitrosamines. *In;* W. Nakahara, S. Takayama, T. Sugimura, and S. Odashima (eds.), Topics in Chemical Carcinogenesis, pp. 259–275, University of Tokyo Press, Tokyo and University Park Press, Baltimore, 1972.
7. Lawley, P. D. Some chemical aspects of dose-response relationships in alkylation mutagenesis. Mutat. Res., *23*: 283–295, 1974.
8. Swann, P. F. and Magee, P. N. Nitrosamine induced carcinogenesis. The alkylation of nucleic acids of the rat by N-methyl-N-nitrosourea dimethylnitrosamine, dimethylsulphate and methyl methanesulphonate. Biochem. J., *110*: 39–47, 1968.
9. Swann, P. F. and Magee, P. N. Nitrosamine induced carcinogenesis. The alkylation of N-7 of guanine of nucleic acids of the rat by diethylnitrosamine, N-ethyl-N-nitrosourea and ethyl methanesulphonate. Biochem. J., *125*, 841–847, 1971.

10. Schoental, R.   Lack of correlation between the presence of 7-methylguanine in deoxyribonucleic acid and ribonucleic acid of organs and the localisation of tumours after a single carcinogenic dose of N-metyl-N-nitrosourethane. Biochem. J., *114*: 55P–56P, 1969.

11. Lijinsky, W. and Ross, A. E.   Alkylation of rat liver nucleic acids not related to carcinogenesis by N-nitrosamines. J. Natl. Cancer Inst., *42*: 1095–1100, 1969.

12. McLean, A. E. M. and Magee, P. N.   Increased renal carcinogenesis by dimethyl-nitrosamine in protein deficient rats. Brit. J. Exp. Pathol., *51*: 587–590, 1970.

13. Swann, P. F. and Magee, P. N.   Induction of rat kidney tumours by ethyl methane-sulphonate and nervous tissue tumours by methyl methanesulphonate and ethyl methanesulphonate. Nature, *223*: 947–948, 1969.

14. Kleihues, P., Mende, C., and Reucher, W.   Tumours of the peripheral and central nervous system induced in BD-rats by prenatal application of methyl methane-sulphonate. Eur. J. Cancer, *8*: 641–645, 1972.

15. Loveless, A.   Possible relevance of O-6 alkylation of deoxyguanosine to the muta-genicity and carcinogenicity of nitrosamines and nitrosamides. Nature, *223*: 206–207, 1969.

16. Lawley, P. D. and Shah, S. A.   Reaction of alkylating mutagens and carcinogens with nucleic acids: Detection and estimation of a small extent of methylation at O-6 of guanine in DNA by methyl methanesulphonate *in vitro*. Chem.-Biol. Interact., *5*: 286–288, 1972.

17. Gerchman, L. L. and Ludlum, D. B.   The properties of O^6-methylguanine in templates for RNA polymerase. Biochim. Biophys. Acta, *308*: 310–316, 1973.

18. Ludlum, D.   The properties of 7-methylguanine-containing templates for ribonucleic acid polymerase. J. Biol. Chem., *245*, 477–482, 1970.

19. Schoental, R.   The mechanisms of action of the carcinogenic nitroso and related compounds. Brit. J. Cancer, *28*: 436–439, 1973.

20. Fahmy, O. G. and Fahmy, M. J.   Genetic properties of N-α-acetoxymethyl-N-methylnitrosamine in relation to the metabolic activation of N,N-dimethylnitro-samine. Cancer Res., *35*: 3780–3785, 1975.

21. Montesano, R. and Magee, P. N.   Comparative metabolism *in vitro* of nitrosamines in various animal species including man. *In;* R. Montesano and L. Tomatis (eds.), Chemical Carcinogenesis Essays, pp. 39–56, International Agency for Research on Cancer, Lyon, 1974.

22. Weekes, U. and Brusick, D.   *In vitro* metabolic activation of chemical mutagens. II. The relationships among mutagen formation, metabolism and carcinogenicity for dimethylnitrosamine and diethylnitrosamine in the livers, kidneys and lungs of BALB/cJ, C_{57}BL/6J and RF/J mice. Mutat. Res., *31*: 175–183, 1975.

23. Weekes, U. Y.   Metabolism of dimethylnitrosamine to mutagenic intermediates by kidney microsomal enzymes and correlation with reported host susceptibility to kidney tumours. J. Natl. Cancer Inst., *55*: 1199–1201, 1975.

24. Goth, R. and Rajewsky, M. F.   Persistence of O^6-ethylguanine in rat brain DNA: Correlation with nervous system-specific carcinogenesis by ethylnitrosourea. Proc. Natl. Acad. Sci. U.S., *71*: 639–643, 1974.

25. Goth, R. and Rajewsky, M. F.   Molecular and cellular mechanisms associated with pulse-carcinogenesis in the rat nervous system by ethylnitrosourea: Ethylation of nucleic acids and elimination rates of ethylated bases from the DNA of different tissues. Z. Krebsforsch., *82*: 37–64, 1974.

26. Kleihues, P. and Margison, G. P. Carcinogenicity of N-methyl-N-nitrosourea: Possible role of excision repair of O⁶-methylguanine from DNA. J. Natl. Cancer Inst., *53*: 1839–1841, 1974.

27. Margison, G. P. and Kleihues, P. Chemical carcinogenesis in the nervous system. Preferential accumulation of O⁶-methylguanine in rat brain deoxyribonucleic acid during repetitive administration of N-methyl-N-nitrosourea. Biochem. J., *148*, 521–525, 1975.

28. Nicoll, J. W., Swann, P. F., and Pegg, A. E. Effect of dimethylnitrosamine on persistence of methylated guanines in rat liver and kidney DNA. Nature, *254*: 261–262, 1975.

29. Magee, P. N. and Barnes, J. M. Induction of kidney tumours in the rat with dimethylnitrosamine (N-nitroso-dimethylamine). J. Pathol. Bacteriol., *84*: 19–31, 1962.

30. Swann, P. F. and McLean, A. E. M. Cellular injury and carcinogenesis. The effect of a protein-free high-carbohydrate diet on the metabolism of dimethylnitrosamine in the rat. Biochem. J., *124*: 283–288, 1971.

31. Lawley, P. D. and Brookes, P. Further studies on the alkylation of nucleic acids and their constituent nucleotides. Biochem. J., *89*: 127–138, 1963.

32. Craddock, V. M. Stability of deoxyribonucleic acid methylated in the intact animal by administration of dimethylnitrosamine. Biochem. J., *111*: 497–502, 1967.

33. Kirtikar, D. M. and Goldthwait, D. A. The enzymatic release of O⁶-methylguanine and 3-methyladenine from DNA reacted with the carcinogen N-methyl-N-nitrosourea. Proc. Natl. Acad. Sci. U.S., *71*: 2022–2026, 1974.

Discussion of Paper of Drs. Magee et al.

DR. MIWA: Is there any information on the removal of O⁶-methylguanine? Is it a demethylation or DNA breakage and rejoining?

DR. MAGEE: We have assumed that the O⁶-methylguanine is removed rather than demethylation but do not yet have evidence for this.

DR. SUGIMURA: In your experiment in which 20 mg of dimethylnitrosamine (DMN) was administered, the rate of removal of methylated base of DNA is certainly faster in the kidney than in the liver. However, the actual amount which remained 96 hr after the administration is just about same in both organs. The actual amount remaining may be important, as the rate of removal is variable.

DR. MAGEE: I think you mean that the rate of removal of O⁶-methylguanine was faster in the liver than in the kidney after the larger dose of DMN. What you say about the final level of alkylation remaining in the liver and kidney at the end of the period is true. It may be, of course, that the level in the liver might have declined more quickly than that in the kidney if the experiment had been continued for a longer time.

DR. KONDO: The rate of disappearance of methylation from DNA becomes almost zero between 1 and 2 days after the drug administration. Does this parallel the depression of DNA replication? Is the mitotic index in kidney about 5%? How big was the overshoot in DNA replication after the depression of the mitotic index by the drug administration?

DR. MAGEE: Cell division is very infrequent in the resting liver and kidney but the frequency is increased as a result of the damage caused by the DMN. We do not have data on the relationship between the induced replication of DNA in the two organs and the rates at which the O⁶-methylguanine is removed from their DNA.

DR. RAJEWSKY: Dr. Magee, by your term "independent" dose (last slide) did you mean an additive effect of two irreversible single doses?

DR. MAGEE: The results were that when the second dose of DMN was given 16 or 32 days after the first the incidence of kidney tumors obtained was that expected if the two doses were completely independent, that is about 14%. When the two doses were given simultaneously, that is combined, at the start of the experiment, the kidney tumor incidence was 53% and this was described as the two doses being completely cumulative. I would emphasize that this experiment is still in progress and the data are those obtained after 80 weeks.

DR. WEISBURGER: Following the comment of Dr. Okada, can we offer an alternative explanation? The cumulative effect may be due to the fact that the liver does not metabolize the double dose as rapidly and thus the kidneys are exposed to higher level of carcinogen. With the fractionated single dose, the liver has recovered, metabolizes DMN more completely, and thus the kidneys are exposed to smaller doses. Have you measured the metabolites in binding under these conditions to check this binding?

DR. MAGEE: No, I have not done that. The results shown were received from Dr. Mohr only about three weeks ago.

DR. GOLDTHWAIT: Perhaps the data which we would like to see involves this persistence of the O^6-methylguanine from the first to the 8th or 16th day. Do you have any further experiments on the late disappearance of O^6-methylguanine? Also are there any investigators examining the presence or persistence of O^4-methylthymine?

DR. MAGEE: We do not yet have data on persistence of O^6-methylguanine on the 8th and 16th day after DMN administration. It would certainly be interesting. The question on methylthymine was referred to Dr. Craddock. She had not found this methylated base in liver DNA of rats treated with DMN.

DR. TANOOKA: Do your data indicate that the removal of the damaged site on DNA occurs during the first few days? Our data on the mouse skin irradiated with beta rays indicate the latent and yet potential carcinogenic alteration persists in the tissue from 10 to 400 days without change.

DR. MAGEE: The biochemical data do indicate that 7-methylguanine and O^6-methylguanine are removed from the DNA of the liver and kidney during the first few days after giving DMN, but the removal from the kidney after the higher dose of DMN, which was carcinogenic for this organ, was considerably delayed. The tumor incidence data cannot, of course, be directly related to events occurring in DNA. They do indicate, however, that after the 16th day the kidney incidence was almost exactly that expected if the two doses were acting completely independently.

DR. BOOTSMA: I should like to make a more general comment on the genetic characterization of the transformed character of cells upon treatments with chemical carcinogens. Prof. H. Harris et al. (Oxford) have presented evidence for the suppression of the malignant character of mouse tumor cells *in vitro* following fusion of these cells with normal diploid cells. Loss of specific chromosomes in these hybrids during further growth could be correlated with the renewed expression of malignancy.

Cell fusion might also be applied in these studies to investigate the genetic basis of cell transformation by fusion of cells that have been made malignant by different carcinogens. It might be interesting to see if complementation of the malignant character can be obtained in specific combinations of cancer cells in hydrids.

FUNDAMENTALS IN CANCER PREVENTION, P. N. MAGEE ET AL. (EDS.),
UNIV. OF TOKYO PRESS, TOKYO / UNIV. PARK PRESS, BALTIMORE, PP. 293–311, 1976

Replication and Repair of DNA in Liver of Rats Treated with Dimethylnitrosamine and with Methyl Methanesulphonate

Valda M. Craddock

Toxicology Unit, MRC Laboratories, Woodmansterne Road, Carshalton, Surrey, U.K.

Abstract: Tissues with a high capacity for repair of genetic damage may become malignant after treatment with carcinogens only if the initial damage is rapidly converted into a stable inheritable form. Possibly this "fixation" occurs during replication of DNA. To assess the concept that replication of DNA must occur before the initial damage has been repaired, it is necessary to study replication, repair, and induction of cancer in the same system, preferably in a one-shot system for inducing cancer. Treatment of rats with dimethylnitrosamine (DMN) during the period of restorative hyperplasia following partial hepatectomy provides such a system for study of carcinogenesis in liver.

The relevance of DNA replication was suggested by the fact that the highest incidence of tumors was induced when DMN was given during the time of maximum DNA synthesis. Analysis of DNA suggested that the difference between regenerating and intact liver was not in the nature, extent or persistence of damage caused by alkylation but in the fact that, in regenerating liver, DNA was stimulated to replicate. Although the replicative response to partial hepatectomy was reduced after treatment with DMN, DNA synthesis occurred at a rate greater than in intact liver.

To determine whether this synthesis represented *de novo* or repair-type replication, repair replication was studied *in vivo* using a new technique. The method depends on the fact that nuclei enlarge during S-phase, and therefore may be separated from nuclei of noncycling cells by rate zonal centrifugation. Incorporation of ^{3}H-TdR into S-phase nuclei represents *de novo* replication, while incorporation into noncycling nuclei represents excision repair. Treatment of intact animals with DMN induced repair-type replication. After partial hepatectomy DNA synthesis, although reduced by DMN treatment, is still stimulated, and part at least of this is *de novo* replication. Therefore replication of DNA before excision repair had taken place could be responsible for carcinogenesis.

I think by now a good deal of evidence exists for the idea that cancer is initiated in different tissues in different ways depending on their rate of cell replication and also on their potential for repair of genetic damage. In tissues which apparently have a low capacity for repair, such as brain (1, 2) and kidney (3), the initial damage may persist for a considerable time, and be responsible *per se* for malignant changes in cell behaviour. Other tissues, including liver (1–3), may have a high potential for repair, at least for certain lesions. In these tissues, cancer may ensue only if the initial damage is rapidly converted into a stable inheritable form, such as a change in base sequence. This so-called "fixation" could be brought about during replication of DNA, if this took place before the damage had been repaired. In a situation of this kind, the incidence of induced tumors could be increased either by an increase in the rate of DNA replication or by a decrease in the rate of repair. To try to assess the concept, it is necessary to study replication, repair, and induction of cancer in the same system, preferably in a one-shot system for inducing cancer. I would like to describe some work I have done using a system of this kind which relates liver cell replication and DNA replication with carcinogenesis, and then to describe results given by a new method for studying repair-type replication of DNA *in vivo* in liver of animals given dimethylnitrosamine (DMN).

Cell Replication and Carcinogenesis

In common with other carcinogens, DMN does not usually induce cancer in liver of adult rats after a single administration (4). This may be due to the low level of cell replication in normal adult liver (5), coupled with a high activity of repair enzyme systems. An obvious way of testing the relevance of cell replication was to find the effect of a stimulus for cell division on the response to a single treatment with DMN. An appropriate stimulus is surgical removal of 2/3 of the liver mass. After partial hepatectomy, a wave of DNA synthesis begins in the paren-

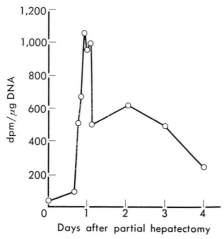

FIG. 1.   Labelling of DNA 1 hr after injection of ³H-TdR, 100 μCi/200 g rat, given at different times after partial hepatectomy.

TABLE 1.   Liver Cell Tumors Induced in Female Rats by a Single Treatment with Alkylating Agents Given after Partial Hepatectomy (PH)

Alkylating agent	Body wt. at start (g)	Time of administration after PH	Dose (mg/kg)	Tumor incidence among survivors
DMN	200	No PH	9	0/12
		2–6 hr	6–9	2/25
		24 hr	9	4/10
		31 hr	9	2/12
DMN	100	No PH	8.4–12.0	0/10
		2 hr	8.4–13.2	0/8
		24 hr	9.6–15.6	5/13
NMU	200	6 hr	90	0/13
		24 hr	45–90	16/38
		31 hr	90	2/8
MMS	200	No PH	66–88	0/6
		0–2 hr	,,	0/12
		24 hr	,,	0/10

chymal cells at about 18 hr, peaks around 24 hr, and remains high for some days (Fig. 1). Animals received one injection of DMN either in the prereplicative stage, or at 24 hr, or later during the time of extensive mitoses.

After 1–2 years, a significant number of animals treated in this way had developed malignant invasive liver cell tumors, some of which had metastasised to the lungs (6–9) (Table 1). With DMN and with nitrosomethylurea (NMU) the highest incidence of liver tumors was induced when the carcinogen was given 24 hr after the operation. Methyl methanesulphonate (MMS), a methylating agent which damages DNA in a similar but not identical way to DMN and NMU (10, 11), did not induce liver tumors. The results suggest of course that not only are DNA damage and cell replication necessary for initiation of cancer, but that the genetic damage must be of a certain type.

Cell Replication and Reaction of DMN with DNA

The partial hepatectomy-DMN system is a useful one-shot method for inducing liver cell cancer, as it can be exploited to find out how DMN acts. The question sounds deceptively simple: what happens in regenerating liver that does not happen in intact liver when the appropriate animals are treated with DMN? Possible differences which merited examination were in the extent, nature or persistence of damage to the genetic material. The major reaction product formed in DNA after treatment with DMN is 7-methylguanine. Within the experimental limits of the methods used, the amount of this base formed in DNA was similar when DMN was given 6 hr or 24 hr after partial hepatectomy, or when the same dose, 9 mg/kg, was given to intact animals (11, 12) (Fig. 2). Also, the rate of disappearance of this base was similar under the different conditions shown here, as well as in intact liver (13, 14).

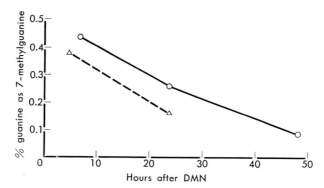

FIG. 2.   Methylation of liver DNA after treatment with DMN, 9 mg/kg, given at 6 hr (△) or 24 hr (○) after partial hepatectomy.

TABLE 2.   Methylated Purines in DNA[a]

Base	Intact liver DMN		Regenerating liver DMN		Partially hepatectomised animal kidney DMN	Intact animal liver MMS
	5 hr	24 hr	7 hr	24 hr	7 hr	4 hr
			(Time after injection)			
3-Me-guanine	0.7	0.4	0.9	0.7	0.6	0.9
7-Me-guanine	84.8	87.5	84.7	86.9	85.2	91.3
O^6-Me-guanine	9.0	11.0	9.8	10.6	9.5	0.0
3-Me-adenine	5.1	1.0	4.4	1.5	4.2	7.2
1-Me-adenine	0.4	0.0	0.2	0.3	0.6	0.6

[a] Expressed as percent of total methylated purines after administration of DMN to intact animals (30 mg/kg) or to animals 24 hr after partial hepatectomy (9 mg/kg) and after treatment of intact animals with MMS (120 mg/kg).

The relative amounts of the different methylated bases formed in DNA of regenerating liver were not detectably different from those formed in intact liver DNA, although only total unfractionated DNA was studied (13) (Table 2). As the relative amounts changed in the same way with time in regenerating as in intact liver, the different bases must be lost at the same rates in the two situations. Evidence suggests that excision of 7-methylguanine is nonenzymatic, while removal of 3-methyladenine and O^6-methylguanine is enzymatic (15). Apparently neither type of excision is inhibited in regenerating liver. Therefore it seems that the difference between regenerating and intact liver may not be in the nature of the initial genetic damage or in the extent or persistence of the damage but in the fact that in the regenerating liver the damaged DNA is stimulated to replicate.

Effect of DMN and MMS on Replication of DNA

1.   *Treatment during the prereplicative stage*
        The next step was therefore to find out whether replication of DNA did in fact

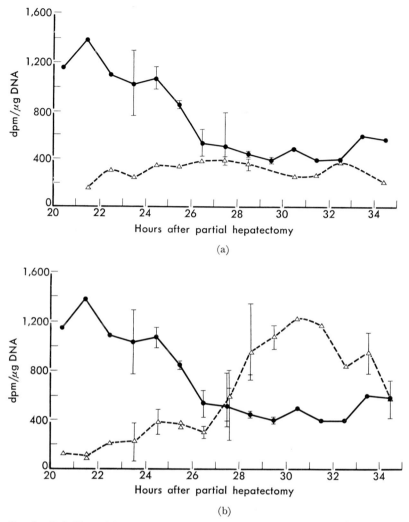

FIG. 3. Labelling of DNA 1 hr after injection of ^{3}H-TdR given at different times after partial hepatectomy (PH). (a) Treatment with DMN, 9 mg/kg, 6 hr after PH. ● PH, untreated; △ DMN 6 hr after PH. (b) Treatment with MMS, 66 mg/kg, 6 hr after PH. ● PH, untreated; △ MMS 6 hr after PH.

take place when partially hepatectomised rats were treated with DMN, or whether it was inhibited by the carcinogen. DMN given early in the prereplicative stage reduced the wave of DNA synthesis which would otherwise have occurred (Fig. 3a). Although the extent of replication was reduced, it was still greater than that of normal intact liver. Replication remained greater than in intact liver during the next week, while the liver weight and total amount of DNA per liver returned to normal (Fig. 4). However, the methylated bases formed in DNA by the carcinogen which had been given at 6 hr would have largely disappeared before the period of elevated DNA synthesis. Therefore mispairing at replication as a consequence

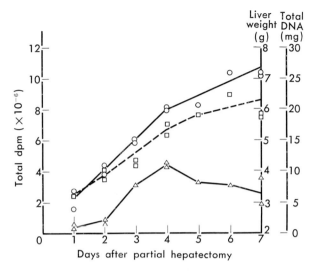

FIG. 4.   Liver regeneration after partial hepatectomy, treatment with DMN, 9 mg/kg, at 6 hr. Total dpm refers to total radioactivity incorporated during 1 hr following injection of ³H-TdR.   ○ liver weight ; □ total DNA ; △ total dpm.

of the presence of O^6-methylguanine probably did not take place. This correlates with the low incidence of tumors resulting from DMN treatment of 6 hr.

MMS, 80 mg/kg, given 6 hr after the operation also reduced DNA synthesis initially, but instead of its continuing at a low level for a week as after treatment with DMN, a well-defined wave of replication occurred with a peak about 8 hr later than normal (Fig. 3b). This difference in response to DMN and MMS is possibly not due to a quantitative difference in the extent of genetic damage, that is, it is not an effect of dose level, but is due to a difference in the type of damage. This is suggested by the fact that an increase in dose of DMN caused a progressive increase in inhibition of DNA synthesis, *i.e.*, the peak values go down (Fig. 5a). By contrast, an increase in dose of MMS caused a progressive delay in replication; the peak moved to the right (Fig. 5b).

This difference in response to DMN and MMS might be due to the fact that while both compounds damage the template in a way which slows the progress of the polymerase, MMS-induced damage might be repaired more rapidly than DMN-induced damage (*16*). However, there is another factor to be considered. Before the wave of DNA synthesis which normally follows partial hepatectomy can take place, induction of synthesis of the necessary enzymes, polymerases, thymidine kinase, and others, must take place. There is evidence that DMN inhibits enzyme induction (*17*). It therefore appeared possible that the template may have been repaired after treatment with DMN, but that replication of DNA could not increase owing to lack of essential enzymes.

To study this possibility, we examined DNA polymerase activity in animals given DMN, 9 mg/kg, or MMS, 80 mg/kg, 6 hr after partial hepatectomy. The animals were killed at 24 hr, by which time there would normally have been a large

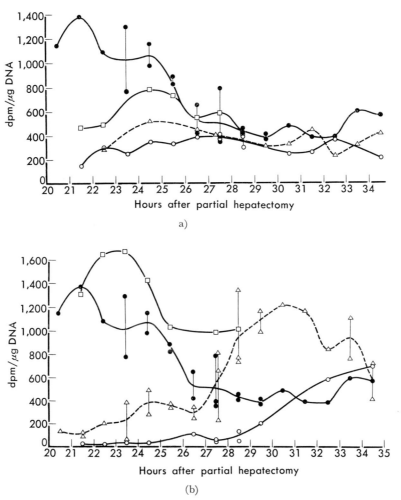

FIG. 5. Labelling of DNA 1 hr after injection of ³H-TdR given at different times after partial hepatectomy (PH).   (a) Treatment with DMN 2, 4 or 9 mg/kg, 6 hr after PH.   ● untreated ; □ 2 ; △ 4 ; ○ 9 mg/kg.   (b) Treatment with MMS 33, 66 or 80 mg/kg, 6 hr after PH.   ● untreated ; □ 33 ; △ 66 ; ○ 80 mg/kg.

increase in DNA polymerase activity. A supernatant fraction of liver was used, as evidence suggests that polymerases found in the supernatant are concerned in *de novo* replication of DNA, while repair polymerases remain bound to the nuclei (*18*). Activated calf thymus DNA was used as primer-template. The results (Fig. 6) suggest that both DMN and MMS inhibit induction of the polymerase. Comparison of polymerase activity measured at different times after treatment of partially hepatectomised animals with DMN or MMS with the time course of DNA synthesis in the intact animal suggests that lack of polymerase correlates with inhibition of DNA synthesis.

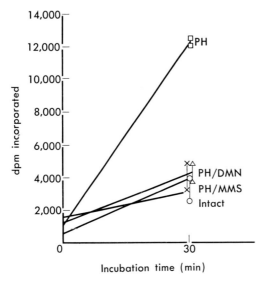

FIG. 6. DNA polymerase activity, *in vitro* assay, using activated calf thymus DNA as primer-template. Incorporation of ^{3}H-thymidine-5′-triphosphate (^{3}H-TTP) into acid-insoluble material. PH; partial hepatectomy. DMN, 9 mg/kg, 6 hr after PH ; MMS, 80 mg/kg, 6 hr after PH. All animals killed 24 hr after PH.

2. Treatment during S-phase

In the experiments described above, DMN was given early in the prereplicative stage, a treatment which induces a low incidence of tumors. When given later, during the period of extensive DNA synthesis, DMN reduced the rate of DNA replication (Fig. 7a). However, the fact to stress is that there was still a considerable residual amount of synthesis during the period following injection of DMN, when alkylation of DNA by the carcinogen was taking place. Thus replication of damaged DNA could have occurred. This correlates with the high incidence of tumors which is induced when DMN is given at this time.

MMS given during S-phase produced a more rapid extensive reduction of DNA synthesis, but again there was simultaneous replication and damage of DNA. However, in the case of MMS, damage to DNA does not include formation of the mispairing base, O^6-methylguanine. Possibly this explains why treatment with MMS did not induce tumors.

In summary, these experiments show that although DNA synthesis in regenerating liver was reduced by DMN treatment, synthesis continued at a higher rate than that of intact animals, and this occurred at a time when damage caused by alkylation was present. It is the DNA which is synthesised under these conditions which could be relevant in carcinogenesis. Obviously it was of interest to study the nature of the DNA replication, especially to distinguish between *de novo* and repair replication. We have therefore studied repair-type replication in the intact animal using the technique described below.

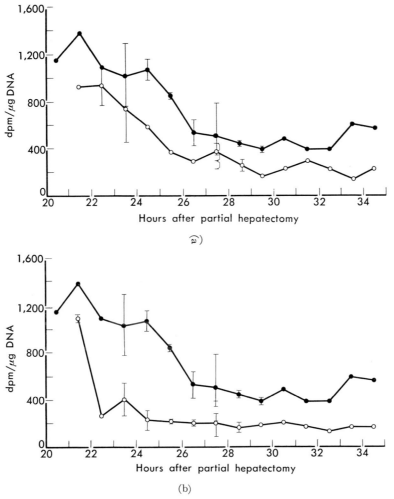

Fig. 7.   Labelling of DNA 1 hr after injection of ³H-TdR given at different times after partial hepatectomy (PH).   (a) Treatment with DMN, 9 mg/kg, at 21 hr. ● control PH ; ○ DMN at 21 hr.   (b) Treatment with MMS, 66 mg/kg, at 21 hr.   ● control PH ; ○ MMS at 21 hr.

Measurement of Repair-type Replication of DNA in the Intact Animal

To correlate repair replication or lack of repair with carcinogenesis, it is necessary to measure repair *in vivo* under conditions which will and will not cause cancer. However, the methods currently used for measuring repair replication, autoradiography and bromodeoxyuridine (BUdR) techniques, are not suitable for measuring the rate of repair as it occurs in the intact animal. The method we have used is based on the fact that during cell replication the nuclei enlarge as a result of an influx of acidic proteins from the cytoplasm (*19*). The increase in size of the replicating nuclei causes them to sediment faster in a sucrose gradient (*20*). After centrifugation of a

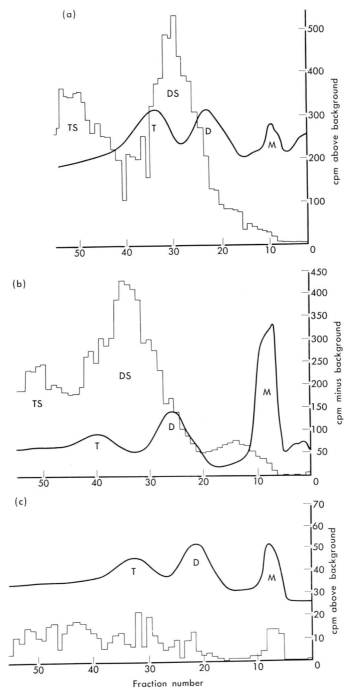

FIG. 8. Fractionation of a preparation of liver nuclei on a sucrose gradient using a zonal rotor, animals killed 1 hr after injection of ^{3}H-TdR. Curved profile, O.D.; step-wise profile, acid-insoluble ^{3}H. D, diploid nuclei; T, tetraploid nuclei; DS, diploid nuclei in S-phase; TS, tetraploid nuclei in S-phase; M, membrane fraction. (a) 300 g rat (b) 200 g rat (c) 200 g rat after treatment with HU, 500 mg/kg, given at the same time as ^{3}H-TdR.

preparation of liver nuclei in a zonal rotor, the optical density of the effluent was recorded as the nuclei were pumped out (Fig. 8a). The optical density (O.D.) profile shows the light membrane fraction, which is probably composed of plasma membranes (21), and fractions containing diploid and tetraploid nuclei. The animals were injected with ³H-TdR 1 hr before they were killed. The acid-insoluble ³H in the effluent reveals the location of the S-phase nuclei. Diploids in S-phase move faster than noncycling diploids, and tetraploid nuclei in S-phase sediment faster than noncycling tetraploids. There is a higher proportion of diploids to tetraploids in younger animals (Fig. 8b).

    In contrast to this behaviour of replicating nuclei, repair replication apparently does not involve nuclear swelling, and so nuclei in which repair replication is taking place might be expected to sediment with nonreplicating nuclei. Before testing this, we reduced *de novo* replication by injection of hydroxyurea (HU), given at the same time as the ³H-TdR. Incorporation of ³H was reduced to a very low level (Fig. 8c).

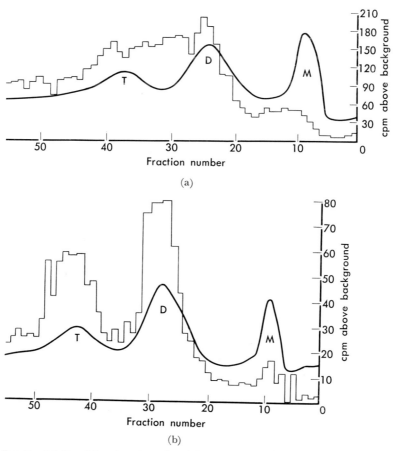

Fig. 9.   (a) Zonal fractionation of nuclei of animal treated with MMS, 120 mg/kg, 15 min before injection of ³H-TdR.   (b) Repeat of 9(a) with administration of MMS, 80 mg/kg, and of HU at the same time as ³H-TdR. Description as for Fig. 8.

Treatment with MMS by itself reduced incorporation of ^{3}H-TdR, and resulted in a broad peak of labelled nuclei over replicating and nonreplicating diploids and tetraploids (Fig. 9a). However, when injection of MMS was followed by treatment with HU with the ^{3}H-TdR, S-phase synthesis was reduced further, and incorporation of ^{3}H into nonreplicating nuclei was revealed (Fig. 9b). It is this HU-resistant non-S-phase synthesis which I suggest represents repair replication.

A similar effect occurred after treatment with DMN. Given by itself, DMN reduced incorporation of ^{3}H-TdR into S-phase nuclei (Fig. 10a), but when HU was given at the same time as the ^{3}H-TdR, a repair-type profile was revealed (Fig. 10b). This was studied at varying times after treatment with DMN and at different dose levels.

To make a quantitative measure of the results, we determined the concentration of nuclei in selected fractions of the effluent using a haemocytometer, and

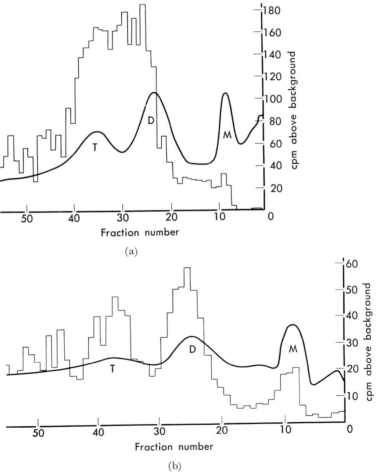

FIG. 10.   (a) Zonal fractionation of nuclei of animals treated with DMN, 30 mg/kg, 2hr before injection of ^{3}H-TdR.   (b) Repeat of 10(a) with administration of HU at the same time as ^{3}H-TdR. Description as for Fig. 8.

TABLE 3. Repair-type Replication of DNA

Compound administered	Dose (mg/kg)	Time before treatment with HU and ^{3}H-TdR (hr)	dpm/10^8 nuclei	
			Diploids	Tetraploids
DMN	30	0	2,035	4,070
		2	4,941	10,488
		16	2,160	4,135
	20	2	3,216	8,230
		16	1,531	3,275
	10	2	3,093	5,666
	2·5	2	2,850	9,156
	0.5	2	2,250	4,736

calculated ^{3}H incorporation as dpm/10^8 nuclei (Table 3). In each case there is approximately twice as much incorporation in tetraploids as in diploids, with one inexplicable exception. If the extent of repair per nucleus depends on the amount of damaged DNA per nucleus, and if the damage is uniformly distributed, then one might expect this result. Repair-type incorporation also shows the time dependence one might expect, allowing time for metabolism of DMN and damage to DNA. There is more methylation of DNA at 2–3 hr than at 0–1 hr, and less at 16–17 hr. Also there is a dose dependence, if the effects of different doses are compared 2 hr after treatment.

Different results were obtained with MMS (Table 4). The specific activity of the tetraploids is sometimes far more than twice that of the diploids; this occurs when there is a higher proportion of tetraploids to diploids than is usual, either because an older animal had been used, or for unknown reasons. It may be that the higher ratio of tetraploids to diploids results from a high rate of replication of tetraploids, which could correlate with high rate of repair replication. We are looking further into the effect of ploidy on the response to carcinogens. In common with some other systems used for studying repair replication (22), there is apparently an absence of a dose response. This may be due to the fact that MMS methylates protein in proportion to nucleic acid to a greater extent than does DMN (23). A

TABLE 4. Repair-type Replication of DNA

Compound administered	Dose (mg/kg)	Time before treatment with HU and ^{3}H-TdR	dpm/10^8 nuclei	
			Diploids	Tetraploids
MMS	120	15 min	1,920	91,350[a]
		,,	2,954	8,541[b]
		,,	2,835	5,370
		2 hr	1,376	2,716
	80	15 min	2,937	4,762
		16 hr	2,320	3,293
	40	15 min	1,864	6,580

[a] High proportion of tetraploids to diploids present. [b] 300 g male rat. All other experiments employed 200 g female rats.

high dose of MMS may therefore inhibit repair enzymes, as well as cause more DNA damage.

To test further the validity of the method for measuring repair-type replication, we studied the effect of inhibition of DNA replication by means other than direct damage to DNA. A suitable agent appeared to be cycloheximide, as this compound is thought to inhibit DNA synthesis indirectly by inhibiting synthesis of protein at the translation stage (24). Possibly it acts by inhibiting synthesis of histones or of initiator proteins. Treatment of animals with cycloheximide by itself (Fig. 11a) or with HU (Fig. 11b) did not induce repair-type replication. Evidence therefore suggests that the HU-resistant non-S-phase incorporation of ³H-TdR caused by alkylating agents represents repair-type replication.

We have started to apply this method to study repair in partially hepatectomised animals treated with DMN. When treated with DMN at 6 hr, the DNA replication which occurred 24 hr after partial hepatectomy was mainly *de novo* syn-

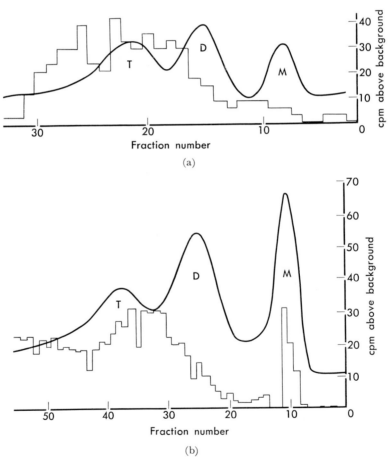

(a)

(b)

FIG. 11. (a) Zonal fractionation of nuclei of animal treated with cycloheximide, 40 mg/kg, 15 min before injection of ³H-TdR. (b) Repeat of 11(a) with administration of HU at the same time as ³H-TdR. Description as for Fig. 8.

thesis. The result shows that *de novo* replication occurred before the alkylation damage had been repaired.

The zonal method is being used also for studying the effect of diethylnitrosamine administration in the diet on the activity of repair enzymes. In addition, the technique should be useful for studying the mechanism of action of compounds whose direct action if any on DNA is not well understood as, for example, in the case of ethionine and thioacetamide. Finally, I think the method could provide a screening test for genotoxic compounds, especially in cases where other methods have not given clear results in intact animals.

To conclude, I think the experiments described above in general agree with work with azo dyes (*25*), urethan (*26–28*) and dimethylbenzanthracene (*29*) which suggests that regenerating liver is more sensitive to carcinogens, that replication does not affect the nature or extent or persistence of binding to DNA and that, although the carcinogens reduce DNA synthesis (*13, 30, 31*), replication of damaged DNA could take place to a greater extent than in the intact animal. However, increased reaction of carcinogen with replicating DNA (*32, 33*) could be a relevant factor. The system merits further study. In particular, it now seems necessary to study the molecular mechanisms of replication and repair of DNA during the critical period when initiation of cancer must be taking place.

REFERENCES

1. Goth, R. and Rajewsky, M. F.   Molecular and cellular mechanisms associated with pulse-carcinogenesis in the rat nervous system by nitrosoethylurea: ethylation of nucleic acids and elimination rates of ethylated bases from DNA of different tissues. Zeit. Krebs, *82*: 37–64, 1974.
2. Margison, G. P. and Kleihuis, P.   Chemical carcinogenesis in the nervous system. Preferential accumulation of O^6-methylguanine in rat brain DNA during repetitive administration of nitrosomethylurea. Biochem. J., *148*: 521–525, 1975.
3. Nicoll, J. W., Swann, P. F., and Pegg, A. E.   Effect of dimethylnitrosamine on persistence of methylated guanines in rat liver and kidney DNA. Nature, *254*: 261–262, 1975.
4. Magee, P. N. and Barnes, J. M.   Carcinogenic nitroso compounds. Adv. Cancer Res., *10*: 163–246, 1967.
5. Post, J. and Hoffman, J.   Changes in the replication times and patterns of the liver cell during the life of the rat. Exp. Cell Res., *36*: 111–123, 1964.
6. Craddock, V. M.   Liver carcinomas induced in rats by single administration of dimethylnitrosamine after partial hepatectomy. J. Natl. Cancer Inst., *47*: 889–907, 1971.
7. Craddock, V. M.   Induction of liver tumours in rats by a single treatment with nitroso compounds given after partial hepatectomy. Nature, *245*: 386–388, 1973.
8. Craddock, V. M. and Frei, J. V.   Induction of liver cell adenomata in the rat by a single treatment with N-methyl-N-nitrosourea given at various times after partial hepatectomy. Brit. J. Cancer, *30*: 503–511, 1974.
9. Craddock V. M.   Effect of a single treatment with the alkylating carcinogens dimethylnitrosamine, diethylnitrosamine and methyl methanesulphonate, on liver re-

generating after partial hepatectomy. I. Test for induction of liver carcinomas. Chem.-Biol. Interact., *10*: 313–321, 1975.

10. O'Connor, P. J., Capps, M. J., and Craig, A. W.   Comparative studies of the hepatocarcinogen dimethylnitrosamine *in vivo*: reaction sites in rat liver DNA and the significance of their relative stabilities. Brit. J. Cancer, *27*: 153–166, 1973.

11. Craddock, V. M.   The pattern of methylated purines formed in DNA of intact and regenerating liver of rats treated with the carcinogen dimethylnitrosamine. Biochim. Biophys. Acta, *312*: 202–210, 1973.

12. Craddock, V. M.   Stability of DNA methylated in the intact animal by administration of dimethylnitrosamine. Biochem. J., *11*: 497–502, 1969.

13. Craddock, V. M.   Effect of a single treatment with the alkylating carcinogens dimethylnitrosamine, diethylnitrosamine and methyl methanesulphonate, on liver regenerating after partial hepatectomy. II. Alkylation of DNA and inhibition of DNA replication. Chem.-Biol. Interact., *10*: 323–332, 1975.

14. Capps, M. J., O'Connor, P. J., and Craig, A. W.   The influence of liver regeneration on the stability of 7-methylguanine in rat liver DNA after treatment with dimethylnitrosamine. Biochim. Biophys. Acta, *331*: 33–40, 1973.

15. Lawley, P. D. and Orr, D. J.   Specific excision of methylation products from DNA of *E. coli*, treated with N-methyl-N'-nitro-N-nitrosoguanidine. Chem.-Biol. Interact., *2*: 154–157, 1970.

16. Damjanov, I., Cox, R., Sarma, D. S. R., and Farber, E.   Patterns of damage and repair of liver DNA induced by carcinogenic methylating agents *in vivo*. Cancer Res., *33*: 2122–2128, 1973.

17. Shank, R. C.   Effect of dimethylnitrosamine on enzyme induction in rat liver. Biochem. J., *52*: 843–849, 1968.

18. Hecht, N. B.   Relationship between two murine DNA dependent DNA polymerases from the cytosol and the low molecular weight DNA polymerase. Biochim. Biophys. Acta, *383*: 388–398, 1975.

19. Merriam, R. W.   Movement of cytoplasmic proteins into nuclei induced to enlarge and initiate DNA or RNA synthesis. J. Cell Soc., *5*: 333–349, 1969.

20. Haines, M. E., Johnston, I. R., and Mathias, A. P.   The role of rat liver nuclear DNA polymerase and its distribution in various classes of liver nuclei. FEBS Lett., *10*: 113–116, 1970.

21. Wisher, M. H. and Evans, W. H.   Functional polarity of the rat hepatocyte surface membrane. Biochem. J., *146*: 375–388, 1975.

22. Thielmann, H. W., Vosberg, H. P., and Reygers, U.   Carcinogen-induced DNA repair in nucleotide-permeable *E. coli* cells. Eur. J. Biochem., *56*: 433–447, 1975.

23. Lawley, P. D., Orr, D. J., and Jarman, M.   Isolation and identification of products from alkylation of nucleic acids: ethyl and isopropyl-purines. Biochem. J., *145*: 73–83, 1975.

24. Brown, R. F., Umeda, T., Takai, S. I., and Lieberman, I.   Effect of inhibitors of protein synthesis on DNA formation in liver. Biochim. Biophys. Acta, *209*: 49–53, 1970.

25. Warwick, G. P.   Covalent binding of metabolites of tritiated 2-methyl-4-dimethylaminoazobenzene to rat liver nucleic acids and proteins, and the carcinogenicity of the unlabelled compound in partially hepatectomised rats. Eur. J. Cancer, *3*: 227–233, 1967.

26. Pound, A. W.   Carcinogenesis and cell proliferation. N. Z. Med. J., *67*: 88–95, 1968.

27. Hollander, C. F. and Bentvelzen, P.   Enhancement of urethane induction of hepatomas in mice by prior hepatectomy. J. Natl. Cancer Inst., *41*: 1303–1306, 1968.

28. Chernozemski, I. N. and Warwick, G. P.   Liver regeneration and induction of hepatomas in B6AF₁ mice by urethan. Cancer Res., *30*: 2685–2690, 1970.

29. Marquardt, H., Sternberg, S. S., and Philips, F. S.   7,12-Dimethylbenz(α)anthracene and hepatic neoplasia in regenerating rat liver. Chem.-Biol. Interact., *2*: 401–403, 1970.

30. Hwang, K. M., Murphree, S. A., and Sartorelli, A. C.   Effect of urethan on the incorporation of thymidine-³H into DNA and the activities of some enzymes required for DNA biosynthesis in rat regenerating liver. Cancer Res., *33*: 2149–2155, 1973.

31. Marquardt, H. and Philips, F. S.   Effects of 7,12-dimethylbenz(α)anthracene on the synthesis of nucleic acids in rapidly dividing hepatic cells in rats. Cancer Res., *30*: 2000–2006, 1970.

32. Marquardt, H., Philips, F. S., and Bendich, A.   DNA binding and inhibition of DNA synthesis after 7,12-dimethylbenz(α)anthracene administered during the early pre-replicative phase of regenerating rat liver. Cancer Res., *32*: 1810–1813, 1972.

33. Pound, A. W. and Lawson, T. A.   Effects of partial hepatectomy on carcinogenicity, metabolism and binding to DNA of ethyl carbamate. J. Natl. Cancer Inst., *53*: 423–429, 1974.

Discussion of Paper of Dr. Craddock

DR. MAGEE: A major difference between the patterns of alkylation of bases in DNA by dimethylnitrosamine (DMN) and by methyl methanesulphonate (MMS) is the formation of O^6-methylguanine by DMN and the much smaller or absent formation of O^6-methylguanine by MMS. Ethyl methanesulphonate (EMS), however, does alkylate DNA on the O^6-position of guanine. Have you studied EMS in your systems?

DR. CRADDOCK: Yes, because of the formation of O^6-ethylguanine by EMS we tested the possible carcinogenic effect of one treatment with EMS given 24 hr after partial hepatectomy. No liver tumors were induced. However, we have not measured the extent of formation of O^6-ethylguanine in liver DNA under these conditions, or the effect of EMS on DNA replication.

DR. HOFSTATTER: In your experiment on the decrease of DNA polymerase after MMS and DMN treatment, respectively, the amount of decrease was the same in both cases. Does that correlate with the amount of DNA alkylation?

How do you explain the observation that this decreased DNA replication practically immediately while not affecting repair replication?

DR. CRADDOCK: The inhibition of DNA synthesis by MMS and by DMN is different at doses of carcinogens which give about the same amount of 7-methylguanine. Sixty-six mg/kg MMS gives approximately the same level of alkylation as 4 mg/kg DMN. As seen from the dose-response curves, 4 mg/kg DMN inhibits the wave of DNA synthesis for at least 34 hr, while 66 mg/kg MMS delays the peak for only about 8 hr, and when it does occur it is as high as in intact animals. Possibly this is because MMS-induced damage is repaired more rapidly than DMN-induced damage.

DMN given during the period of increased DNA synthesis, 24 hr after partial hepatectomy, reduces DNA synthesis after only a short delay. This effect seems likely to be due to damage of the template, although we have no direct evidence for this. The damage would cause rather than inhibit repair replication.

DR. KOIKE: You indicated that MMS inhibits the *de novo* synthesis of DNA polymerase. Is there a possibility that DNA polymerase activity itself is inhibited under such conditions? Do you have further evidence on the *de novo* synthesis of polymerase? For instance, RNA synthesis?

DR. CRADDOCK: I do not think that MMS can be inhibiting DNA polymerase activity by a direct effect on the enzyme. MMS was given 6 hr after partial hepatectomy, and at this time polymerase activity is very low. Induced synthesis of enzyme does not begin for some hours, and by the time synthesis of the enzyme starts, unreacted MMS would have disappeared from the animal. Enzyme activity was measured 24 hr after partial hepatectomy.

DR. LIEBERMAN: There are now three well-defined polymerases in eukaryotes (see A. Weissbach, *Cell*, *5*: 101–108, 1975). I worry about looking at "total" polymerase. I think all of us must be much more rigorous in applying results and techniques in cell and molecular biology to our systems in studying carcinogenesis.

DR. CRADDOCK: Yes, I agree. We have in fact made a start at fractionating the cytoplasmic and nuclear DNA polymerases on phosphocellulose by the method of Hecht, to study the effect of carcinogens in more detail. However, it was necessary first to find out what effect, if any, treatment with DMN and MMS had on the DNA polymerase activity which has previously been shown by other workers to increase after partial hepatectomy.

FUNDAMENTALS IN CANCER PREVENTION, P. N. MAGEE ET AL. (EDS.),
UNIV. OF TOKYO PRESS, TOKYO / UNIV. PARK PRESS, BALTIMORE, PP. 313–334, 1976

Molecular and Cellular Mechanisms in Nervous System-specific Carcinogenesis by N-Ethyl-N-nitrosourea

Manfred F. Rajewsky,[*1] Regine Goth,[*2] Ole D. Laerum,[*3]
Harald Biessmann,[*4] and Dieter F. Hülser[*5]

Abteilung Physikalische Biologie, Max-Planck-Institut für Virusforschung, Tübingen, Germany

Abstract: A single pulse of N-ethyl-N-nitrosourea (ENU), applied to BDIX rats during the perinatal age, specifically results in a high incidence of neuroectodermal neoplasms in the central and peripheral nervous system (NS). The pronounced sensitivity of the developing NS suggests a dependence of the carcinogenic effect on the proliferative and/or differentiative state of the target cells at the time of the ENU pulse. The specificity of ENU for the NS cannot be due to tissue variations in the degree of carcinogen-cell interactions, since the reactive, electrophilic ethyl cation is produced by rapid, nonenzymatic decomposition of ENU indiscriminately in all tissues. Correspondingly, the initial molar fractions of ethylated purine bases are similar in the DNA of "high-risk" (perinatal brain) and "low-risk" tissues (*e.g.*, liver; adult brain). However, while the respective half lives in DNA of N^7-ethylguanine and N^3-ethyladenine show only minor differences for both types of tissues, the mutagenic ethylation product O^6-ethylguanine is removed from brain DNA very much more slowly than from the DNA of other tissues. Together with their high rate of DNA replication during the perinatal age, the incapacity of rat brain cells for enzymatic elimination of O^6-alkylguanine from their DNA could account for an increased probability of neoplastic conversion, and hence for the NS specificity of ENU in the rat.

Dissociated fetal (18th day of gestation) BDIX-rat brain cells (FBC), transferred to long-term cell culture at 20–90 hr after a transplacental pulse of ENU (75 μg/g body weight), contrary to untreated FBC became tumorigenic after *ca.* 200 days (as assayed by reimplantation into baby BDIX rats). The multiclonal

---

[*1] Present address: Institut für Zellbiologie (Tumorforschung), Universität Essen, D-4300 Essen, Germany.

[*2] Present address: Laboratory of Radiobiology, School of Medicine, University of California San Francisco, San Francisco, California, U.S.A.

[*3] Present address: The Gade Institute, Department of Pathology, University of Bergen, Bergen, Norway.

[*4] Present address: Department of Biochemistry, School of Medicine, University of California San Francisco, San Francisco, California, U.S.A.

[*5] Present address: Institut für Biologie, Universität Stuttgart, D-7000 Stuttgart, Germany.

proliferation of neoplastic neurogenic cells was preceded by a characteristic sequence of phenotypic alterations of the cultured FBC. This *"in vivo-in vitro* system" may represent a model for analysis of the unclarified interval between primary carcinogen-cell interaction and the onset of malignant growth on the one hand, and for characterization of the type and differentiated state of the particular FBC that undergo neoplastic transformation by ENU on the other.

   One of the few signposts in the present labyrinth of approaches to the problem of carcinogenesis remains the notion that direct interactions of carcinogenic chemicals with informational macromolecules, and with genetic material in particular, can apparently be necessary prerequisites for initiation of the process of neoplastic transformation (*1–3*). There is evidence indicating a mostly covalent binding to DNA of many carcinogens, or rather of their reactive, generally electrophilic metabolic derivatives ("ultimate carcinogens") (*1, 2*). Furthermore, most carcinogens prove to be mutagenic when tested in appropriate microbial and eukaryote systems (*4*). Extensive analyses, however, of both the metabolic activation of oncogenic agents (*5*) as well as the physicochemical nature of their primary interactions with various cellular constituents (*2, 3*) have thus far failed to provide unequivocal correlations between the extent and types of initial reactions on the one hand, and the carcinogenic effect on the other.
   Until recently, surprisingly little attention has been given to the question whether specific phenotypic properties of cells coming into play after the initial carcinogen-cell interaction might perhaps have an equally important influence on the probability of neoplastic transformation. Of particular relevance in this context may be the rate of target cell proliferation, since repeated rounds of DNA replication and cell division seem to be required for the "fixation" and phenotypic expression of carcinogen-induced genome alterations (*3, 6–10*) and the capacity of target cells to eliminate and correctly replace (repair) carcinogen-modified, potentially mutagenic molecular structures in their DNA (*11–20*). This would shift the emphasis towards the differentiative state and functional behavior of target cells and, accordingly, require characterization of possibly small subpopulations of "high-risk cells" contained in the target tissues with their generally complex cellular composition. A lead in this direction may be provided by the pronounced tissue specificity of the tumorigenic effect of certain chemical carcinogens in those cases where this specificity is not a "secondary" one, *i.e.*, not due to tissue differences in the activity of enzymes required for the formation of their ultimate reactive forms (*18, 19*).

Nervous System (NS)-specific Carcinogenic Effect of ENU in the Rat

   A "model carcinogen" that fulfils the above condition is the ethylating agent N-ethyl-N-nitrosourea (ENU) (*21*). Alkylation of nucleic acid constituents in relation to mutagenesis and carcinogenesis has recently received much attention (*2–5, 22, 23*). Under *in vivo* conditions, ENU decomposes heterolytically (*i.e.*, without

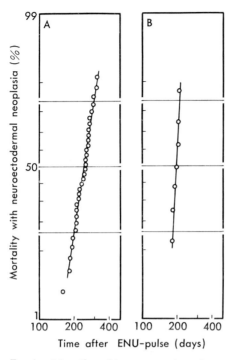

FIG. 1.   Mortality with neuroectodermal tumors in the offspring of BDIX rats treated with a single, transplacental intraperitoneal (i.p.) injection of either 25 or 75 mg of ENU/kg body wt., on the 18th day of gestation. Each point represents one animal. Note normal distribution of times until death with tumors. Horizontal lines (probits) indicate 1 standard deviation of the T_{50} values, respectively (probability grid). Y represents the percentage of animals with macroscopically detectable neoplasms (27). A: ENU, 25 mg/kg ; T_{50}, 240 days$\pm$19% (S.D.) ; Y, 89%.   B: ENU, 75 mg/kg ; T_{50}, 195 days$\pm$8% (S.D.) ; Y, 89%.   The corresponding values for BDIX rats treated with a single i.p. injection of 75 mg of ENU/kg body wt. at the age of 10 days, were $T_{50}=291$ days$\pm$22% (S.D.), and $Y=95\%$, respectively (18, 19).

enzyme involvement) with a half life of $t_{1/2}\leqq8$ min (24). The ultimate reactant, an electrophilic ethyl cation, is thus produced indiscriminately in all tissues. In spite of this fact, a single pulse of ENU, when applied to rats during the perinatal age, specifically results in a very high incidence of neuroectodermal neoplasms in the central and peripheral NS (21, 25, 26), after a dose-dependent "latency period" (Fig. 1) (18, 19, 27). The panel of ENU-induced rat tumors encompasses mixed glioma-, astrocytoma-, oligodendroglioma-, glioblastoma-, and ependymoma-like neoplasms in the brain; and neurinoma- or Schwannoma-like tumors in the peripheral NS (21, 26, 27). The particular sensitivity of the developing NS suggests that the carcinogenic effect may be related to the proliferative and/or differentiative state of the target cells at the time of the ENU pulse (18, 19). In the rat NS, the perinatal age is characterized by the presence of highly proliferative matrices, particularly in the subependymal area of the brain (Fig. 2) (18, 19, 28, 29).

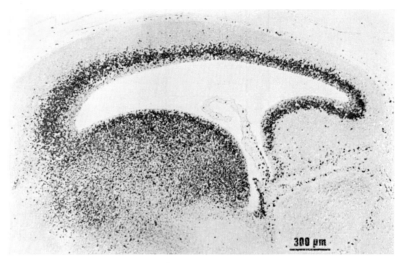

FIG. 2.   High DNA-synthetic activity in the subependymal proliferative matrix of the fetal (18th day of gestation) BDIX-rat brain. Feulgen-stained sagittal section. Autoradiogram (Ilford K5 enulsion; exposure time, 15 days) prepared after a transplacental pulse of thymidine-methyl-³H (spec. act., 15 Ci/mmole; 3 μCi/g body wt.). ³H-labeled, DNA-synthesizing nuclei: black spots (19).

Molecular Mechanisms

1.   Initial degree of DNA ethylation by ENU

As a result of their equal exposure to the ENU-derived ethyl cation, the initial (at 1 hr after the ENU pulse) extent of base ethylation in the DNA of both "high-risk" and "low-risk" tissues could be expected to be of similar magnitude. To test this assumption, [1-¹⁴C]-ENU (specific activity, 5.72 Ci/mole; Farbwerke Hoechst AG, Frankfurt/Main, Germany) was applied to fetal (18th day of gestation), 10-day-old, and adult rats of the BDIX strain (30) *in vivo*, and DNA was then isolated from brain, liver, and other pooled tissues with a modified Kirby method (24). After mild hydrolysis of DNA in 0.1 N HCl at 37°C for 20 hr (31), and addition of nonradioactive ethylated purine bases as "markers," radiochromatography was performed on Sephadex G-10 (Fig. 3), with 0.05 M ammonium formate buffer, pH 6.8 (32). The molar fractions of the ethylated bases were calculated from the integral ¹⁴C-activity of the corresponding chromatographic peaks, considering their specific ¹⁴C-activity as identical with that of the [1-¹⁴C]-ENU applied. The amounts of guanine (G) and adenine (A) were derived from the UV-extinction coefficients, at neutral pH, of $\varepsilon_{260} = 7,200$ for G, and $\varepsilon_{260} = 13,300$ for A (33).

The initial (1 hr after injection of 75 μg of [1-¹⁴C]-ENU/g) molar fractions of N⁷-ethylguanine (N⁷-EtG/G), O⁶-ethylguanine (O⁶-EtG/G) and N³-ethyladenine (N³-EtA/A) in the DNA of "high risk" (fetal and 10-day-old brain) and "low risk" (*e.g.*, liver; adult brain) tissues were indeed similar (~ 1–2×10^{-5}) (18, 19). The relative initial frequencies of these ethylation products in DNA were $\sim 55\%$ (N⁷-EtG), $\sim 28\%$ (O⁶-EtG), and $\sim 17\%$ (N³-EtA), respectively. The same relative

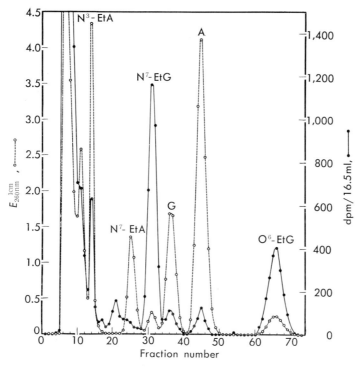

Fig. 3. Separation of bases from brain DNA by radiochromatography on Sephadex G-10, at 4 hr after ethylation *in vivo* by an i.p. pulse of 75 μg of [1-^{14}C]-ENU/g body wit. to 10-day-old BDIX rats. Nonradioactive N^3-EtA, N^7-EtG, and 0^6-EtG were added as "markers" (*18, 19*).

base ethylation frequencies were found after incubation of rat liver DNA with [1-^{14}C]-ENU for 1 hr at 37°C in 25 mM potassium phosphate buffer, pH 7.2 (*19*). Therefore, the initial degree of purine base ethylation in DNA *per se* does not provide an explanation for the NS specificity of the carcinogenic effect. It was, however, of interest to find that O^6-EtG is a major product of ethylation by ENU *in vivo* and *in vitro*. Among the different possible substitutions of purine bases in DNA, O^6-alkylguanine is particularly likely to cause miscoding and anomalous base-pairing during subsequent DNA replication, and represents a mutagenic and thus potentially carcinogenic event (*23, 34, 35*). Formation of O^6-alkylguanine in DNA after *in vivo* administration of alkylating N-nitroso carcinogens primarily of the "S_N1-type" (*36*) has recently been reported by several authors (*18, 19, 31, 37–40*). The relative yield of O^6-EtG obtained in the present analyses was *ca.* 4 times higher than the corresponding O^6-methylguanine value reported for the less carcinogenic (*41*) methylating homologue of ENU, N-methyl-N-nitrosourea (MNU) (*39*). Furthermore, the same molar fractions of N^7-EtG/G, O^6-EtG/G and N^3-EtA/A were obtained in fetal DNA, when ENU was administered during temporary reduction of the rate of fetal DNA replication to ∼ 1% of the control value by hydroxyurea (500 μg/g body weight, injected 1 hr prior to the ENU pulse) (*19*). Correspondingly, significant differences in the degree of base ethylation were neither observed in fetal or 10-day-old *versus* adult rat tissues nor in liver DNA, when the ENU pulse was placed into the "prereplicative phase" (at 11 hr) *versus* the phase of maximum DNA replication (at 24 hr) after partial hepatectomy (*19*). With respect to O^6-G, this indicates that ethylation is not restricted to a situation where this position is not "protected" by hydrogen bonding (*i.e.*, replicating DNA).

In the present analyses of DNA ethylated by ENU *in vivo* or *in vitro*, only 20–30% of the total ^{14}C-activity in the Sephadex G-10 radiochromatograms was due to ethylated purine bases (*18, 19*). Most of the remaining ^{14}C-activity eluted immediately after the void volume (Fig. 3). Although this "early peak" (*19*) includes ethylated pyrimidine nucleotides (not investigated in this study), there is evidence suggesting that its major component are phosphotriesters formed by reaction of the ENU-derived ethyl cation with the phosphodiester groups of DNA (*19, 42–45*). These appear to be relatively stable in DNA (*40*), and could cause alterations of conformation (*46*) and molecular interactions (*17*), possibly resulting in a reduced susceptibility of DNA to enzymatic hydrolysis (*43*). Phosphotriester formation in DNA has recently been proposed to be a potentially important molecular event in the process of carcinogenesis by alkylating agents (*23, 45*).

2.   Elimination rates of ethylated purine bases from the DNA of "high-risk" and "low-risk" rat tissues

Since cellular repair processes for structurally modified DNA involve the removal of altered bases from DNA (*11–20*), the tissue-specific carcinogenic effect of ENU could possibly result from tissue differences in the elimination rates of potentially mutagenic ethylated bases from DNA. Measurements were, therefore, performed over a period of 240 hr following the ENU pulse of the elimination rates

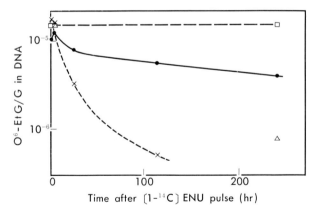

FIG. 4.   Kinetics of the elimination of O^6-EtG from the DNA of different tissues of 10-day-old BDIX rats *in vivo*. Molar fraction of O^6-EtG/G in DNA of brain, liver, and other pooled tissues (intestine, kidney, lung, muscle, spleen), as a function of time after an i.p. pulse of 75 μg of [1-^{14}C]-ENU/g body wt. For comparison : O^6-EtG/G in the DNA of pooled tissues (isolated at 4 hr after an [1-^{14}C]-ENU pulse *in vivo*, and dissolved in 25 mM potassium phosphate buffer, 0.02% sodium azide, pH 7.2), incubated *in vitro* at 37°C for 240 hr (*18*).   □ *in vitro* ; ● brain ; × liver ; △ other tissues pooled.

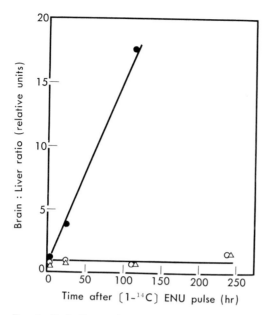

FIG. 5.   Brain-liver ratio for the molar contents in DNA of O⁶-EtG/G (●) and N⁷-EtG/G (○), respectively, and for the "early peak" specific ¹⁴C-activity (expressed as dpm/mg of input DNA ; compare Fig. 3) in the Sephadex G-10 radiochromatograms (△ Goth and Rajewsky, unpublished results), as a function of time after an i.p. pulse of 75 μg of [1-¹⁴C]-ENU/g body wt. to 10-day-old BDIX rats. Initial values at 1 hr after the carcinogen pulse, normalized to 1.0 (*18*, *19*).

of N⁷-EtG, O⁶-EtG and N³-EtA from the DNA of different tissues of 10-day-old BDIX rats (*17–19*). The data obtained by these analyses revealed a remarkable difference between brain on the one hand, and liver and a number of other "low-risk" tissues on the other. O⁶-EtG disappeared from brain DNA very much more slowly ($t_{1/2} \sim 229$ hr) than from liver DNA ($t_{1/2} \sim 36$ hr) or from the DNA of several other (pooled) tissues (kidney, lung, spleen, intestine, muscle; $t_{1/2} \sim 54$ hr); and also more slowly than N⁷-EtG and N³-EtA whose respective half lives were similar in brain and liver DNA (Figs. 4 and 5, Table 1). Equally similar for brain and liver DNA were the half lives ($t_{1/2} \sim 115$ hr and 99 hr, respectively) of the integral ¹⁴C-activity of the "early peaks" (mainly attributed to ethylphosphotriesters) (*19*, *23*, *45*) in the Sephadex G-10 radiochromatograms (Fig. 5). Incubation for 240 hr *in vitro* of DNA previously ethylated by ENU *in vivo*, showed complete stability of O⁶-EtG in DNA, while the half lives of N⁷-EtG and N³-EtA in DNA were $t_{1/2} \sim 225$ hr and $t_{1/2} \sim 33$ hr, respectively (Table 1) (*19*). In view of the mutagenic potential of guanine-O⁶ alkylation (*22*, *23*, *34*, *35*), it appears conceivable that the selective persistence of O⁶-EtG in brain DNA, together with the high rate of DNA replication and cell division at this developmental stage of the rat NS, could increase the probability of malignant transformation. This, in turn, might provide an explanation for the NS specificity of the carcinogenic effect of ENU. In the same context, it remains to be investigated whether, and in which way, the presence in DNA of

TABLE 1.   Half Lives (hr) of Ethylated Purine Bases in the DNA of Different Tissues, after an Intraperitoneal Pulse of [1-^{14}C]-ENU to 10-day-old BDIX Rats (18–20)

Tissue	In vivo/in vitro	N^3-EtA	N^7-EtG	O^6-EtG
Brain	In vivo	16[a]	89[b]	229[b]
Liver	In vivo	12[a]	64[b]	36[c]
Other tissues (pooled)	In vivo	Not measured	60[d]	54[d]
DNA (ethylated in vivo)	In vitro[e]	33[f]	225[f]	Stable[f]

[a] Observation period: 1–25 hr after [1-^{14}C]-ENU pulse.   [b] Observation period: 25–240 hr after [1-^{14}C]-ENU pulse.   [c] Observation period: 25–114 hr after [1-^{14}C]-ENU pulse.   [d] Based on measurements at 1, 4, and 240 hr after [1-^{14}C]-ENU pulse.   [e] 25 mM potassium phosphate buffer (0.02% sodium azide); pH 7.2; 37°C.   [f] Observation period: 1–240 hr after the beginning of incubation.

alkylated purines such as O^6-EtG could also impair interactions of DNA with regulatory proteins involved in the control of gene expression (48–50).

The observed differences in the elimination rates from DNA of O^6-EtG are unlikely to result from differential dilution of this ethylation product in DNA due to different rates of DNA replication and cell division in the respective tissues. If this were the case, the elimination rates, e.g., of N^7-EtG from brain versus liver DNA, should differ by a factor similar to that found for the half lives of O^6-EtG, unless large differences existed in these tissues with regard to intranuclear conditions for the hydrolysis of glycosidic linkages leading to release of N^7-EtG from DNA. Rather, the data strongly argue for the existence of a specific enzymatic mechanism for the recognition and elimination of O^6-alkylguanine from DNA, which is either lacking or substantially less effective in rat brain (18, 19). Such a mechanism could basically operate according to the scheme of excision repair (11), involving specific enzymes for recognition and elimination of modified bases, and subsequent repair of the resulting apurinic sites. A mammalian enzyme selectively releasing O^6-alkylguanine from DNA has thus far not been identified. However, recent data from several laboratories (51–56) suggest that this may soon be the case.

Selective persistence in the DNA of rat brain has recently also been demonstrated for O^6-methylguanine (O^6-MeG), when the predominantly NS-specific carcinogen MNU was applied over a period of 35 days (57, 58). Since kidney tumors are known to develop occasionally after single high doses of MNU (59), it is of interest that a low degree of accumulation of O^6-MeG was also found in kidney DNA. Extending these analyses to the dialkylnitrosamines, it was further shown (60, 61) that after a single high dose of 20 µg of dimethylnitrosamine (DMN)/g to adult rats (which induces tumors of the kidney but not of the liver) (62), O^6-MeG is much more slowly eliminated from kidney DNA, than after a low (not kidney-tumorigenic) dose (2.5 µg of DMN/g) or from liver DNA after either dose. This suggests that the enzyme system responsible for the elimination of O^6-alkylguanine from DNA, either has only a limited capacity or can be inhibited by high doses of the alkylating carcinogen.

Neoplastic Transformation of Fetal Rat Brain Cells in Culture after Exposure to ENU in Vivo

The above data have been obtained on whole tissues; *i.e.*, they do not provide information on the differentiative and proliferative properties of the particular (precursor?) brain cells undergoing neoplastic transformation after exposure to ENU. Furthermore, the interval between primary carcinogen-cell interaction and the onset of clonal tumor growth remains a largely unclarified phase in the process of carcinogenesis. Yet this period may involve a characteristic sequence of phenotypic and functional alterations of the presumptive cancer cells. Investigation of these problems *in vivo* is hampered by the complex composition of intact tissues, together with the fact that apparently only a minor fraction of their constituent cells undergo the changes ultimately resulting in expression of a "malignant phenotype." On the other hand, cultured cells as target populations for oncogenic agents (*3, 63*) have obvious limitations as substitutes for the highly controlled cell systems *in vivo* with their distinct subcompartments of proliferating and differentiating cells (*27*). Furthermore, by the capacity for "unlimited" proliferation acquired by established cell cultures, part of the process of carcinogenesis might be anticipated.

We have recently shown (*27*) that these limitations of *in vitro* systems may in part be circumvented if a tissue-specific carcinogen (ENU) is administered *in vivo*, prior to transfer of the respective target cells (fetal BDIX-rat brain cells; FBC) into long-term cell culture. This "*in vivo-in vitro* system" (Fig. 6) combines several favorable features: (1) The target cells are exposed to the carcinogen under physiological conditions *in vivo*. (2) The sequence of events subsequently monitored *in vitro*, occurs in a cell population derived from the very cell system giving rise to neuroectodermal tumors *in vivo* after an ENU pulse at the perinatal age. (3) Fetal rat cells appear to undergo "spontaneous" neoplastic transformation in culture less frequently than embryonic cells from other rodent species (*64*). (4) With the aid of different markers (*65–69*), the resulting neoplastic cell lines can be analyzed for phenotypic expression of NS-specific properties. (5) Under standardized conditions, the system may be applicable to assay the transformation frequency of preselected subpopulations of FBC.

Single cell suspensions of FBC, transferred to long-term monolayer cell culture at 20–90 hr after a pulse of 75 μg of ENU/g body weight administered on the 18th day of gestation, became tumorigenic after $\sim$ 200 days (as assayed by reimplantation into baby BDIX rats) (*27, 70*). This time interval is similar to the average period of time ($\sim$ 195 days) until death with neuroectodermal tumors, in the offspring of BDIX rats injected with the same dose of ENU at the same stage of gestation (*19, 27*). Acquisition of tumorigenicity in culture was preceded by a characteristic sequence of phenotypic alterations, termed "Stages I–IV" (Figs. 6 and 7; Table 2). During early primary culture (Stage I), both ENU and untreated control cultures exhibited stationary glia-like cells on a growing layer of flat, epithelioid (possibly glial precursors) (*27, 70*) and few fibroblastoid cells. Stage II ($\sim$ 10th–40th day) was characterized by a constant proportion of glia-like cells in the ENU cultures, and their gradual disappearance in the controls. During Stage III ($\sim$ 40th–100th day), slowly-proliferating glia-like cells in the ENU cultures formed

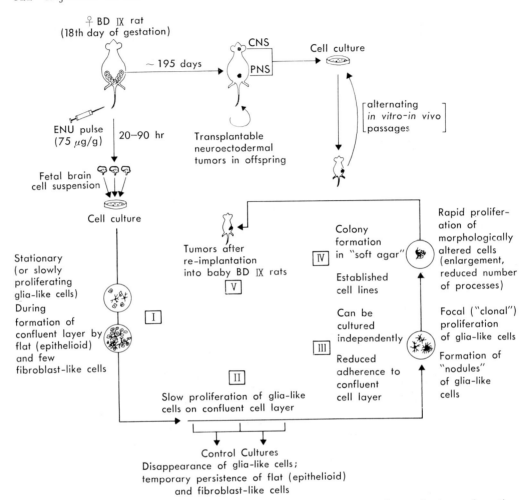

FIG. 6.   Diagrammatic representation of the *in vivo-in vitro* system for neoplastic transformation of fetal BDIX-rat brain cells by ENU. CNS, central nervous system ; PNS, peripheral nervous system (*27*).

→ FIG. 7 (a-f).   Phenotypic alterations of FBC (18th day of gestation) during neoplastic transformation in culture, after a transplacental pulse of 75 μg of ENU/g body wt. *in vivo* (phase contrast micrographs) (*27*).   (a) Secondary FBC (untreated control ; 19th day in culture). Glia-like cells on dense layer of flat, epithelioid and few fibroblast-like cells.   (b) Later appearance of FBC culture shown in (a) ; 3rd culture passage. Glia-like cells have disappeared, but the flat epithelioid cell layer persists for sometimes up to 10 months (!).   (c) Primary culture (8th day) of FBC exposed to ENU *in vivo*. Multiple glia-like cells on dense layer of flat, epithelioid and few fibroblast-like cells (Stage II, see Fig. 6).   (d) FBC exposed to ENU *in vivo* (4th culture passage). Multifocal proliferation of glia-like cells with long cytoplasmic processes. Piled-up foci (Stage III, see Fig. 6).   (e) Glia-like cells shown in (d), after separation from underlying cell layer and further subculture (advanced Stage III, see Fig. 6). Strong resemblance to astrocytes ; note apparent intercellular communication.   (f) FBC exposed to ENU *in vivo* (7th culture passage). Rapid, disordered proliferation of "morphologically transformed" cells (shorter and fewer cytoplasmic processes per cell ; Stage IV, see Fig. 6).

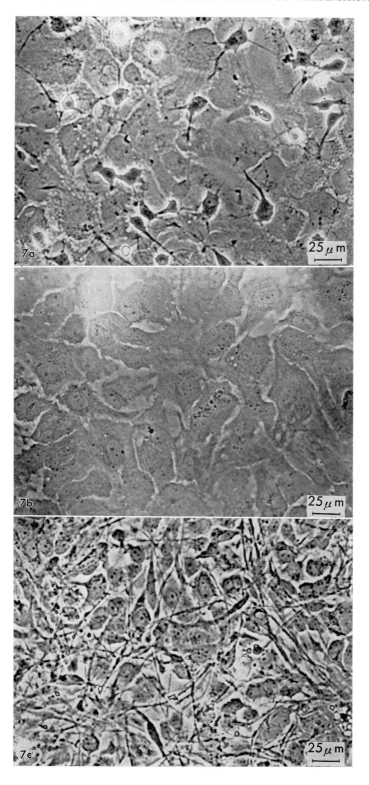

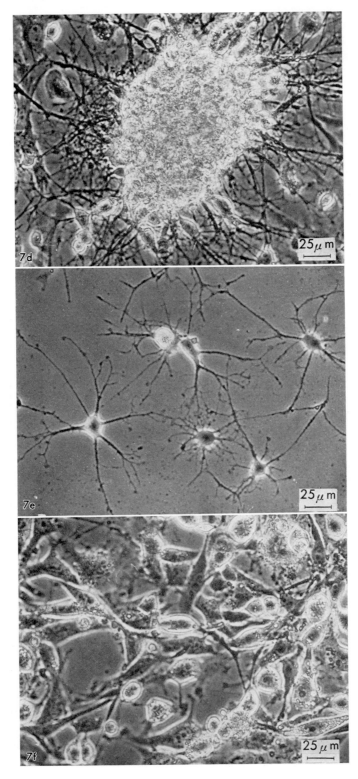

TABLE 2. *In Vivo-in Vitro* System for Neoplastic Transformation of Fetal (18th Day of Gestation) BDIX-rat Brain Cells in Culture, after Exposure to ENU *in Vivo*

	$t_M{}^{a)}$		$t_A{}^{b)}$		$t_T{}^{c)}$	
	Days	Passage number	Days	Passage number	Days	Passage number
Mean ($\pm$S.E.)	98 ($\pm$20)	4 ($\pm$0.7)	138 ($\pm$19)	6 ($\pm$2)	199 ($\pm$28)	12 ($\pm$2)

Average time intervals between transplacental ENU pulse (75 μg of ENU/g body wt.) and first observation of " morphological transformation " (t_M), ability to form colonies in semi-solid agar medium (t_A), and tumorigenicity upon reimplantation into isogeneic hosts (t_T). Mean values ($\pm$S.E.) for 7 independent sets of experiments. Cell suspensions from 6–10 pooled fetal brains per experiment ($\geqq$10 separate cultures; 1–2$\times$10^6 viable cells per 100 mm Falcon plastic dish or 250 ml plastic flask; Eagle-Dulbecco medium, 10% inactivated bovine serum; gassed with 5% CO_2 in humidified air) (27). [a] Time interval between ENU pulse *in vivo* and first observation of morphological transformation. [b] Time interval between ENU pulse *in vivo* and first observation of ability to form colonies in semisolid agar medium. Initial cloning efficiency of 10^4 viable cells seeded into 30 ml of 0.15% agar medium, 0.9$\pm$ 0.3% (S.E.). [c] Time interval between ENU pulse *in vivo* and first observation of tumorigenicity. The time interval from subcutaneous reimplantation of 10^6 cells into baby BDIX rats, until the first tumors became palpable, was 48$\pm$13 days (S.E.). However, much longer latency intervals ($\leqq$10 months) were occasionally recorded.

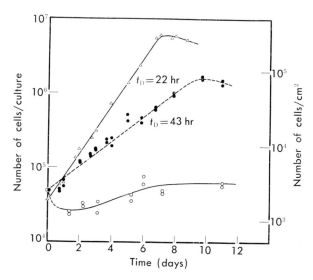

FIG. 8. Growth curves for the (neoplastic) neurogenic cell line BT5C during culture passages 8 (Stage IV ; see Fig. 6) and 25 (Stage V ; Fig. 6), respectively. Population doubling times (t_D) and maximum cell densities were t_D=43 hr (8$\times$10^4 cells/cm^2) during the 8th passage, and t_D=22 hr (30$\times$10^4 cells/cm^2) during the 25th passage, respectively. A curve for secondary FBC (19th day of gestation ; untreated control) is given for comparison (27). $\triangle$ BT5C (25th passage) ; $\bullet$ BT5C (8th passage) ; $\bigcirc$ fetal brain cells.

"piled-up" foci. These could be removed and cultured separately. Transition to Stage IV (*ca.* 100th–200th day) was marked by proliferation of morphologically transformed cells, which formed colonies in semi-solid agar, and finally became tumorigenic (Stage V; see Fig. 8 for comparison of proliferation rates during Stages IV and V, and Table 2 for average time intervals between the different stages). The solid tumors developed upon subcutaneous reimplantation of the resulting neoplastic neurogenic cell lines ("BT lines") (70) into baby BDIX rats, appeared histologically as neurinoma-, glioma-, or glioblastoma-like, and frequently pleiomorphic neoplasms. Although exhibiting a more atypical cellular morphology, these tumors resembled the different types of neuroectodermal rat neoplasms induced by ENU *in vivo*. Like several neurogenic cell culture lines ("V lines") (70) derived from ENU-induced, neuroectodermal BDIX-rat tumors (27, 70–73), the BT lines contained multipolar, glia-like cells, but also flatter cells with shorter and fewer cytoplasmic processes, and occasionally giant cells. The pluriclonal "parental" BT and V lines exhibited different degrees of aneuploidy, and contained multiple subpopulations of cells, as reflected by plurimodal DNA distributions recorded by pulse-cytophotometry (Fig. 9) (70, 74, 75). All parental lines and their (cloned) sublines (total number > 30) expressed, to a varying extent, the NS-specific "mark-

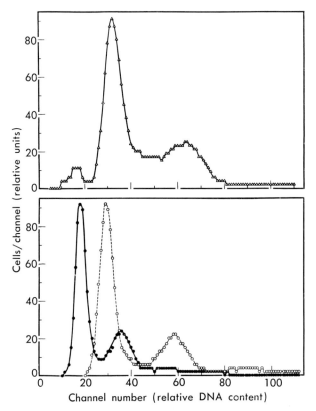

Fig. 9.   Pulse-cytophotometric DNA distributions of the original ("parental") neoplastic, neurogenic "V line" (27, 70) NV1C (125th culture passage ; above), and of 2 NV1C-derived, cloned sublines (NV1Cb, ○ ; and NV1Cc, ●) in their 43rd and 40th culture passage, respectively (below). Data for 5–10 × 10⁴ ethidium bromide-stained, log-phase cells, respectively. Euploid log-phase BDIX-rat embryo cells had a relative modal G_1-DNA value corresponding to channel No. 16. Pulse-cytophotometer ICP 11 (PHYWE AG, Göttingen, Germany). Note the unimodal DNA distributions of the cloned sublines, as opposed to the plurimodal distribution of the parental line (70, 74, 75).

er" protein S-100, which is virtually absent in FBC (*65, 70*). There was no indication of more than borderline neurotransmitter activity (acetylcholinesterase, choline acetyltransferase, L-glutamate decarboxylase I) (*67, 70*), nor has electrical membrane excitability thus far been detected (*76*). Serological analyses in the Ouchterlony test, of selected BT and V lines gave no evidence for the presence of group-specific(gs) interspecies oncornaviral antigens (by courtesy of Prof. W. Schäfer of this institute) (*27, 70, 77*).

To this date, this "*in vivo-in vitro* system" has not permitted subpopulations of probable "high-risk" FBC to be defined with certainty. Yet, the glia-like morphology of the particular cells that underwent "morphological transformation" and the demonstration, in the resulting neoplastic cell lines, of the predominantly glial S-100 marker protein (with the lack of evidence for expression of neuronal properties) (*27, 70, 76*), make glia cells, or rather their (proliferative) precursors potential candidates (*18, 27, 70*). The latter would be in accordance with the assumption that the risk of malignant transformation may vary with the stage of the target cells in their differentiative pathway at the time of interaction with a carcinogen (*9, 18, 19, 27*). For example, the probability of a genetic "fixation" of carcinogen-induced modifications of DNA may depend on the number of rounds of DNA replication that target cells would still (be programmed to?) undergo, before reaching a terminally differentiated, nonproliferative state (with much reduced risk of neoplastic conversion).

Neuroglia and neurons are, however, believed to have common neuroepithelial precursors (*78*); and immature cells of neuronal lineages were certainly not absent from the present FBC cultures initially. Therefore, neoplastic clones expressing both glial and/or neuronal properties might, in principle, have been expected to develop. However, during rat brain development, and on an overall scale, neurons precede the glial cell populations with respect to proliferation and differentiation (*28*). Hence, at the developmental stage chosen for the ENU pulse (18th day of gestation), the precursor compartments may predominantly contain glial precursors. This, in turn, might explain the prevalence of neoplastic cells with phenotypic traits of glial cells. It may, however, be noted, that some neoplastic cell lines expressing neuron-like properties have recently been derived from neuroectodermal BDIX-rat tumors induced by application of ENU on the 15th day of gestation (*73*).

ACKNOWLEDGMENTS

This work was supported in part by the Deutsche Forschungsgemeinschaft (Ra 119/5–6). O.D.L. was a Research Training Fellow of the International Agency for Research on Cancer, Lyon (France), during this investigation. Thanks for valuable technical help are due to Mrs. I. Arndt, Miss I. Klein, Mrs. H. Rajewsky, Miss I. Reber, Mr. A. Wälder, and Mr. D. Webb.

REFERENCES

1. Miller, J. A.   Carcinogenesis by chemicals: An overview. Cancer Res., *30*: 559–576, 1970.

2. Miller, E. C. and Miller, J. A.   Biochemical mechanisms of chemical carcinogenesis. *In;* H. Busch (ed.), The Molecular Biology of Cancer, pp. 377–402, Academic Press, New York-London, 1974.

3. Heidelberger, C.   Chemical carcinogenesis. Annu. Rev. Biochem., *44*: 79–121, 1975.

4. Montesano, R., Bartsch, H., and Tomatis, L. (eds.). Screening Tests in Chemical Carcinogenesis, IARC Scientific Publications No. 12, International Agency for Research on Cancer, Lyon, 1976.

5. Magee, P. N.   Activation and inactivation of chemical carcinogens and mutagens in the mammal. *In;* P. N. Campbell and F. Dickens (eds.), Essays in Biochemistry, vol. 10, pp. 105–136, Academic Press, London, 1974.

6. Sachs, L.   An analysis of the mechanism of carcinogenesis by polyoma virus, hydrocarbons, and X-irradiation. *In;* H. Holzer and A. W. Holldorf (eds.), Molekulare Biologie des malignen Wachstums, pp. 242–255, Springer-Verlag, Berlin-Heidelberg-New York, 1966.

7. Rajewsky, M. F.   Changes in DNA synthesis and cell proliferation during hepatocarcinogenesis by diethylnitrosamine. Eur. J. Cancer, *3*: 335–342, 1967.

8. Warwick, G. P.   Effect of the cell cycle on carcinogenesis. Fed. Proc., *30*: 1760–1765, 1971.

9. Rajewsky, M. F.   Proliferative parameters of mammalian cell systems and their role in tumor growth and carcinogenesis. Z. Krebsforsch., *78*: 12–30, 1972.

10. Kakunaga, T.   Requirement for cell replication in the fixation and expression of the transformed state in mouse cells treated with 4-nitroquinoline-1-oxide. Int. J. Cancer, *14*: 736–742, 1974.

11. Howard-Flanders, P. DNA repair. Annu. Rev. Biochem., *37*: 175–200, 1968.

12. Roberts, J. J., Crathorn, A. R., and Brent, T. P.   Repair of alkylated DNA in mammalian cells. Nature, *218*: 970–972, 1968.

13. Stich, H. F., San, R. H. C., and Kawazoe, Y.   DNA repair-synthesis in mammalian cells exposed to a series of oncogenic and non-oncogenic derivatives of 4-nitroquinoline-1-oxide. Nature New Biol., *229*: 416–419, 1971.

14. Cleaver, J. E.   DNA repair with purines and pyrimidines in radiation- and carcinogen-damaged normal and Xeroderma pigmentosum human cells. Cancer Res., *33*: 362–369, 1973.

15. Sarma, D. S. R., Rajalakshmi, S., and Farber, E.   Chemical carcinogenesis: Interactions of carcinogens with nucleic acids. *In;* F. Becker (ed.), Cancer, vol. 1, pp. 235–287, Plenum Press, New York, 1975.

16. Cleaver, J. E. and Bootsma, D.   Xeroderma pigmentosum: Biochemical and genetic characteristics. Annu. Rev. Genet., *9*: 19–38, 1975.

17. Rajewsky, M. F., Goth, R., and Laerum, O. D.   Pulse-carcinogenesis by ethylnitrosourea in the rat nervous system. I. Target cell proliferation and the elimination rates of ethylated bases from DNA as possible determinants in the process of malignant transformation. Abstr. VIth Meet., European Study Group for Cell Proliferation (ESGCP), p. 48, U.S.S.R. Academy of Sciences, Moscow, 1973.

18. Goth, R. and Rajewsky, M. F.   Persistence of O^6-ethylguanine in rat-brain DNA: Correlation with nervous system-specific carcinogenesis by ethylnitrosourea. Proc. Natl. Acad. Sci. U.S., *71*: 639–643, 1974.

19. Goth, R. and Rajewsky, M. F.   Molecular and cellular mechanisms associated with pulse-carcinogenesis in the rat nervous system by ethylnitrosourea: Ethylation of

nucleic acids and elimination rates of ethylated bases from the DNA of different tissues. Z. Krebsforsch., *82*: 37–64, 1974.

20. Rajewsky, M. F. and Goth, R. Nervous system-specificity of carcinogenesis by N-ethyl-N-nitrosourea in the rat: Possible significance of O^6-guanine-alkylation and DNA repair. *In;* R. Montesano, H. Bartsch, and L. Tomatis (eds.), Screening Tests in Chemical Carcinogenesis, IARC Scientific Publications No. 12, pp. 593–600, International Agency for Research on Cancer, Lyon, 1976.

21. Ivankovic, S. and Druckrey, H. Transplacentare Erzeugung maligner Tumoren des Nervensystems. I. Äthylnitrosoharnstoff (ÄNH) an BD IX-Ratten. Z. Krebsforsch., *71*: 320–360, 1968.

22. Lawley, P. D. Some chemical aspects of dose-response relationships in alkylation mutagenesis. Mutat. Res., *23*: 283–295, 1974.

23. Singer, B. The chemical effects of nucleic acid alkylation and their relation to mutagenesis and carcinogenesis. *In;* W. Cohn (ed.), Prog. Nucl. Acid. Res. and Mol. Biol., vol. 15, pp. 219–284 and appendix pp. 330–332, Academic Press, New York-San Francisco-London, 1975.

24. Goth, R. and Rajewsky, M. F. Ethylation of nucleic acids by ethylnitrosourea-1-^{14}C in the fetal and adult rat. Cancer Res., *32*: 1501–1505, 1972.

25. Druckrey, H., Schagen, B., and Ivankovic, S. Erzeugung neurogener Malignome durch einmalige Gabe von Äthyl-Nitrosoharnstoff (ÄNH) an neugeborene und junge BD IX-Ratten. Z. Krebsforsch., *74*: 141–161, 1970.

26. Wechsler, W., Kleihues, P., Matsumoto, S., Zülch, K. J., Ivankovic, S., Preussmann, R., and Druckrey, H. Pathology of experimental neurogenic tumors chemically induced during prenatal and postnatal life. Ann. N.Y. Acad. Sci., *159*: 360–408, 1969.

27. Laerum, O. D. and Rajewsky, M. F. Neoplastic transformation of fetal rat brain cells in culture after exposure to ethylnitrosourea *in vivo.* J. Natl. Cancer Inst., *55*: 1177–1187, 1975.

28. Altman, J. DNA metabolism and cell proliferation. *In;* A. Lajtha (ed.), Handbook of Neurochemistry, vol. II, pp. 137–182, Plenum Press, New York-London, 1969.

29. Bosch, D. A., Gerrits, P. O., and Ebels, E. J. The cytotoxic effect of ethylnitrosourea and methylnitrosourea on the nervous system of the rat at different stages of development. Z. Krebsforsch., *77*: 308–318, 1972.

30. Druckrey, H. Genotypes and phenotypes of ten inbred strains of BD-rats. Arzneimittel-Forschung, *21*: 1274–1278, 1971.

31. Lawley, P. D. and Thatcher, C. J. Methylation of deoxyribonucleic acid in cultured mammalian cells by N-methyl-N'-nitro-N-nitrosoguanidine. Biochem. J., *116*: 693–707, 1970.

32. Lawley, P. D. and Shah, S. A. Methylation of ribonucleic acid by the carcinogens dimethyl sulfate, N-methyl-N-nitrosourea and N-methyl-N'-nitro-N-nitrosoguanidine. Biochem. J., *128*: 117–132, 1972.

33. Beaven, G. H., Holiday, E. R., and Johnson, E. A. Optical properties of nucleic acids and their components. *In;* E. Chargaff, and J. N. Davidson (eds.), The Nucleic Acids, vol. I, pp. 493–553, Academic Press, New York-London, 1955.

34. Loveless, A. Possible relevance of O^6-alkylation of deoxyguanosine to the mutagenicity and carcinogenicity of nitrosamines and nitrosamides. Nature, *223*: 206–207, 1969.

35. Gerchman, L. L. and Ludlum, D. B. The properties of O^6-methylguanine in templates for RNA polymerase. Biochim. Biophys. Acta, *308*: 310–316, 1973.

36. Ingold, C. K.   Structure and Mechanism in Organic Chemistry, Cornell University Press, Ithaca-New York, 1953.

37. Frei, J. V.   Tissue-dependent differences in DNA methylation products of mice treated with methyl-labelled methylnitrosourea. Int. J. Cancer, 7: 436–442, 1971.

38. Craddock, V. M.   The pattern of methylated purines formed in DNA of intact and regenerating liver of rats treated with the carcinogen dimethylnitrosamine. Biochim. Biophys. Acta, 312: 202–210, 1973.

39. Kleihues, P. and Magee, P. N.   Alkylation of rat brain nucleic acids by N-methyl-N-nitrosourea and methylmethanesulfonate. J. Neurochem., 20: 595–600, 1973.

40. O'connor, P. J., Capps, M. J., and Craig, A. W.   Comparative studies of the hepatocarcinogen N, N-dimethylnitrosamine in vivo: Reaction sites in rat liver DNA and the significance of their relative stabilities. Brit. J. Cancer, 27: 153–166, 1973.

41. Druckrey, H., Ivankovic, S., and Gimmy, J.   Cancerogene Wirkung von Methyl- und Äthylnitrosoharnstoff (MNH und ÄNH) nach einmaliger intracerebraler bzw. intracarotidaler Injektion bei neugeborenen und jungen BD-Ratten. Z. Krebsforsch., 79: 282–297, 1973.

42. Rhaese, H.-J. and Freese, E.   Chemical analysis of DNA alterations. IV. Reactions of oligodeoxynucleotides with monofunctional alkylating agents leading to backbone breakage. Biochim. Biophys. Acta, 190: 418–433, 1969.

43. Miller, P. S., Fang, K. N., Kondo, N. S., and Ts'o, P. O. P.   Syntheses and properties of adenine and thymine nucleoside alkyl phosphotriesters, the neutral analogs of dinucleoside monophosphates. J. Am. Chem. Soc., 93: 6657–6665, 1971.

44. Bannon, P. and Verly, W.   Alkylation of phosphates and stability of phosphate triesters in DNA. Eur. J. Biochem., 31: 103–111, 1972.

45. Sun, L. and Singer, B.   The specificity of different classes of ethylating agents toward various sites of HeLa cell DNA in vitro and in vivo. Biochemistry, 14: 1795–1802, 1975.

46. Kan, L. S., Barrett, J. C., Miller, P. S., and Ts'o, P. O. P.   Proton magnetic resonance studies of the conformational changes of dideoxynucleoside ethyl phosphotriesters. Biopolymers, 12: 2225–2240, 1973.

47. Miller, P. S., Barrett, J. C., and Ts'o, P. O. P. Synthesis of oligodeoxyribonucleotide ethyl phosphotriesters and their specific complex formation with transfer ribonucleic acid. Biochemistry, 13: 4887–4896, 1974.

48. Biessmann, H. and Rajewsky, M. F.   Nuclear protein patterns in developing and adult rat brain and in ethylnitrosourea-induced neuroectodermal tumors of the rat. J. Neurochem., 24: 387–393, 1975.

49. Augenlicht, L. H., Biessmann, H., and Rajewsky, M. F. Chromosomal proteins of rat brain: Increased synthesis and affinity for DNA following a pulse of the carcinogen ethylnitrosourea in vivo. J. Cell. Physiol., 86: 431–438, 1975.

50. Biessmann, H. and Rajewsky, M. F. The synthesis of brain chromosomal proteins after a pulse of the nervous system-specific carcinogen N-ethyl-N-nitrosourea to the fetal rat. J. Neurochem., 1976, in press.

51. Kirtikar, D. M. and Goldthwait, D. A.   The enzymatic release of O^6-methylguanine and 3-methyladenine from DNA reacted with the carcinogen N-methyl-N-nitrosourea. Proc. Natl. Acad. Sci. U.S., 71: 2022–2026, 1974.

52. Maher, V. M., Douville, D., Tomura, T., and Van Lancker, J. L. Mutagenicity of reactive derivatives of carcinogenic hydrocarbons: Evidence of DNA repair. Mutat. Res., 23: 113–128, 1974.

53. Verly, W. G. Maintenance of DNA and repair of sites without base. Biomedicine, *22*: 342–347, 1975.

54. Thielmann, H. W., Vosberg, H.-P., and Reygers, U. Carcinogen-induced DNA repair in nucleotide-permeable *Escherichia coli* cells. Eur. J. Biochem., *56*: 433–447, 1975.

55. Lindahl, T. New class of enzymes acting on damaged DNA. Nature, *259*: 64–66, 1976.

56. Kirtikar, D. M., Kuebler, J. P., Dipple, A., and Goldthwait, D. A. Endonuclease II of *Escherichia coli* and related enzymes. This volume, pp. 349–362.

57. Kleihues, P. and Margison, G. P. Carcinogenicity of N-methyl-N-nitrosourea: Possible role of repair excision of O^6-methylguanine from DNA. J. Natl. Cancer Inst., *53*: 1839–1841, 1974.

58. Margison, G. P. and Kleihues, P. Chemical carcinogenesis in the nervous system. Biochem. J., *148*: 521–525, 1975.

59. Druckrey, H., Preussmann, R., Ivankovic, S., and Schmähl, D. Organotrope carcinogene Wirkung bei 65 verschiedenen N-Nitroso-Verbindungen an BD-Ratten. Z. Krebsforsch., *69*: 103–201, 1967.

60. Nicoll, J. W., Swann, P. F., and Pegg, A. E. Effect of dimethylnitrosamine on persistence of methylated guanines in rat liver and kidney DNA. Nature, *254*: 261–262, 1975.

61. Magee, P. N., Nicoll, J. W., Pegg, A. E., and Swann, P. F. Alkylating intermediates in nitrosamine metabolism. Biochem. Soc. Trans., *3*: 62–65, 1975.

62. Swann, P. F. and Magee, P. N. Nitrosamine-induced carcinogenesis. The alkylation of nucleic acids of the rat by N-ethyl-N-nitrosourea, dimethyl-nitrosamine, dimethylsulfate and methyl methanesulfonate. Biochem. J., *110*: 39–47, 1968.

63. Heidelberger, C. Chemical oncogenesis in culture. Adv. Cancer Res., *18*: 317–366, 1973.

64. Sanford, K. K. "Spontaneous" neoplastic transformation of cells *in vitro*: Some facts and theories. Natl. Cancer Inst. Monogr., *26*: 387–418, 1967.

65. Herschman, H. R., Levine, L., and De Vellis, J. Appearance of a brain-specific antigen (S-100 protein) in the developing rat brain. J. Neurochem., *18*: 629–633, 1971.

66. Eng, L. F., Vandershaeghen, J. J., Bignami, A., and Gerstl, B. An acidic protein isolated from fibrous astrocytes. Brain Res., *28*: 351–354, 1971.

67. Wilson, S. H., Schrier, B. K., Farber, J. L., Thompson, E. J., Rosenberg, R. N., Blume, A. J., and Nirenberg, M. W. Markers for gene expression in cultured cells from the nervous system. J. Biol. Chem., *247*: 3159–3169, 1972.

68. Schachner, M. NS-1 (nervous system antigen-1), a glial-cell-specific antigenic component of the surface membrane. Proc. Natl. Acad. Sci. U. S., *71*: 1795–1799, 1974.

69. Fields, K. L., Gosling, C., Megson, M., and Stern, P. L. New cell surface antigens in rat defined by tumors of the nervous system. Proc. Natl. Acad. Sci. U.S., *72*: 1296–1300, 1975.

70. Laerum, O. D., Rajewsky, M. F., Schachner, M., Stavrou, D., Haglid, K. G., and Haugen, Å. Phenotypic properties of neoplastic cell lines developed from fetal rat brain cells in culture after exposure to ethylnitrosourea *in vivo*. Unpublished.

71. Benda, P., Someda, K., Messer, J., and Sweet, W. H. Morphological and immunological studies of rat glial tumors and clonal strains propagated in culture. J. Neurosurg., *34*: 310–323, 1971.

72. Pfeiffer, S. E. and Wechsler, W. Biochemically differentiated neoplastic clone of Schwann cells. Proc. Natl. Acad. Sci. U. S., *69*: 2885–2889, 1972.

73. Schubert, D., Heinemann, S., Carlisle, W., Tarikas, H., Kimes, B., Patrick, J., Steinbach, J. H., Culp, W., and Brandt, B. L. Clonal cell lines from the rat central nervous system. Nature, *249*: 224–227, 1974.

74. Laerum, O. D. and Hansteen, I. L. Chromosome analysis and cytofluorometric DNA measurements on malignant neurogenic cell lines in culture. *In;* C. A. M. Haanen, H. F. D. Hillen, and J. M. C. Wessels (eds.), Pulse-Cytophotometry, pp. 172–181, European Press-Medicon, Ghent, 1975.

75. Hanke, K. and Rajewsky, M. F. Proliferative characteristics of neoplastic cell systems: Pulse-cytophotometric analyses of subpopulations derived from tumor cell clones in semisolid agar medium. *In;* C. A. M. Haanen, H. F. D. Hillen, and J. M. C. Wessels (eds.), Pulse-Cytophotometry, pp. 182–191, European Press-Medicon, Ghent, 1975.

76. Laerum, O. D., Hülser, D. F., and Rajewsky, M. F. Electrophysiological properties of ethylnitrosourea-induced, neoplastic neurogenic cell lines cultured *in vitro* and *in vivo*. Cancer Res., *36*: 2135–2161, 1976.

77. Schäfer, W., Pister, L., Hunsmann, G., and Moennig, V. Comparative serological studies on type C viruses of various mammals. Nature New Biol., *245*: 75–77, 1973.

78. Langman, J., Shimada, M., and Haden, C. Formation and migration of neuroblasts. *In;* D. C. Pease (ed.), Cellular Aspects of Neural Growth and Differentiation, UCLA Forum in Medical Sciences, No. 14, pp. 33–59, University of California Press, Berkeley-Los Angeles-London, 1971.

Discussion of Paper of Drs. Rajewsky et al.

DR. SUGIMURA: You demonstrated so beautifully the importance of O^6-ethylated guanine. May I ask a question on protein rather than on DNA? I am sure ethylation was produced in proteins, including chromatin proteins. Do you have any information on half lives of ^{14}C-ethylated protein in brain and liver?

We previously reported dibutyl-cAMP produced the maturation of *in vitro* cultured glioblastoma of mice. If you add cAMP, would you think that the malignant transformation step would be prevented?

DR. RAJEWSKY: We have measured the specific ^{14}C-activity of total DNA, RNA and protein in BDIX-rat brain and liver, as a function of time after a pulse of $[1\text{-}^{14}C]$-ENU, and in BDIX-rat liver after a pulse of $[1\text{-}^{14}C]$-diethylnitrosoamine (see R. Goth and M. F. Rajewsky, Z. Krebsforsch., *82*: 37–64, 1974). The respective half lives were of a similar order. With regard to chromosomal proteins (CP), we have recently found that neoplastic neurogenic cell lines derived from ENU-induced neuroectodermal tumors of the BDIX rat contained two nonhistone CP, which occur specifically in the fetal and adult rat brain, respectively (H. Biessmann and M. F. Rajewsky, J. Neurochem., *24*: 387–393, 1975). Furthermore, the brain cells of ENU-treated, 10-day-old BDIX rats exhibited both an increased rate of CP synthesis and affinity of the newly synthesized CP for brain DNA of both control and carcinogen-treated animals, at 120 hr after the ENU pulse (L. H. Augenlicht, H. Biessmann, and M. F. Rajewsky, J. Cell. Physiol., *86*: 431–438, 1975).

With respect to your second question, I can at present only say that my colleagues Drs. Laerum and Haugen have confirmed data of R. Lim, K. Mitsunobu, and W. K. P. Li (Exp. Cell Res., *79*: 243–246, 1973) on the morphological maturation-stimulating effect of adult rat brain extracts, on the flat, epithelioid cells in the fetal rat brain cell cultures I had mentioned in my description of our *in vivo-in vitro* system, which we suspect to contain precursor cells of glial cell lineages. Experiments are underway to investigate a possible interference of early maturation-stimulation with the process of neoplastic transformation.

DR. CRADDOCK: The idea that brain cells are especially vulnerable to ENU during the perinatal period because the cells are dividing is an attractive hypothesis but many other cells in the neonatal animal are also dividing. Why should brain be especially susceptible?

DR. RAJEWSKY: It appears conceivable that the high rate of DNA replication and cell division of rat brain cells during the perinatal age, together with their incapacity to (enzymatically) remove a potentially mutagenic alkylation product, *i.e.*, O^6-alkylguanine, might result in an increased probability of neoplastic transformation in this cell system. DNA replication appears to be a prerequisite for the "fixation" of genome alterations, such as brought about, *e.g.*, by anomalous base pairing in replicating DNA containing O^6-alkylguanine.

DR. BOOTSMA: Did you try to induce the transformation of normal brain cells *in vitro* by treating the cells with ENU?

DR. RAJEWSKY: Yes, we have begun such experiments, but we have no clear-cut and reproducible results yet.

DR. SATO: Have you checked for the existence of S-100 protein in transformed cells *in vitro*? Is there any change in the content of S-100 in these cells?

DR. RAJEWSKY: During rat brain development, the S-100 protein appears essentially after birth (H. R. Herschman, L. Levine, and J. de Vellis, J. Neurochem., *18*: 629–633, 1971). It is present, to varying degrees and in varying proportions of the cells, in all our neoplastic neurogenic cell lines, *i.e.*, both in the lines originating from long-term cultures of brain cells from fetal rats treated with ENU on the 18th day of gestation *in vivo*, and in lines derived from autochthonous neuroectodermal BDIX-rat tumors.

DR. TAKEBE: In your discussion of accessibility of repair enzymes, were you going to say that the defects in repair could be due to defects in accessibility of the repair enzymes, or that the repair enzymes may be inactivated so they cannot repair the damage in DNA?

DR. RAJEWSKY: I think that the present state of our knowledge about the molecular mechanisms of DNA repair in relation to carcinogen binding to DNA in general and to base alkylation in particular is so poor that many possibilities may be considered.

DR. LAUFS: Most of the rats carry type-C viruses. Did you exclude the presence of oncornaviruses in your cultures?

DR. RAJEWSKY: Prof. W. Schäfer of our Institute could not find any evidence for the presence of gs-interspecies RNA tumor virus antigens in a number of our neoplastic neurogenic lines, both derived from ENU-induced neuroectodermal BDIX-rat tumors, and from fetal BDIX-rat brain cells in culture, after exposure to ENU *in vivo* (Laerum and Rajewsky, J. Natl. Cancer Inst., *55*: 1975). However, this does, of course, not entirely exclude a role of such viruses in the process of carcinogenesis in this system.

FUNDAMENTALS IN CANCER PREVENTION, P. N. MAGEE ET AL. (EDS.),
UNIV. OF TOKYO PRESS, TOKYO / UNIV. PARK PRESS, BALTIMORE, PP. 335–348, 1976

Removal of Bound Acetylaminofluorene from the DNA of Mammalian Cells in Culture

Michael W. Lieberman,* David E. Amacher, John A. Elliott, and
Shiu L. Huang

*Somatic Cell Genetics Section, Environmental Mutagenesis Branch, National Institute of Environmental
Health Sciences, National Institutes of Health, Research Triangle Park, North Carolina, U.S.A.*

Abstract: The disappearance of radioactive label from the DNA of 6 types of
mammalian cells was investigated after exposing them to 10^{-6} M [9-^{14}C]-N-acetoxy-
2-acetylaminofluorene. In 24 hr human fibroblasts removed 25% of the acetylaminofluorene (AAF) adducts from DNA while for fibroblasts from a xeroderma
pigmentosum patient (Group D) the amount of removal was 13%. The percentage
of label lost in 24 hr for other cell types was: Balb/c 3T3 (mouse) cells, 27%; 3rd
passage Swiss mouse embryo cells, 46%; 5th passage guinea pig embryo cells, 37%;
Potorous (rat kangaroo) cells, 67%. Initial levels of binding ranged from one
molecule of carcinogen/30,000 to 1/120,000 bases. The removal of adducts was most
rapid during the first 12 hr, but continued for at least 48 hr. These data suggest that
the same enzymatic mechanism responsible for removal of pyrimidine dimers in
normal cells (and absent or reduced in xeroderma cells) is responsible for the
removal of bound AAF adducts. Alternatively different repair processes for these
two different types of damage may be under similar genetic control. Mouse cells
remove AAF moieties about as well as human cells, although previous studies using
ultraviolet radiation (pyrimidine dimers) have estimated the repair capacity of
murine cells to be only 10–15% of human cells.

Several developments over the past few years have stimulated interest in the
analysis of the removal of bound carcinogen from DNA during the repair process.
First, DNA repair in response to ultraviolet radiation (UVR) is now well characterized in mammalian cells and serves as a convenient standard of comparison:
analysis of unscheduled DNA synthesis, repair "replication," and pyrimidine dimer
removal as well as host cell reactivation have all been examined in a variety of
human and nonhuman mammalian cells in culture (1–5). In addition, the availability of a variety of repair-deficient mutant strains (xeroderma pigmentosum

---

* Present address: Department of Pathology, Washington University School of Medicine, St. Louis,
Missouri, U.S.A.

(XP) strains) as well as some rodent cell types with relatively less repair synthesis than normal human cells has heightened interest in comparative cell biology and biochemistry and especially in the analysis of the role repair processes in neoplasia (6–9). Some studies, especially those relating to repair synthesis have been carried out following treatment of cells with chemical carcinogens (10–13); however, to our knowledge, no extensive comparative study of the removal of bound carcinogen has been attempted (however, see Ref. 14). In this paper we present some of our preliminary findings on the extent of removal of adducts of the carcinogen N-acetoxy-2-acetylaminofluorene (NA-AAF) from the DNA of cultured mammalian cells.

In designing our experiments we have used confluent cells to reduce physiologic variation and to simplify analysis. Work was done with a low concentration of carcinogen to allow high cell survival (colony-forming ability) and to reduce artifacts resulting from possible saturation of repair mechanisms. NA-AAF was chosen because its reaction products with nucleotides are partially characterized (15) and thought to be relatively stable chemically. In addition, repair synthesis induced by NA-AAF appears to be similar to that induced by UVR (11, 13, 16). Although cell culture may not be strictly comparable to in vivo systems for examining neoplasia, NA-AAF is a potent inducer of neoplastic transformation in vitro (17, 18).

Adduct Formation after Treatment with 9-^{14}C-NA-AAF

In a typical experiment cells are grown to confluence in 150 mm plastic petri dishes; 9-^{14}C-NA-AAF is added in anhydrous dimethylsulfoxide (DMSO). Fifteen minutes later either the cells are harvested (by scraping) or the medium is replaced by nonradioactive conditioned medium, and the cells are harvested at some future time. DNA is prepared from crude nuclei by CsCl equilibrium centrifugation (16, 19). Under these conditions the DNA and the radioactivity co-band indicating binding of the carcinogen to DNA (Fig. 1) (20). The stability of the products and the lack of intercalated acetylaminofluorene (AAF) moieties have been demonstrated in several ways: (1) rebanding in CsCl does not change the specific activity; (2) heat denaturation of DNA and rebanding in CsCl results in no loss of label; (3) results of column chromatography on Sephadex G-15 with or without 2.5% sodium dodecylsulfate (SDS) indicate that all of the radioactivity co-chromatographs with the DNA in the void column. This latter technique has been effective in removing a variety of loosely bound chemicals from DNA (21, 22). Furthermore, data from XP (Group D) cells show much less loss of bound carcinogen from DNA than do normal human fibroblasts (see below): the most straightforward interpretation of this finding is that loss of label is equivalent to the excision of covalently bound carcinogen. Thus because the cells are confluent (and therefore not making DNA) and the products are stable, changes in specific activity may be related directly to DNA repair processes.

At the present time we have followed the disappearance of radioactivity from cellular DNA although efforts are underway to identify the nature of the adducts. In the text we refer to AAF adducts of DNA as a convenient shorthand without

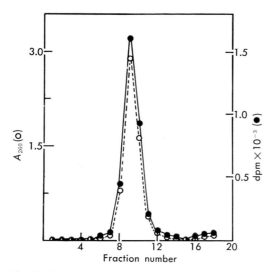

FIG. 1.   Preparation of cellular DNA and co-banding of radioactivity and DNA after treatment with [9-¹⁴C]-NA-AAF. In this example, confluent 5th passage guinea pig embryo cells were treated with 10^{-6} M [9-¹⁴C]-NA-AAF at 37°C. Fifteen minutes later cells were harvested and the DNA was prepared from crude nuclei by equilibrium CsCl centrifugation. Fractions (0.4 ml) were diluted with 2.0 ml H_2O before measurement of absorbance. The entire sample was counted in Instagel (Packard).

meaning to imply actual chemical identification of products. The problem of product identification of fluorenyl hydroxamic acid derivatives of DNA is a difficult one (23). In a sense, the use of cultured cells and NA-AAF should be a simpler system than in vivo organ experiments (liver, kidney, etc.) since many of the metabolic pathways which alter fluorenyl hydroxamic acids are probably absent in fibroblasts (23–25).

Survival Data

To be physiologically meaningful, removal studies must be done under conditions which allow a high proportion of the cells to survive. The data presented in Fig. 2 indicate that human fibroblasts treated in confluent cultures show high levels of survival (relative colony-forming ability) after treatment with 2×10^{-6} M NA-AAF or less. Preliminary experiments with radioactive NA-AAF indicated that reliable measurements of binding were difficult to obtain when cells were treated with less than 10^{-6} M NA-AAF. This dose produced about 80% survival (Fig. 2) and was used in all binding experiments. Actually the data from survival experiments and binding studies are only roughly comparable because in the former case cells were treated for 1 hr in 15% serum while in the latter they were treated for 15 min in 10% serum. Studies of survival of both human cells and the other cells used to study removal (Table 1) are now in progress. In addition, inspection of cell cultures by phase microscopy revealed no sloughing or changes in cell morphology during the course of experiments.

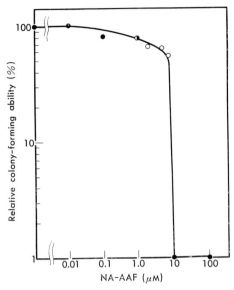

FIG. 2. Relative colony-forming ability of human fibroblasts treated with NA-AAF. MI TEN cells were obtained from American Type Culture Collection (ATCC) (CRL 1113) while FU was derived from a foreskin at NIEHS. Cells were grown to confluence in Ham's F10 with 15% fetal calf serum in either 60 mm petri dishes (MI TEN, ●) or 150 mm petri dishes (FU, ○) and treated with unlabeled NA-AAF dissolved in dry DMSO. After 1 hr cells were trypsinized and replated at low density in fresh medium. Colonies were scored at 13 days. Absolute plating efficiency was approximately 33%. The MI TEN data are from one experiment done on a single day. The FU data points were done individually over several months and represent the average of two or three determinations.

TABLE 1. Binding and Removal of AAF Moieties from the DNA of Cultured Mammalian Cells

Name	Source	μmole AAF / Mole DNA-P	AAF molecules bound / Bases	% carcinogen removed (24 hr)
FU	Human foreskin	8.9	1/112,000	25
Cay Wen	XP (Group D) ATCC CRL-1157	23.5	1/42,500	13
Balb/c 3T3	Mouse " fibroblast " ATCC CCL-163	11.0	1/790,000	27
ME	NIH Swiss mouse embryo 3rd passage	18.8	1/53,000	46
GP	Guinea pig embryo (Hartley) 5th passage	32.4	1/31,000	37
Pt-K2	*Potorous tridactylis* ATCC CCL-56	18.9	1/53,000	67

All cells were treated at confluence with 10^{-6} M [9-^{14}C]-NA-AAF as described in the text.

Extent of Removal of Bound Carcinogen

In order to evaluate the removal of bound products on a comparative basis, low levels of damage must be analyzed. At high levels saturation of repair systems may occur and obscure results. Treatment of cells with 10^{-6} M [^{14}C]-NA-AAF results in approximately one bound carcinogen molecule per 30,000 to 112,000 bases (Table 1) (20).

TABLE 2. Comparison of Removal of Bound AAF and Pyrimidine Dimers[a]

	AAF molecules bound Bases	% removed (24 hr)	Fluence (erg/mm²)	% dimers	Dimers Bases	% removed (24 hr)
Human						
FU	1/112,000	25				
WI-38			100	0.05	1/6,600	80
Fibroblast[b]			50			80 (20 hr)
Fibroblast[c]				0.06		~50%
FL (amnion)[c]				0.06	1/5,500[e]	~50%
Potorous						
Pt-K2	1/53,000	67	100	0.0425	1/7,800	79
Mouse						
Balb/c 3T3	1/90,000	27	200	0.11	1/3,000	" None "
3T3[b]			50			10 (20 hr)
NIH Swiss embryo 3rd passage	1/53,000	46				
L5178Y[d]			110	0.023–0.03	1/14,000– 1/11,000[e]	13–16 (6 hr)
			220	0.04	1/8,200[e]	0 (6 hr)

[a] All data from Amacher, Elliott, and Lieberman (*20*) except where indicated. [b] Data of Setlow *et al.* (*30*). [c] Data of Takebe *et al.* (*9*). [d] Data of Lehmann (*29*). [e] Our calculations based on cited data.

This amount of damage is substantially less than that usually analyzed after exposure to UVR. In the latter instance 100 erg/mm² (10 J/m²) is often used to produce pyrimidine dimers. In our laboratory, this exposure results in 0.05% dimers or about one dimer/6,600 bases (see also Table 2). From one point of view, approximately 1 molecule of carcinogen per 50,000 bases is a relatively small amount in that it allows high cell survival (see above). However, in terms of number of hits per diploid genome it is large: if diploid mammalian cells contain roughly 12.8×10^9 bases (*26, 27*), then there are about 250,000 hits/dipolid genome.

To date, we have evaluated 6 cell types for the ability to remove bound carcinogen (Table 1); these include a normal human strain (FU), a Group D XP strain (*8*), Balb/c 3T3 cells, 3rd passage mouse embryo cells, 5th passage guinea pig embryo cells, and rat kangaroo cells. In most cases the time course of binding and removal was examined (*e.g.*, Fig. 3, Table 3). This type of study is somewhat more difficult with chemical carcinogens than with UVR, because the attack is not instantaneous and early time points may reflect two competing events—binding and removal. Thus the maximal extent of binding is probably somewhat underestimated by this method because removal may start before binding is completed.

From such studies a number of interesting conclusions may be drawn (Table 1). Even at low levels of damage, human foreskin cells are not very effective at removing bound carcinogen, while the XP strain is even less effective. FU cells remove approximately 25% of the bound carcinogen in 24 hr; this corresponds to the removal of 30,000 molecules/cell in 24 hr ! The Group D XP cells remove about half as much carcinogen as the FU cells; this latter number is not a firm one, however, since the experiment has been done only once and the precision of this

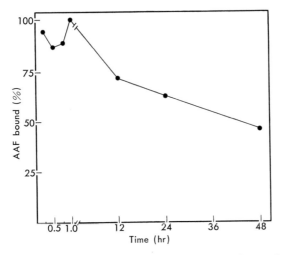

FIG. 3.   Time course of removal of bound carcinogen from guinea pig embryo cells. Confluent cell cultures were treated with 10^{-6} M [9-^{14}C]-NA-AAF as described in the text and the legend to Fig. 1. At varying times after treatment the DNA was prepared from cultured cells (see Fig. 1). The 100% value (*i.e.*, maximal amount of binding) occurred at 1 hr and equals 32.4 μmoles AAF/mole DNA-P. Note change in abscissa scale.

TABLE   3.   Time Course of Removal of Bound AAF

	% carcinogen removed		
	12 hr	24 hr	48 hr
Balb/c 3T3	33	53	65
GP	28	37	54
Pt-K2	69	69	85

determination must be investigated. Interestingly, Group D cells have been reported to have 25–50% as much unscheduled DNA synthesis as normal cells following exposure to 300 erg/mm² UVR (*28*). The reduced amount of carcinogen removal in these XP cells lends support to the conclusion that the disappearance of radioactivity from cellular DNA is an active cellular process and not the result of chemical decomposition or selective removal of injured cells. It appears that the same enzyme or enzymes are responsible for the removal of both pyrimidine dimers and AAF moieties from DNA in human cells although it is possible that in XP a whole series of repair enzymes (as opposed to a single set) have been deleted or are not expressed.

Of interest also is that both mouse Balb/c 3T3 cells and 3rd passage embryo cells remove substantial amounts of carcinogen (roughly as much as is removed by human cells). A number of previous studies which looked at the removal of dimers and/or repair synthesis suggested that mouse cells had only 10–15% of the repair capability of human cells (*7, 29, 30*). (We exclude from the present discussion recent data of Ben-Ishai and Peleg which suggests that mouse primary cultures may have repair rates similar to human strains (4).) In general, these UVR studies were done with UVR fluences of 50–200 erg/mm² and produced significantly greater amounts of DNA damage than that produced by 10^{-6} M NA-AAF. Table 2 presents a summary of our data and some literature values for the extent of damage and amount of removal after exposure of cells to UVR or NA-AAF. They illustrate that human cells and Potorous cells are effective at removing not only damage in the range of one hit/50,000 bases produced by 10^{-6} M NA-AAF, but also the larger amounts of damage produced by UVR. On the other hand, mouse cells (Balb/c 3T3, L5178Y, and 3T3 cells) are less efficient at removing the increased amounts of damage produced by 50–200 erg/mm² UVR. One explanation for this finding is that these amounts of damage are saturating for the mouse cell—either the mouse cell has fewer "repair" enzymes/cell or for some reason they are less efficient. The final resolution of the problem awaits enzyme purification and kinetic studies; however, it is clear that amount of damage must be carefully assessed if one is to make quantitative judgments about repair capacity.

Guinea pig embryo cells and Potorous cells are also able to remove bound carcinogen. We included the Pt-K2 since photoreaction has been easier to demonstrate in these cells than in placental mammals, and we were curious to know if presence of an efficient photoreactivating system reduced the efficiency of the excision repair system. Clearly this is not the case.

Time Course of Removal of Bound AAF Derivatives

Most *in vitro* studies of repair synthesis have tended to emphasize the rapidity with which damage is repaired. Investigators have looked at the removal of products over the first 6–12 hr after damage (14, 19, 31), and analyses of repair synthesis have indicated that the repair process begins to plateau by 9–12 hr (7, 10, 19). However, more precise measurements have demonstrated unscheduled DNA synthesis at longer time periods (Fig. 4) (32, 33).

Examination of several cell types for removal of carcinogen over a 48-hr period was carried out. Table 3 summarizes our removal data: it is apparent that, although removal is most rapid during the first 12 hr, substantial removal also occurs between 12–24 hr and 24–48 hr. At the present time it is not clear if the type of damage being removed during the later time period is the same or qualitatively different from that being removed during the early stages of repair.

In general these results are similar to those from *in vivo* studies. Szafarz and Weisburger (34) and Witschi et al. (35) studied the disappearance of radioactivity from rat liver DNA after the injection of [9-¹⁴C]-N-hydroxy-2-acetylaminofluorene. The first workers found that roughly 75% of the radioactivity was lost over a 48-hr period, while the result from the second laboratory was about 25%. Kriek, on the other hand, reported the presence of two products, one which was removed at a somewhat slower rate than that found by Witschi et al. and a second which apparently was not removed at all (36). The chemical structures of the adducts from either *in vivo* or *in vitro* experiments have not been identified with certainty. In fact,

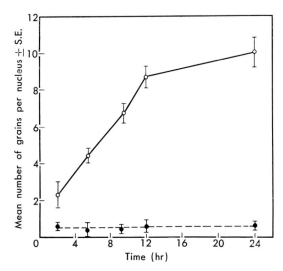

Fig. 4. Time course of DNA repair synthesis in WI-38 human diploid fibroblasts after treatment with 10^{-5} M NA-AAF. For details see Ref. *33*; this figure is reprinted with permission.

the great versatility of liver in metabolizing hydroxamic acids and related compounds (*23–25*), as well as the use of different AAF derivatives *in vitro* and *in vivo*, suggest the need to identify the adducts formed in culturde cells treated with NA-AAF (see Note Added in Proof).

Comparison of Results with Data on the Removal of Adducts of 7-Bromomethylbenz(a)-anthracene and 4-Nitroquinoline 1-Oxide (4NQO)

Two previous investigations have looked at the removal of methylbenz-anthracene adducts from cultured human lymphocyte DNA, following treatment with [³H]-7-bromomethylbenz(a)anthracene (*19, 31*). Lieberman and Dipple found that 15–17% of the bound carcinogen was removed by 12 hr (the earliest time point investigated) when one molecule of carcinogen was bound per 25,000–30,000 bases. Slor extended these findings by demonstrating that lymphocytes from two XP patients removed only 1–2% of the damage by 6 hr while those from normal donors removed 15–19%. These findings are in general agreement with those presented in Table 1; however, careful quantitative comparison must await analysis of removal of the same carcinogen from both lymphocytes and fibroblasts of the same origin. It would be of great interest to determine if these different cell types removed different amounts of known adducts—similar to the results of Goth and Rajewsky (*37*).

Recently Ikenaga, Ishii, Tada, Kakunaga, Takebe, and Kondo have investigated the removal of DNA damage produced by 4NQO in cultured mammalian cells (I thank Dr. Y. Ishii for making me aware of their findings) (*38*). These investigators looked at the removal of 4NQO-purine products and 4-aminoquinoline 1-oxide (4AQO) products from human amnion cells, XP cells, and mouse 3T3 cells.

The 4NQO-purine products were not removed by the XP cells, but, by 24 hr, the human amnion cells had removed about 60% of the damage and the 3T3 cells about 40% of the damage. These findings are in concert with our finding: *i.e.*, the mouse cells are roughly as efficient as human cells at removing low levels of chemical damage, and XP cells remove less damage. 4AQO is interesting since it evidently may be removed by XP cells but is removed more rapidly by normal human strains.

CONCLUSIONS

Our results illustrate that a variety of cultured mammalian cells can remove bound AAF from their DNA. To obtain quantitative measurements of removal, levels of damage should be kept low to prevent artifacts resulting from the possible saturation of repair processes. Comparison of data from XP cells and normal human cells suggest that the same process or processes under similar genetic control are involved in the removal of dimers and AAF moieties. In the past rodent cells have been reported to have much less excision repair capacity than human cells: however, we have found that mouse cells are about as efficient as human cells in removing AAF damage. Although removal of bound carcinogen is most rapid in the first few hours after treatment, the process occurs over an extended period of time (at least 48 hr) in cultured cells.

NOTE ADDED IN PROOF

Using a thin layer chromatographic system developed by Kriek (*36*), we have found that about 80% of the radioactivity in the DNA extracted from Balb/c 3T3 cells treated with [9-^{14}C] NA-AAF co-chromatographs with N-(deoxyguanosin-8-yl)-2-acetylaminofluorene. The remainder of the radioactivity chromatographs in the region of Kriek's other product, *i.e.*, with an R_f 0.5 (*36*).

ACKNOWLEDGMENTS

D.E.A. was a recipient of a U.S.P.H.S. postdoctoral fellowship (award number F22 Ca00334) and J.E.A. was also a recipient of the same fellowship (award number F22-ES01741) during this investigation.

REFERENCES

1. Beers, R. F., Herriott, R. M., and Tilghman, R. C. (eds.). Molecular and Cellular Repair Mechanisms. The Johns Hopkins University Press, Baltimore, 1972.
2. Day, R. S. Studies on repair of adenovirus 2 by human fibroblasts using normal, xeroderma pigmentosum and xeroderma pigmentosum heterozygous strains. Cancer Res., *34*: 1965–1970, 1974.
3. Cleaver, J. E. Repair processes for photochemical damage in mammalian cells. Adv. Radiat. Biol., *4*: 1–75, 1974.
4. Hanawalt, P. C. and Setlow, R. B. (eds.). Molecular Mechanisms for the Repair of DNA, Plenum Press, New York, 1975.

5. Lieberman, M. W.   Approaches to the analysis of fidelity of DNA repair in mammalian cells. Int. Rev. Cytol., 1975, *46*: 1–23, 1976.

6. Kleijer, W. J., De Weerd-Kastelein, E. A., Sluyter, M. L., Keijzer, W., De Wit, J., and Bootsma, D. UV induced DNA repair synthesis in cells of patients with different forms of xeroderma pigmentosum and of heterozygotes. Mutat. Res., *20*: 417–428, 1973.

7. Hart, R. W. and Setlow, R. B.   Correlation between deoxyribonucleic acid excision repair and life-span in a number of mammalian species. Proc. Natl. Acad. Sci. U.S., *71*: 2169–2173, 1974.

8. Robbins, J. H., Kraemer, K. H., Lutzner, M. A., Festoff, B. W., and Coon, H. G. Xeroderma pigmentosum: An inherited disease with sun sensitivity, multiple cutaneous neoplasms, and abnormal DNA repair. Ann. Intern. Med., *80*: 221–248, 1974.

9. Takebe, H., Nii, S., Ishii, M. I., and Utsumi, H.   Comparative studies of host-cell reactivation, colony forming ability and excision repair after UV irradiation of xeroderma pigmentosum, normal human and some other mammalian cells. Mutat. Res., *25*: 383–390, 1974.

10. Lieberman, M. W., Baney, R. N., Lee, R. E., Sell, S., and Farber, E.   Studies on DNA repair in human lymphocytes treated with proximate carcinogens and alkylating agents. Cancer Res., *31*: 1297–1306, 1971.

11. Stich, H. F., San, R. H. C., Miller, J. A., and Miller, E. C. Various levels of DNA repair synthesis in xeroderma pigmentosum cells exposed to the carcinogens N-hydroxy and N-acetoxy-2-acetylaminofluorene. Nature New Biol., *238*: 9–10, 1972.

12. Cleaver, J. E.   DNA repair with purines and pyrimidines in radiation- and carcinogen-damaged normal and xeroderma pigmentosum human cells. Cancer Res., *33*: 362–369, 1973.

13. Regan, J. D. and Setlow, R. B.   Two forms of repair in the DNA of human cells damaged by chemical carcinogens and mutagens. Cancer Res., *34*: 3318–3325, 1974.

14. Roberts, J. J., Pacsoe, J. M., Smith, B. A., and Crathorn, A. R.   Quantitative aspects of the repair of alkylated DNA in cultured mammalian cells. II. Non-semiconservative DNA synthesis ("repair synthesis") in HeLa and Chinese hamster cells following treatment with alkylating agents. Chem.-Biol. Interact, 3: 49–68, 1971.

15. Kriek, E., Miller, J. A., Juhl, U., and Miller, E. C.   8-(N-2-Fluorenylacetamido)-guanosine, an arylamidation reaction product of guanosine and the carcinogen N-acetoxy-N-2-fluorenylacetamide in neutral solution. Biochemistry, *6*: 177–182, 1967.

16. Lieberman, M. W. and Poirier, M. C.   Deoxyribonucleotide incorporation during DNA repair of carcinogen-induced damage in human diploid fibroblasts. Cancer Res., *33*: 2097–2103, 1973.

17. Di Paolo, J. A., Takano, K., and Popescu, R. C. Quantitation of chemically induced neoplastic transformation of Balb/3T3 cloned cell lines. Cancer Res., *32*: 2686–2695, 1972.

18. Ishii, Y. and Lieberman, M. W. Unpublished.

19. Lieberman, M. W. and Dipple, A.   Removal of bound carcinogen during DNA repair in nondividing human lymphocytes. Cancer Res., *32*: 1855–1860, 1972.

20. Amacher, D. E., Elliott, J. A., and Lieberman, M. W.   Unpublished.

21. Levine, A. F., Fink, L. M., Weinstein, I. B., and Grunberger, D. Effect of N-2-acetylaminofluorene modification on the conformation of nucleic acids. Cancer Res., *34*: 319–327, 1974.

22. Müller, W. Personal communication.

23. Weisburger, J. H. and Weisburger, E. K. Biochemical formation and pharmacologi-

cal, toxicological, and pathological properties of hydoxylamines and hydroxamic acids. Pharmacol. Rev., *25*: 1–66, 1973.

24. King, C. M. and Phillips, B.   N-Hydroxy-2-fluorenylacetamide: Reaction of the carcinogen with guanosine, ribonucleic acid, deoxyribonucleic acid and protein following enzymatic deacetylation or esterification. J. Biol. Chem., *244*: 6209–6216, 1969.

25. Kriek, E.   Carcinogenesis by aromatic amines. Biochim. Biophys. Acta, *355*: 177–203, 1974.

26. Mann, T.   The Biochemistry of Semen and the Male Reproductive Tract. p. 147, Wiley, New York, 1964.

27. McCarthy, B. J.   The evolution of base sequences in polynucleotides. Prog. Nucl. Acid Res. Mol. Biol., *4*: 129–160, 1965.

28. Kraemer, K. H., Coon, H. G., Petinga, R. A., Barrett, S. F., Rahe, A. E., and Robbins, J. H. Genetic heterogeneity in xeroderma pigmentosum: Complementation groups and their relationship to DNA repair rates. Proc. Natl. Acad. Sci. U.S., *72*: 59–63, 1975.

29. Lehmann, A. R. Post replication repair of DNA in ultraviolet-irradiated mammalian cells. Eur. J. Biochem., *31*: 438–445, 1972.

30. Setlow, R. B., Regan, J. D., and Carrier, W. L. Different levels of excision repair in mammalian cell lines. Biophys. Soc. Abstr., *12*: 19a, 1972.

31. Slor, H. Induction of unscheduled DNA synthesis by the carcinogen 7 bromomethyl-benz(a)anthracene and its removal from the DNA of normal and xeroderma pigmentosum lymphocytes. Mutat. Res., *19*: 231–235, 1973.

32. Robbins, J. H. and Kraemer, K. H. Prolonged ultraviolet-induced thymidine incorporation into xeroderma pigmentosum lymphocytes: Studies on the duration, amount, localization and relationship to hydroxyurea. Biochim. Biophys. Acta, *277*: 7–14, 1972.

33. Harris, C. C., Connor, R. J., Jackson, F. E., and Lieberman, M. W.   Intranuclear distribution of DNA repair synthesis induced by chemical carcinogens or ultraviolet light in human diploid fibroblasts.   Cancer Res., *34*: 3461–3468, 1974.

34. Szafarz, D. and Weisburger, J. H. Stability of the binding of label from N-hydroxy-N-fluorenylacetamide to intranuclear targets, particularly deoxyribonucleic acid in rat liver. Cancer Res., *29*: 962–968, 1969.

35. Witschi, H., Epstein, S. M., and Farber, E. Influence of liver regeneration on the loss of fluorenylacetamide derivative bound to liver DNA. Cancer Res., *31*: 270–273, 1971.

36. Kriek, E.   Persistent binding of a new reaction product of the carcinogen N-hydroxy-N-2-acetylaminofluorene with guanine in rat liver DNA *in vivo*. Cancer Res., *32*: 2042–2048, 1972.

37. Goth, R. and Rajewsky, M. F.   Molecular and cellular mechanisms associated with pulse-carcinogenesis in the rat nervous system by ethylnitrosourea: Ethylation of nucleic acids and elimination rates of ethylated bases from the DNA of different tissues. Z. Krebsforsch., *82*: 37–64, 1974.

38. Ikenaga, M., Ishii, Y., Tada, M., Kakunaga, T., Takebe, H., and Kondo, S.   Excision repair of 4-nitroquinoline-1-oxide damage responsible for killing, mutation and cancer. *In;* P. C. Hanawalt and R. B. Setlow (eds.), Molecular Mechanisms for the Repair of DNA, pp. 763–771, Plenum Press, New York, 1975.

Discussion of Paper of Drs. Lieberman et al.

DR. KURODA: Have you tried to determine the difference in the binding ability of cells for carcinogen at different phases of cell cycle?

DR. LIEBERMAN: No, we have not looked at this problem. It is difficult for us to do that because of the large number of cells we would need.

DR. BOOTSMA: In addition to the previous remark, I would like to draw your attention to the techniques of premature chromosome condensation which can be induced by fusion of cells in metaphase with cells in mitosis. This technique allows the investigation of the repair at the chromosomal level and its dependence in the progression through the cell cycle.

DR. LIEBERMAN: Thank you very much for this suggestion. I agree that this would be interesting to investigate especially if a carcinogen with a high specific activity of ^{3}H were used.

DR. FARBER: As you are no doubt aware, Dr. Kriek in the Netherlands has reported at least two forms of bound acetylaminofluorene (AAF) in rat liver DNA—one form that is removed fairly quickly (2–3 weeks) and another which seems not to be removed to any significant degree even after weeks. Have you carried out your time studies for a sufficiently long period of time to test this in your *in vitro* systems?

DR. LIEBERMAN: We have not looked at periods of time greater than 48 hr. We are now in the process of analyzing the adducts formed *in vitro* by treatment of cells with N-acetoxy-2-acetylaminofluorene (NA-AAF). Because of the great metabolic capability of liver, it may be that administration of N-hydroxy-2-acetylamino-fluorene to animals results in a greater variety of adducts than that seen in our experiments. The resolution of this problem will be of great interest to all of us.

DR. IKENAGA: You found about 50% removal of AAF lesions in mouse 3T3 cell line. We also found about 60 to 70% removal of 4-nitroquinoline 1-oxide (4NQO)-induced lesions in a subclone of 3T3. So, I feel that endonuclease working on AAF or 4NQO lesions is different from UV-specific endonuclease. The supporting experimental evidence is the fact that T4 UV endonuclease does not work on 4NQO damage. May I ask your opinion?

DR. LIEBERMAN: It would be interesting to know if the enzymes involved in the removal of these chemical adducts and dimers are the same or different. In mammalian cells I don't think we have enough data at present. Whether or not the T4 endonuclease data will be a useful guide remains to be seen.

DR. MAHER: You stressed in your presentation that repair studies measuring removal of dimers or of AAF residues should be carried out over periods of longer and longer times. It is also most important that the doses used be as low as possible. Your one slide showing the removal of AAF residues was with 10 μM NA-AAF which gives only 1% survival.

DR. LIEBERMAN: Yes, I agree. The slide I presented were old data from C. Harris et al. (Cancer Res., 34: 3461–3468, 1974). I used these data merely to point to the importance of looking at longer time periods in the older literature. All of our removal studies have been done with 1 μM NA-AAF which result in high survival (80% in human liver).

DR. OKADA: Could you tell us how the rate of AAF removal is affected when the confluent cells are stimulated to enter DNA synthesis?

DR. LIEBERMAN: We have not done this experiment. Data in vivo on the removal of AAF adducts from rat liver DNA indicate that partial hepatectomy does not change the rate of removal (H. Witschi, S. M. Epstein, and E. Farber, Cancer Res., 31: 270, 1971).

DR. TAKEBE: Mr. Watanabe and Dr. Horikawa at Kanazawa University have been studying cell-cycle dependence of DNA damage and its repair. What they have found so far, published in Mutation Research I believe, is that the amount of damage caused by UV or 4NQO depends on cell cycle, but the rate of repair stays constant throughout the cell cycle.

If I remember correctly, the difference in sensitivity of colony-forming ability between normal and xeroderma pigmentosum cells was much greater for UV than for AAF. Therefore it may be reasonable to assume that the DNA damage caused by AAF might behave differently to excision repair system.

DR. LIEBERMAN: I think at this stage, we should leave open the question of the similarity or differences in the repair systems which deal with these two types of damage.

DR. RAJEWSKY: Could I ask Dr. Magee whether he interprets the finding of Nicoll et al. (Nature, 254: 261, 1975) on the low and high rate of O^6-alkylguanine removal from kidney DNA after a high and low dose, respectively, in a similar way as suggested by Dr. Lieberman for high or low level of NA-AAF adduct formation in mouse DNA?

DR. MAGEE: I think it possible that similar mechanisms may apply to the rat kidney *in vivo* after larger and smaller doses of dimethylnitrosamine (DMN) as those postulated by Dr. Lieberman to explain his observations *in vitro*. However, as I emphasized yesterday, in rats treated with DMN *in vivo*, particularly after the higher dose, the liver is severely damaged and the kidney is also damaged to a lesser extent. It is, therefore, difficult to relate events *in vivo* to those observed *in vitro*.

FUNDAMENTALS IN CANCER PREVENTION, P. N. MAGEE ET AL. (EDS.),
UNIV. OF TOKYO PRESS, TOKYO / UNIV. PARK PRESS, BALTIMORE, PP. 349–362, 1976

Endonuclease II of *Escherichia coli* and Related Enzymes

Dollie M. Kirtikar,[*1] J. Philip Kuebler,[*1] Anthony Dipple,[*2] and
David A. Goldthwait[*1]

*Department of Biochemistry, Case Western Reserve University, Cleveland, Ohio, U.S.A.[*1] and Chester
Beatty Research Institute, Fulham Road, U.K.[*2]*

Abstract : 1) Endonuclease II of *Escherichia coli*, active on DNA treated with methyl
methanesulfonate (MMS), methylnitrosourea (MNU), 7-bromomethyl-12-methyl-
benz[a]anthracene (7-BMMB), and γ-irradiation, has been separated from an
endonuclease active on depurinated DNA. 2) The mutant AB3027 lacks endonuclease II while the mutant BW2001 lacks the apurinic acid endonuclease. 3)
Endonuclease II has a molecular weight of approximately 33,000, has no divalent
metal requirement but is stimulated by Mg^{2+}. The products of phosphodiester bond
hydrolysis in MMS DNA are 3′-hydroxyls and 5′-phosphates. 4) Endonuclease II
hydrolizes phosphodiester bonds and also releases 3-methyladenine, but not 7-
methylguanine from DNA treated with dimethylsulfate. From MNU-treated DNA,
the enzyme releases O^6-methylguanine and 3-methyladenine as well as 1-methyl-
and 7-methyladenine. 3-Methyladenine is released at approximately 4 times the
rate of the other derivatives. 5) DNA treated with 7-BMMB is a substrate for
endonuclease II. The enzyme hydrolyzes phosphodiester bonds and releases the
N^6-adenyl and N^2-guanyl derivatives. The adenine base derivative is released at
approximately 4 times the rate of the guanine base derivative. 6) Phorbol ester
inhibits both phosphodiester bond hydrolysis and base release from 7-BMMB-
treated DNA catalyzed by endonuclease II. Phorbol ester does not inhibit the
apurinic acid endonuclease. 7) Endonuclease II recognizes damage in DNA due to
γ-irradiation. Enzyme-sensitive sites can be increased in the DNA by a preincubation at 37°C for 4 hr in the presence of nitrogen after the irradiation. 8) An endonuclease specific for apurinic acid has been purified from calf liver. A comparison
of some of the properties of this enzyme with the enzyme from calf thymus suggests
that they are isoenzymes.

Endonuclease II of *Escherichia coli* is now defined as an enzyme which re-

---

[*2] Present address: Frederick Cancer Research Center, Frederick, Maryland, U.S.A.

cognizes distortions in the DNA molecule due to alkylating agents (*1*) as well as due to an aralkylating agent (*2*) and γ-irradiation (*3*). This enzyme is different from the enzyme active on depurinated DNA which will be referred to as the apurinic acid endonuclease.

Separation of Endonuclease II of E. coli from the Apurinic Acid Endonuclease

For separation of these activities, the *E. coli* cells were broken with glass beads, the high-speed supernatant fraction was treated with 0.8% streptomycin sulfate, a portion of the supernatant fraction was precipitated with $(NH_4)_2SO_4$ between 45 and 80% (*4*). This material was applied to a DEAE column and eluted as shown in Fig. 1. Three peaks of enzyme activity were isolated. Peak I is active primarily on depurinated or depurinated reduced DNA (*5*), and is similar to the enzyme isolated by Verly and Paquette (*6*). The very slight activity on methyl methanc-sulfonate (MMS)-treated DNA may be due to depurination sites in this substrate, although this has not been proved. Peak III is active primarily on MMS-treated DNA and has a low level of activity on depurinated DNA. This rate of degradation is approximately 10% of that on MMS DNA and this percentage remains constant throughout a 3,000-fold purification procedure. Evidence will be presented later to support the concept that this activity on depurinated DNA is an intrinsic activity of endonuclease II. In a previous publication from this laboratory it was concluded erroneously that the activity on depurinated DNA was due to the same enzyme which recognized alkylated DNA (*5*).

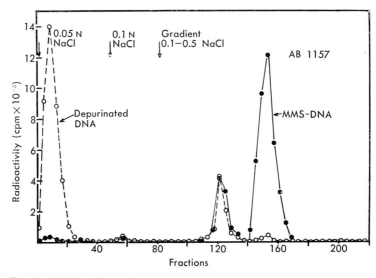

FIG. 1.   DEAE column chromatography of an extract of wild type (AB1157) of *E. coli*.

Different Genes Control Endonuclease II and the Apurinic Acid Endonuclease

A mutant strain of *E. coli*, AB3027, originally isolated by Dr. P. Howard-

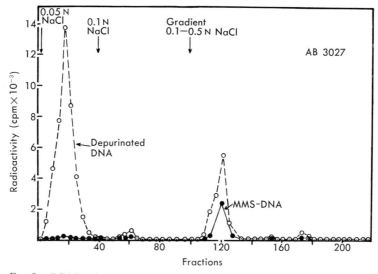

FIG. 2. DEAE column chromatography of an extract of a mutant (AB3027) of *E. coli*.

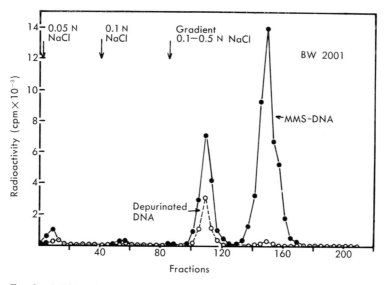

FIG. 3. DEAE column chromatography of an extract of a mutant (BW2001) of *E. coli*.

Flanders because of its sensitivity to MMS, has been shown to be lacking Peak III or endonuclease II as demonstrated in Fig. 2. A mutant, BW2001, isolated by Dr. Weiss (7), on the basis of a decreased endonucleolytic activity on MMS DNA, was also examined as shown in Fig. 3. This mutant is obviously lacking Peak I, the apurinic acid enzyme. The exact nature of Peak II is under investigation. It contains equal amounts of both activities in the wild-type strain and in each of the mutants there is a decrease, but not an absence of the defective enzyme. On re-chromatography, Peak II does not split into Peaks I and III. The possibility of a stable dimer is under investigation.

Properties of Endonuclease II

An approximate molecular weight determined by gel filtrations is 33,000. When examined with MMS DNA, the enzyme has no divalent metal requirement, but is stimulated approximately twofold by Mg^{2+}. It is active in the presence of various chelating agents such as 8-hydroxyquinoline at 6×10^{-4} M. EDTA does inhibit the enzyme activity 71% at 10^{-4} M and 90% at 10^{-3} M. No inhibition was observed with tRNA. The enzyme does have reactive sulfhydryl groups as indicated by its sensitivity to *p*-chloromercurisulfonate. A careful study showed that the enzyme produced one double-strand break in DNA treated with MMS for every 4 single-strand breaks. Since the preparation had limited activity on single-stranded DNA only at high enzyme concentrations, a possible interpretation of these results is that DNA is alkylated nonrandomly (*1*).

The 3,000-fold purified endonuclease II preparation from Peak II hydrolyzes phosphodiester bonds of MMS DNA to produce 3'-hydroxyl and 5'-phosphate residues. This has been determined using snake venom and bovine spleen exonucleases with and without alkaline phosphatase as shown in Fig. 4.

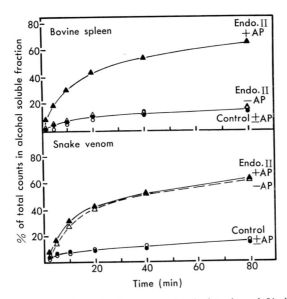

Fig. 4. Evidence for formation of 3'-hydroxyls and 5'-phosphates by endonuclease II.

Release of Methylated Purine Bases by Endonuclease II from DNA Treated with Dimethyl-sulfate or Methylnitrosourea (MNU)

When DNA was reacted with [³H]-dimethylsulfate, and then exposed to an enzyme preparation containing endonuclease II, 3-methyladenine, but not 7-methylguanine was released and could be isolated by paper or column chromatography (*8*). The ratio of 3-methyladenine to 7-methylguanine in DNA treated with dimethylsulfate is approximately 1:4. Thus, the enzyme has some specificity for alkylated bases.

MNU, a strong mutagen and carcinogen, is known to methylate DNA bases to give not only 3-methyladenine and 7-methylguanine, but also O^6-methyl guanine (*9*). Faulty base pairing has been demonstrated with a polymer containing O^6-methylguanine (*10*) and it is this alkylated base that is considered to be mutagenic and therefore probably carcinogenic. A preparation of endonuclease II recognizes altered bases in MNU-treated DNA and makes phosphodiester bond breaks. The enzyme also releases O^6-methylguanine and 3-methyladenine as free bases. The stoichiometry of such a reaction, in which the products were isolated by chromatography on Dowex 50, is shown in Table 1. Smaller amounts of other methylated bases are released and can be analyzed by thin-layer chromatography, as shown in Table 2. When the release of these bases was examined as a function

TABLE 1.   Stoichiometry of the Enzyme Reaction with DNA Alkylated with MNU

| Fractions | Percentage of the total counts in the reaction mixture | | | | | |
| | Alcohol-soluble fraction | | | Alcohol-insoluble fraction | | |
	− enzyme	+ enzyme	Δ	− enzyme	+ enzyme	Δ
O^6-Methylguanine	1.4	6.8	+5.4	7.8	2.8	−5.0
3-Methyladenine	1.8	13.7	+11.9	21.1	7.0	−14.1
7-Methylguanine + 7-methyladenine	7.0	9.0	+2.0	41.8	37.8	−4.0

− enzyme, without endonuclease II in the reaction mixture;   + enzyme, with endonuclease II in the reaction mixture. Details of this work have been published (*8*).

TABLE 2.   The Percent of the Total Counts Present on a Thin-layer Chromatogram Recovered in Different Bases as a Function of Enzyme Concentration

| | Enzyme units | | | |
	0.02 U (% total cpm)	0.04 U (%)	0.08 U (%)	0.20 U (%)
3-Methyladenine	5.0	10.7	14.2	14.8
O^6-Methylguanine	0.5	2.3	3.0	5.5
1-Methyladenine	0.41	0.89	1.2	1.4
7-Methyladenine	0	0.1	1.2	1.4
7-Methylguanine	0.03	0	0	0

Unlabeled T4 DNA (3,000 nmoles) in 2.0 ml was reacted with [³H]-MNU (specific activity 48 mCi/mM) at MNU:DNA nucleotide ratio of 7:1; after alcohol precipitation and washing the alkylated DNA was solubilized in 1.0 ml of 0.05 M Tris-HCl (pH 8.0) at 0°C. For enzymatic hydrolysis, 0.1-ml reaction mixtures containing 20 nmoles of [³H]-MNU-T4 DNA (specific activity 2,500 ³H cpm/nmole of nucleotide, with 23.7 mmoles of [³H]-methyl per mole of DNA nucleotide), 1×10^{-4} M β-mercaptoethanol, 1×10^{-4} M 8-hydroxyquinoline, 5×10^{-2} M Tris-HCl (pH 8.0), and enzyme as indicated were incubated at 37°C for 1 hr. The reactions were terminated with EDTA at a final concentration of 0.02 M. The aliquot of 20 μl (approximately 5,000 ³H cpm), supplemented with methylated bases, from each sample was chromatographed separately on thin-layer sheets. The total counts recovered from all the sections of the thin-layer plate were taken as 100%. Details of this work have been published (*8*).

of time, 3-methyladenine appeared at a rate which was approximately four times the rate of release of O^6-methylguanine, 1-methyladenine, or 7-methylguanine. Again in these experiments, the enzymatic release of 7-methylguanine was not observed. This pattern of release of O^6-methylguanine and 3-methyladenine, but not of 7-methylguanine was observed in *E. coli in vivo* by Lawley and Orr (*11*) and is undoubtedly due to the activity of endonuclease II. Again, the experiments with MNU-treated DNA and endonuclease II show that the enzyme has some specificity in base recognition.

DNA Treated with 7-Bromomethyl-12-methylbenz[a]anthracene (7-BMMB) as a Substrate for Endonuclease II

The brominated derivative of 7-methyl-12-methylbenz[a]anthracene (DMBA) is a potent carcinogen in several animal test systems (*12*). It reacts directly with the amino groups of adenine, guanine, and cytosine in DNA both *in vitro* and *in vivo* (*13, 14*). Recent studies with endonuclease II (*2*) have shown that the enzyme makes phosphodiester bond breaks in DNA treated with the hydrocarbon. This is shown in Table 3. Base release by the enzyme was also observed when DNA treated with radioactive 7-BMMB was incubated with the enzyme. The reaction mixture was treated with alcohol to give a precipitate containing DNA and a supernatant fraction with the bases which were liberated. By chromatography of the alcohol-soluble fraction as well as the acid-hydrolized alcohol-insoluble fraction on Sephadex LH20, the release of the hydrocarbon derivatives of adenine and guanine by the enzyme were observed. The stoichiometry of one such experiment is shown in Table 4. Proof that bases rather than nucleosides were released has been obtained by using marker compounds. The rate of release of the hydrocarbon derivative of adenine was approximately 4 times that of the rate of release of the derivative of guanine as observed by separation on thin-layer plates. Thus, endonuclease II recognizes DNA treated with 7-BMMB by hydrolyzing phosphodiester

TABLE 3.   Enzyme-induced Single-strand Breaks in DNA Treated with 7-BMMB

Enzyme units	Single-strand breaks
—	3
0.01	3
0.02	6
0.04	11
0.08	16
0.16	25

[³H]-purine-labeled T7 DNA (specific activity 1960 cpm per nmole DNA nucleotide) was reacted with unlabeled 7-BMMB at a hydrocarbon to DNA nucleotide ratio of 1:10 (*13*). Incubation mixtures (0.25 ml) contained 15 nmoles of hydrocarbon modified DNA nucleotides, 1×10^{-4} M β-mercaptoethanol, 1×10^{-4} M 8-hydroxyquinoline, 5×10^{-2} M Tris-HCl buffer, pH 8.0 and enzyme units as indicated. After 60 min at 37°C, reactions were terminated by adding EDTA and sodium dodecylsulfate at final concentrations of 2×10^{-2} M and 0.25%, respectively. The samples were then incubated in alkali (0.066 M final concentration) at 37°C for 20 min and aliquots were centrifuged through 5–20% alkaline sucrose density-gradient solutions. Single-strand breaks were calculated.

TABLE 4. Enzymatic Release of DMBA Derivatives of DNA Bases

Base derivative	Alcohol-soluble $\Delta(+)$ *vs.* $(-)$ enzyme (cpm)	Alcohol-insoluble $\Delta(+)$ *vs.* $(-)$ enzyme (cpm)
N[6]-DMBA adenine	+22,423	−21,590
N[2]-DMBA guanine	+6,764	−6,757
N[4]-DMBA cytosine	−89	−512

The incubation mixtures (1.0 ml) contained 85 nmoles DNA nucleotide ((^{3}H)-hydrocarbon-salmon sperm DNA, 0.82 mmoles carcinogen per mole DNA nucleotide, specific activity 500 cpm per nmole DNA nucleotide), 1×10^{-4} M β-mercaptoethanol, 5×10^{-2} M Tris-HCl, pH 8 buffer, 1×10^{-4} M 8-hydroxyquinoline, and 0.4 units of enzyme where indicated. After 60 min at 35°C the reaction was terminated, and an alcohol-soluble and an alcohol-insoluble fraction were obtained. The latter was digested to nucleosides (*17*) and hydrolyzed to bases. The hydrolyzed sample as well as the alcohol-soluble material were supplemented with [^{14}C]-labeled markers and chromatographed on Sephadex LH-20 eluted in spectroanalyzed methanol.

bonds and by liberating N[6]-DMBA adenine and N[2]-DMBA guanine. The enzyme does not recognize the cytosine derivative.

Phorbol Ester, an Inhibitor of Endonuclease II

The cocarcinogen phorbol myristate acetate (*15*) inhibits both the hydrolysis of phosphodiester bonds and the release of base derivatives catalyzed by endonuclease II. With both MMS-treated DNA and 7-BMMB-treated DNA as substrates, phorbol ester inhibits the hydrolysis of phosphodiester bonds as shown in Fig. 5. The cocarcinogen does not inhibit phosphodiester bond hydrolysis in depurinated DNA by the apurinic acid enzyme. The enzyme preparation used for this experiment contained both activities. Depurinated sites may be present in the MMS-treated DNA and may account for inability of the phorbol ester to give complete inhibition. The hydrolysis of the hydrocarbon-treated DNA was inhibited at very low levels of the cocarcinogen. For example 95% inhibition was observed with

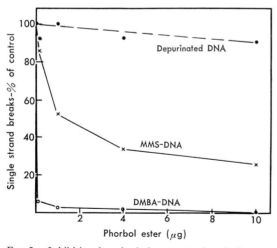

FIG. 5. Inhibition by phorbol ester of phosphodiester bond hydrolysis by endonuclease II.

TABLE 5. Inhibition of Enzymatic Release of DMBA Base by Phorbol Ester

Phorbol ester (μg)	% inhibition
0	0
0.02	51
0.10	92
1.0	96
5.0	99
10.0	99
(1 μg $= 1.66 \times 10^{-6}$ M)	

Incubation mixtures (0.25 ml) contained 60–75 nmoles [^{3}H]-hydrocarbon-treated DNA, 5×10^{-2} M Tris-HCl, pH 8.0 buffer, 1×10^{-4} M β-mercaptoethanol, 1×10^{-4} M 8 hydroxyquinoline, and phorbol ester as indicated. Enzyme (0.06 units for 0.02 and 0.1 μg of phorbol ester and 0.25 units for 1–10 μg) was reacted with phorbol ester 5 min at 0°C prior to addition of substrate. After 45- and 60-min incubation at 36°C with the two enzyme concentrations, reactions were terminated by adding EDTA to final concentration of 2×10^{-2} M. The samples were supplemented with unlabeled T4 DNA (50–100 μg per tube) and unhydrolyzed DNA was precipitated out with alcohol. Alcohol-soluble and alcohol-insoluble radioactivity was determined.

a concentration of 3.3×10^{-7} M. The enzymatic release of bases of DNA treated with 7-BMMB was also inhibited by phorbol ester. In Table 5 the percent inhibition of release as a function of phorbol ester concentration is shown. This reaction shows a similar sensitivity. These experiments were done with the enzyme preparation which contains both the activity on MMS DNA and the activity on depurinated DNA. When the purified endonuclease II, active primarily on MMS DNA, but with a residual activity on depurinated DNA, was incubated with depurinated reduced DNA plus phorbol ester, inhibition of phosphodiester bond hydrolysis was observed. Because the apurinic acid enzyme was not inhibited by phorbol ester, this result indicates that the residual activity of endonuclease II on depurinated DNA is a property of this enzyme and not due to a contamination by the apurinic acid enzyme.

γ-Irradiated DNA, a Substrate for Endonuclease II

Endonuclease II also recognizes damage in DNA due to γ-irradiation (3). The preparation of endonuclease II, free of Peaks I and II, is the fraction responsible. When DNA was irradiated under nitrogen (Fig. 6A) and then preincubated at 37°C in the presence of oxygen (air) for 4 hr, there was both an increase in spontaneous single-strand breaks which are primarily induced by alkali as well as an increase in enzyme-sensitive sites. These enzyme-sensitive sites were not depurinated or depyrimidinated sites because the reaction mixtures with and without enzyme after the incubation were then exposed to 0.066 N NaOH at 37°C for 20 min. This latter treatment cleaves phosphodiester bonds at all depurinated sites so that a chemical depurination by γ-irradiation would appear as a spontaneous, non-enzymatic break. When the DNA was irradiated under nitrogen and the preincubation done also under nitrogen (Fig. 6B) the spontaneous strand breaks are minimal, but the enzyme-sensitive sites increased as in the previous case. If the DNA was irradiated in oxygen and preincubated in oxygen (Fig. 6C), almost all of the breaks

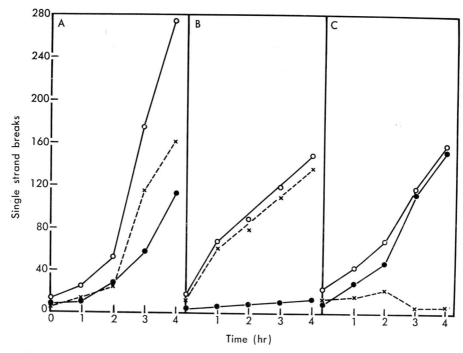

Fig. 6.   The effect of oxygen or nitrogen during a preincubation period at 37°C following the irradiation. [³H] T7DNA was irradiated under N_2 (A and B) or O_2 (C) and then preincubated in O_2 (A and C) or N_2 (B).   ○ total breaks; × enzyme-induced breaks; ● non-enzymatic breaks.

TABLE 6.   The Effect of Addition of $NaBH_4$ or NH_2OH before or after Preincubation of Irradiated DNA on Spontaneous Single-strand Breaks

Preincubation	Additions		Single-strand breaks
	Before preincubation	After preincubation	
+	—	—	47
+	$NaBH_4$	—	4
+	—	$NaBH_4$	11
+	NH_2OH	—	5
+	—	NH_2OH	13
−	—	—	8
−	—	$NaBH_4$	4
−	—	NH_2OH	4

Vials containing [³H]-thymine-labeled T7 DNA (2,900 cpm/nmole of DNA nucleotide) were irradiated under nitrogen at pH 7.0, 0°C, by a ⁶⁰Co γ-ray source with 22.5 krads. The pH was adjusted to 8.5 and some samples were preincubated under nitrogen at 37°C for 4 hr. Additions of $NaBH_4$ at a final concentration of 0.25 M or NH_2OH at a final concentration of 0.2 M were as indicated. Prior to analysis by sucrose-gradient centrifugation all samples were exposed to 0.066 N NaOH at 37°C for 20 min under conditions adequate to hydrolyze phosphodiester bonds at depurinated sites. Details of the conditions have been reported (*3*).

were spontaneous and the enzyme-sensitive sites decreased rather than increased.

The spontaneous breaks can be almost entirely prevented by reduction with $NaBH_4$ or reaction with NH_2OH (Table 6), which suggests that they are depurinated or depyrimidinated sites. Preliminary evidence for the release of radioactivity from both purine- and thymine-labeled DNA has been obtained, but the sensitivity of these sites to the apurinic acid enzyme is under investigation. The nature of the enzyme-sensitive sites is not known. Judging from the specificity of endonuclease II for purine derivatives observed to date, it seems reasonable to assume that altered purine residues may be involved. This is also under investigation.

TABLE 7.   Calf Apurinic Acid Enzymes

Properties	Liver (Kuebler)	Thymus (Lindahl)	Thymus (Kuebler)
Purification	900	830	10–30
pH optimum	9.5	8.5	—
Max. Mg^{2+} stimulation	$1.3\times$	$1,000\times$	$8\times$
Conc. Mg^{2+} for max. stimulation	0.01 mM	3.0 mM	0.5–2.0 mM
50% inhibition by salt	0.023 M	0.2 M	0.12 M
Stimulation by low salt	None	—	>4-fold at 0.01 M
DNA breaks	SS and ds	SS	—
Mol. wt.	29,000	32,000	

An Apurinic Acid Endonuclease from Calf Liver

An endonuclease specific for depurinated DNA has been purified approximately 900-fold from calf liver. The enzyme does not recognize DNA treated with UV irradiation nor does it recognize the sites in γ-irradiated DNA which are seen by endonuclease II. This enzyme is of some interest in that a number of its properties differ from the apurinic acid endonuclease purified from calf thymus by Ljungquist and Lindahl (16). The calf thymus enzyme has also been partially purified 10- to 30-fold. A summary of some of the properties of the calf liver preparation and the calf thymus preparation extensively purified by Ljungquist and Lindahl (16) and partially purified in this laboratory are shown in Table 7. The liver enzyme has a higher pH optimum than the thymus enzyme. It does not show the dependence on Mg^{2+} seen with the thymus enzyme especially in its purified form. The liver enzyme shows a stimulation with Mg^{2+} of 1.3-fold at a concentration of 0.01 M but at levels higher than this there is increasing inhibition. The liver enzyme is very sensitive to ionic strength and it is inhibited 50% by 0.023 M NaCl while the thymus enzyme shows a stimulation by low concentrations of NaCl, and a 50% inhibition only at 0.12–0.2 M NaCl. The liver enzyme can make both single- and double-strand breaks in depurinated reduced DNA while Ljungquist and Lindahl state that the thymus enzyme does not make double-strand breaks. The molecular weights of these two enzymes are similar. The liver enzyme has a molecular weight of approximately 29,000 by gel filtration while the thymus enzyme has a molecualr weight of 32,000. These properties vary enough to support the concept that isoenzymes of the apurinic acid enzyme exist.

ACKNOWLEDGMENTS

This work was supported by grants from the National Institutes of Health (CA11322), the Health Fund of Greater Cleveland, the Cuyahoga Unit of the American Cancer Society, and a contract with ERDA (11-1) 2725. D.A.G. was a recipient of a National Institutes of Health Research Career Award Fellowship (K6-GM-21444) during this investigation.

REFERENCES

1. Friedberg, E. C., Hadi, S. M., and Goldthwait, D. A.   Endonuclease II of *Escherichia coli*: II. Enzyme properties and studies on the degradation of alkylated and native DNA. J. Biol. Chem., *244*: 5879–5889, 1969.

2. Kirtikar, D., Dipple, A., and Goldthwait, D. A. Endonuclease II of *Escherichia coli*: DNA reacted with 7-bromomethyl-12-methylbenz[a]anthracene as a substrate. Biochemistry, *14*: 5548–5553, 1975.

3. Kirtikar, D., Slaughter, J., and Goldthwait, D. A. Endonuclease II of *Escherichia coli*: Degradation of γ-irradiated DNA. Biochemistry, *14*: 1235–1244, 1975.

4. Friedberg, E. C. and Goldthwait, D. A.   Endonuclease II of *E. coli*: I. Isolation and purification. Proc. Natl. Acad. Sci. U.S., *62*: 934–940, 1969.

5. Hadi, S. M. and Goldthwait, D. A.   Endonuclease II of *Escherichia coli*: Degradation of partially depurinated DNA. Biochemistry, *10*: 4986–4994, 1971.

6. Verly, W. S. and Paquette, Y.   An endonuclease for depurinated DNA in *Escherichia coli*. Can. J. Biochem., *50*: 217–224, 1972.

7. Yajko, D. M. and Weiss, B.   Mutations simultaneously affecting endonuclease II and exonuclease III in *Escherichia coli*. Proc. Natl. Acad. Sci. U.S., *72*: 688–692, 1975.

8. Kirtikar, D. M. and Goldthwait, D. A.   The enzymatic release of O⁶-methylguanine and 3-methyladenine from DNA reacted with the carcinogen N-methyl-N-nitrosourea. Proc. Natl. Acad. Sci. U.S., *71*: 2022–2026, 1974.

9. Loveless, A.   Possible relevance of O-6 alkylation of deoxyguanosine to the mutagenicity and carcinogenicity of nitrosamines and nitrosamides. Nature, *223*: 206–207, 1969.

10. Gerchman, L. L. and Ludlum, D. B.   The properties of O-6 methylguanine in templates for RNA polymerase. Biochim. Biophys. Acta, *308*: 310–316, 1973.

11. Lawley, P. D. and Orr, D. J.   Specific excision of methylation products from DNA of *Escherichia coli* treated with N-methyl-N′-nitro-N-nitrosoguanidine. Chem.-Biol. Interact., *2*: 154–157, 1970.

12. Roe, F. J. C., Dipple, A., and Mitchley, B. C. V.   Carcinogenic activity of some benz[a]anthracene derivatives in newborn mice. Brit. J. Cancer, *26*: 461–465, 1972.

13. Rayman, M. P. and Dipple, A.   Structure and activity in chemical carcinogenesis. Comparison of the reactions of 7-bromomethylbenz[a]anthracene and 7-bromomethyl-12-methylbenz[a]anthracene with mouse skin DNA *in vivo*. Biochemistry, *12*: 1202–1207, 1973.

14. Rayman, M. P. and Dipple, A.   Structure and activity in chemical carcinogenesis. Comparison of the reactions of 7-bromomethylbenz[a]anthracene with 7-bromomethyl-12-methylbenz[a]anthracene with DNA *in vitro*. Biochemistry, *12*: 1538–1542, 1973.

15. Hecker, E.   Isolation and characterization of the cocarcinogenic principles from croton oil. Methods Cancer Res., *6*: 439–484, 1971.

16. Ljungquist, S. and Lindahl, T.   A mammalian endonuclease specific for apurinic sites in double stranded DNA. I. Purification and general properties. J. Biol. Chem., *249*: 1530–1535, 1974.

17. Dipple, A., Brookes, P., Mackintosh, D. D., and Rayman, M. P.   Reactions of 7-bromomethylbenz[a]anthracene with nucleic acids, polynucleotides, and nucleosides. Biochemistry, *10*: 4323–4330, 1971.

Discussion of Paper of Drs. Goldthwait et al.

DR. TANOOKA: Endonuclease II seems to have a broad spectrum for various types of chemical damage, compared with T4 endonuclease which possesses a very strict substrate specificity.

DR. GOLDTHWAIT: The T4 endonuclease differs from the bacterial endonuclease in that it can recognize dimers in single-stranded DNA. Perhaps the bacterial cell enzyme also recognizes distortion in the double helix and this type of distortion can be produced by a number of agents.

DR. SUGIMURA: Your findings on phorbol ester are extremely interesting. By the way, does phorbol ester bind with enzyme and/or 7-methyl-12-methylbenz[a]-anthracene (DMBA)-modified part of DNA? Have you ever tried the effect of caffeine on endonuclease II?

DR. GOLDTHWAIT: We have not yet done the proper kinetic experiments to determine the type of inhibition. I suspect there is a binding site on the enzyme for phorbol ester, since preincubation of the enzyme with phorbol ester gives better inhibition than preincubation of the DNA with phorbol ester. Caffeine does not inhibit the enzyme.

DR. FARBER: Dr. Goldthwait, how does the liver enzyme of Tomura and Van Lancker relate to your work in mammalian tissue?

DR. GOLDTHWAIT: We have been looking in liver, thymus and placenta for an enzyme comparable to endonuclease II. To date using the gel assay, we have not been successful in finding a methyl methanesulfonate (MMS) activity. An apurinic acid endonuclease is found in all tissues in the soluble fraction and must not be mistaken for the MMS type of activity.

DR. SUTHERLAND: W. L. Carrier reported a few years ago that he could separate enzyme activities from *Escherichia coli* towards γ- and X-irradiated DNA. Do any of the enzyme peaks from your DEAE column have activity towards X-irradiated DNA?

DR. GOLDTHWAIT: We have not tested this.

DR. TROLL: Did you try the parent alcohol phorbol as inhibitor of endonuclease II?

DR. GOLDTHWAIT: No, we have phorbol, but have not yet tested it.

DR. KONDO: Does your endonuclease II contain exonucleolytic activity?

DR. GOLDTHWAIT: No, we have been able to separate the exonuclease III activity, measured by release of inorganic phosphate, from the MMS activity. Dr. Verly, in a recent J. Biol. Chem. article has purified the apurinic acid activity to homogeneity and this preparation does not have exonucleolytic activity. Therefore, I feel exonuclease III is not an integral part of endonuclease II or the apurinic acid endonuclease. It is possible that some loose complex occurs and accounts for Weiss's results.

DR. KADA: We have isolated a similar enzyme from *Bacillus subtilis*. This enzyme increases the priming activity for DNA-polymerase 1 of γ-irradiated or MMS-treated DNA extracted from T7 but not the UV-irradiated DNA (Biochim. Biophys. Acta, *395*: 284–305, 1975). This primer-activation enzyme is an endonuclease specific to depurinated DNA. Do you know of a mutant strain deficient in your enzyme?

DR. GOLDTHWAIT: Only the *E. coli* mutants noted; I do not know of similar mutants in *B. subtilis*.

FUNDAMENTALS IN CANCER PREVENTION, P. N. MAGEE ET AL. (EDS.), UNIV. OF TOKYO PRESS, TOKYO / UNIV. PARK PRESS, BALTIMORE, PP. 363–382, 1976

Effect of DNA Repair on the Frequency of Mutations Induced in Human Cells by Ultraviolet Irradiation and by Chemical Carcinogens

Veronica M. Maher, Rodger D. Curren, Louis M. Ouellette, and J. Justin McCormick

Michigan Cancer Foundation, Detroit, Michigan, U.S.A.

Abstract: The cytotoxic effect of ultraviolet (UV) radiation and of derivatives of aromatic amide carcinogens and polycyclic hydrocarbons was compared in normally-repairing human cells and in xeroderma pigmentosum (XP) strains either deficient in excision repair or having abnormal postreplication repair by determining the % survival of the cloning ability. The lower survival of the excision-defective XP strains reflected their lower excision capacity. However, cells from XP variants, *i.e.*, patients with clinical manifestations of the disease but normal rates of excision repair of UV lesions, also showed lower survival than normal cells after exposure to these agents. These latter cells exhibit slower rates of postreplication repair of lesions in DNA caused by such carcinogenic agents.

The effect of repair on the frequency of mutations induced by UV or by such carcinogens was investigated by comparing the frequency in XP strains with that found in normal cells. The excision-defective XP strain showed a higher frequency of mutations per UV dose which was directly related to the increased cytotoxic effect of UV. The frequency of mutations per dose induced by the "K-region" epoxides of benzo(a)pyrene, 7,12-dimethylbenz(a)anthracene and dibenz(a,h)-anthracene was also found to be significantly higher in the XP cells than in normal cells and directly related to the increased cytotoxicity. At equicytotoxic doses of UV or hydrocarbons, the frequency of mutations induced in the XP strain which carries out little or no excision repair is essentially equal to that measured in the normal cells which have carried on more extensive excision repair of UV-induced lesions in DNA. These results provide evidence that the processes involved in excision repair of UV damage or "UV-like" hydrocarbon-induced damage to DNA in human cells do not themselves introduce the mutations and support the hypothesis that the cytotoxic and mutagenic effects of exposure to such agents result from lesions in DNA which cells fail to excise. Preliminary investigations with 2-(2-furyl)-3-(5-nitro-2-furyl) acrylamide (AF-2) show that this carcinogen also causes mutations in human cells and does so at a higher frequency in the XP strain than in the normal.

Cells from an XP variant, exhibiting abnormal postreplication repair, also exhibited a higher frequency of UV-induced or carcinogen-induced mutations per dose than did normal cells. Since XP variant patients, like the classical XP patients, exhibit a greatly increased susceptibility to sunlight-induced skin cancer, the fact that their cells also are subject to a higher frequency of mutations induced by UV radiation strengthens the link between mutagenicity and carcinogenicity.

One widely-studied theory to explain the heritable change which transforms normal cells of the body into tumorigenic cells whose progeny cells are all malignant is the somatic mutation hypothesis suggested in 1914 by Boveri (1). Obviously, an alteration of the DNA of a cell caused by the action of a carcinogenic agent could permanently alter the make-up of a cell and such an alteration would be passed on to the cells derived from the original one. For a long time, it was not possible to observe a good correlation between the mutagenic action of chemicals and their carcinogenicity. This is because it was not understood that the majority of chemical carcinogens require metabolic activation to change them into active forms ("ultimate carcinogens") which can react with DNA or other target macromolecules in the cell. The organisms used in standard mutagenicity tests at that time, such as, bacteria, *Neurospora*, *etc.*, were not able to carry on the necessary activation and, thus, gave negative results even with powerful carcinogens.

Pioneer work on the metabolic activation of aromatic amide carcinogens has been carried out by Drs. J. A. and E. C. Miller and their associates at the McArdle Laboratory of the University of Wisconsin (2). In collaboration with them, we investigated the mutagenicity of a series of active derivatives of aromatic amide carcinogens using an *in vitro* system involving transforming DNA isolated from *Bacillus subtilis* (3, 4). In this system, one exposes the compounds directly to highly purified DNA free of extraneous cellular material which might interfere with the chemical reaching the macromolecule target. The carcinogen-treated DNA was examined for the biological effects of the compound by returning the DNA to selected recipient strains which incorporated it into their genome and then assaying them for loss of the transforming ability of the DNA and for the frequency of mutations induced in the incorporated region by means of physically-linked genes (3). Using radioactively-labeled carcinogens, we were the first to show that the active forms of such aromatic amide carcinogens bind covalently to DNA to cause mutations with a frequency directly related to the number of carcinogen residues bound (3–5). We extended this system to demonstrate the mutagenic action of derivatives of polycyclic hydrocarbon carcinogens (6–8). In addition, by using recipient bacteria deficient in excision repair of ultraviolet (UV)-induced DNA damage (pyrimidine dimers), we demonstrated that the covalent binding of derivatives of both of these classes of carcinogens causes lesions in the DNA helix, such that the bacterial endonuclease which recognizes and initiates excision of thymine dimers also recognizes and initiates repair of these lesions. The biological transforming activity of carcinogen-treated DNA was lower in recipient strains that could not carry out excision than in normally repairing strains (3, 8).

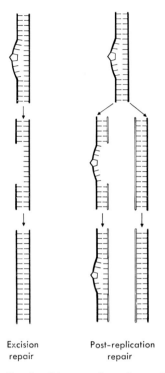

Excision   Post-replication
repair   repair

FIG. 1.   Diagram of two forms of DNA repair.

Because cancer is ultimately a human problem, we wanted to determine whether such physical and chemical carcinogenic agents would exhibit similar effects in human cells. At the time we began our investigation of the mutagenicity of carcinogens in human cells and the role of DNA repair, there already existed evidence from studies on cells from XP patients (9) that human cells possess genetically-determined UV repair capabilities similar to those found in bacteria and that such processes may play an important role in carcinogenesis. Such XP patients suffer from multiple carcinomas of the skin on areas exposed to sunlight (9, 10). Cells from the majority of such patients (classical XP) have been shown to be deficient in excision repair of pyrimidine dimers (9–14). The multiple skin carcinomas caused by exposure of the skin cells of XP patients to UV radiation could well be the result of somatic cell mutations introduced into their DNA *directly during DNA replication*, past unexcised UV lesions or by mistakes made during faulty ("*error-prone*") *excision repair* of such dimers. Alternatively, they could be introduced directly by "*error-prone*" *postreplication repair* processes or indirectly by *failure to complete this latter process*. Figure 1 diagrams these two forms of dealing with UV damage in DNA as they are presently conceived. During excision repair, the distortion in the DNA (caused by the presence of the dimer) is removed and if the opposite DNA strand which serves as the copying template is free of damage errors introduced by the repolymerizing process would not be expected. In contrast, the term postreplication repair refers to a process by which cells are able to by-pass DNA damage, such as dimers, during semi-conservative DNA replication. It has been suggested that when DNA replication occurs past an unexcised dimer, discontinuities are left in the newly-formed daughter strand. Such interruptions are apparently filled in later because the DNA is eventually restored to the size of DNA in unirradiated control cells (*15–19*). However, since the dimer which remains in the parental DNA cannot form hydrogen bonds in the normal manner, errors could be expected to occur if such DNA is used as a template.

Our present investigations into the question of a link between somatic cell mutations and the origin of human cancer, therefore, are directed toward determining *first*, whether excision-defective XP strains exhibit higher frequencies of UV-induced mutations than normally-repairing human cells; *second*, whether excision-defective XP cells exhibit a similar inability to excise damage introduced into their DNA by aromatic amide and polycyclic hydrocarbon carcinogens; *third*, whether exposure to such chemical carcinogens results in mutations in human cells and does so at higher frequencies in XP cells; and *fourth*, whether cells from the class of XP designated "variants" (*20*), which have been shown to have normal rates of excision repair of UV-induced damage (*16, 20*), but to be much slower than normal cells in their ability to convert initially low molecular weight DNA into high molecular weight DNA similar in size to that produced in unirradiated cells (*16*), will also exhibit increased mutation frequencies compared to normal human cells in culture when exposed to such DNA-damaging agents.

share some common defect in excision repair because they fail to complement that

Effect of Excision Repair on Survival Following Exposure to UV

By complementation studies, classical XP patients have recently been shown to fall into five groups, *i.e.*, the cells of patients in each separate group appear to

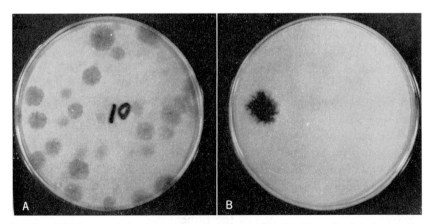

FIG. 2.   (A) Characteristic colonies of normal human skin fibroblasts developed approximately 13 days after plating 100 cells into 60-mm plastic dishes. Cells are fixed with methanol and stained with 2% methylene blue.   (B) Characteristic azaguanine-resistant colony developed *ca.* 23 days in selective azaguanine medium (2×10^{-5} M) (*cf.* Refs. *23, 24*).

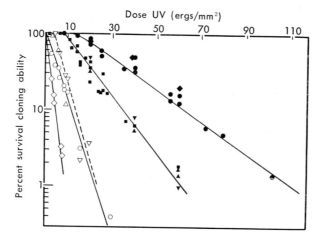

FIG. 3. Percent survival, as a function of UV dose, of the colony-forming ability of various strains of human skin fibroblasts with different capacities for DNA repair. Survival of the cloning ability of irradiated cells divided by that of unirradiated control cultures is expressed as %. Cloning efficiencies for controls ranged from 15–35% for normal cells (NF) ; 10–25% for XP 2, 4, 5, 6, and 13 ; and 5–15% for XP7TA and XP12. Exponential portion of these curves is drawn using the method of least squares. Each symbol represents the value averaged from a series of 8–12 replicate dishes of cells irradiated with the specified dose of UV. Variation in number of colonies found per point for values above 1% survival was smaller than the size of the symbol used. Cells were plated in Ham's F10 supplemented with 15% fetal bovine serum (GIBCO), allowed 10–12 hr to attach, rinsed with phosphate-buffered saline, irradiated, and incubated until macroscopic colonies developed. Cells were protected from photoreactivation for 48–72 hr after irradiation. ● NF (newborns) ; ◆ NF (15 yrs. old) ; ■ XP4BE (variant) ; ▲ XP13BE (variant) ; ▼ XP7TA (variant) ; ○ XP2BE (group C) ; ◇ XP12BE (group A) ; △ XP5BE (group D) ; ▽ XP6BE (group D).

of the other members of their group (21, 22). (The XP variant strains, with normal rates of excision repair, complement all 5 classical groups.) Representatives from the majority of these XP classes were compared with normal human cells for the % survival of their ability to form colonies following exposure to UV irradiation. (An example of the size and of the characteristics of colonies formed is shown in Fig. 2.) The % survival of these various cell strains, as a function of increasing dose of UV irradiation, is shown in Fig. 3. As can be seen, there is a shoulder on some of these survival curves which suggests efficient repair of lesions up to the indicated dose. Note that the XP variants are more sensitive to UV radiation than normal cells. A fourth variant, XP30RO, gave identical results (25). The slope of the survival curve for the XP variants is almost 2 times steeper than the curve for the normal cells. Such a result could not have been predicted since the rate of excision repair in these variants, as measured by physical techniques, appears normal (16, 20). However, the fact that these cells were taken from a patient with XP disease and that we have shown them to be clearly more sensitive to the cytotoxic action of UV than normal cells (25, 26) indicates that they are subject to some kind of defect in handling UV-induced lesions.

Classical XP12BE from group A, reported (*10*) to carry out virtually no excision of UV dimers as determined by physical techniques, is extremely sensitive to the killing effect of UV. XP2BE, a classical XP strain from complementation group C whose rate of excision is reported to be 10–20% of normal (*10*), is less sensitive than the group A strain. XP5BE and XP6BE from group D exhibit a sensitivity very similar to XP2BE, even though group D strains are reported to have a slightly higher rate of excision (25–50% of normal) (*10*). Since their biological sensitivity to UV damage is greater than one would predict from these physical studies, we are currently reinvestigating these strains. The slope of their survival curve and that of XP2BE is approximately 4- to 5-fold steeper than that of normal cells. The curve for XP12BE is 10-fold steeper. Thus, the survival of these various XP strains reflects their capacity for excision repair of UV lesions and indicates that variants cannot be perfectly normal in their handling of UV lesions.

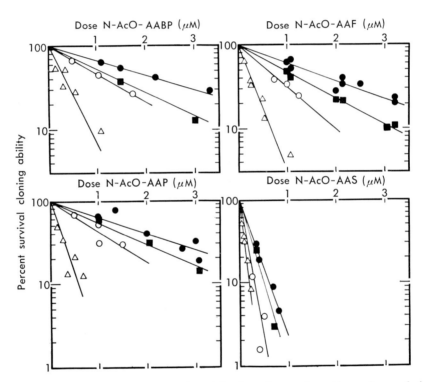

FIG. 4.   Percent survival, as a function of the dose of aromatic amide carcinogen derivative, of the colony-forming ability of four strains of human fibroblasts, each with a different capacity for DNA repair. Procedures used are similar to those given for Fig. 3 except for the following. After 12–16 hr for attachment, the culture medium was removed and the cells given serum-free Ham's F10 medium. Freshly-prepared ethanol solutions of the carcinogens were administered to the individual dishes by micropipette. After 4 hr, the exposure was terminated by removing the medium and replacing it with standard culture medium containing 15% fetal bovine serum.   (From Ref. *26*).   ● NF ; ■ XP4BE ; ○ XP2BE ; △ XP12BE.

Effect of Repair on Survival after Exposure to Carcinogens

The survival of 4 of these strains was then determined as a function of the concentration of an active derivative, the N-acetoxy ester (N-AcO-), of 4 aromatic amide carcinogens, *viz.*, 4-acetylaminobiphenyl (AABP), 2-acetylaminofluorene (AAF), 2-acetylaminophenanthrene (AAP), and 4-acetylaminostilbene (AAS) (*26*). The results are shown in Fig. 4. A similar comparative study was made (*27, 28*) of their % survival following exposure to the "K-region" epoxides of several carcinogenic hydrocarbons, such as, benzo(a)pyrene (BP), 7,12-dimethylbenz(a)anthracene (DMBA) and benz(a)anthracene (BA) with the results shown in Fig. 5. It will be noted that, in contrast to the UV survival curves, there are, apparently, no shoulders on these survival curves. This may simply reflect the fact that we have not yet completed a detailed study of survival at low doses of carcinogens. Alternatively, it may indicate that excision repair of such lesions is carried out less efficiently than repair of UV lesions or that some lesions are not repairable. For each active derivative, the ratio between the slope of the survival curve for the particular XP strain and that determined for the normal fibroblasts is similar and is approximately the same as the ratio of the slopes for the exponential portion of the corresponding UV survival curves. For example, the ratio between the survival curve for

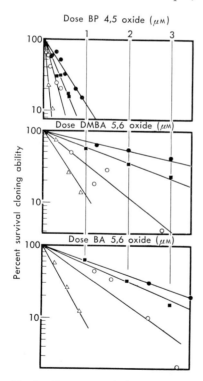

FIG. 5.   Percent survival, as a function of the dose of carcinogenic hydrocarbon epoxide, of the colony-forming ability of the four strains of human fibroblasts. Procedures followed are as outlined in the legends for Figs. 3 and 4.   (From Ref. *27*).   ● NF ; ■ XP4BE ; ○ XP2BE ; △ XP12BE.

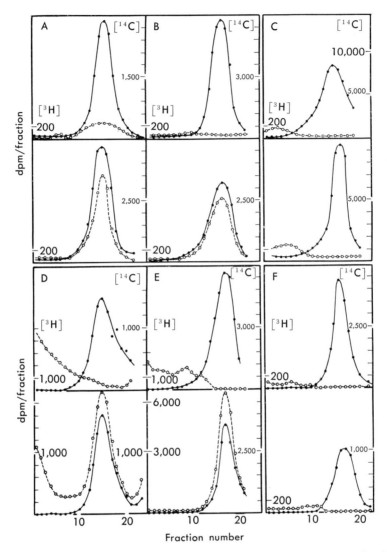

Fig. 6. Physicochemical evidence of DNA excision repair by human fibroblasts following exposure to N-AcO-AAF. The DNA was prelabeled with [^{14}C]-TdR (●) for 20 hr. Fresh serum-free medium supplemented with BrdU (10 μg/ml) was given for 1 hr to density label any replicating DNA molecules. Cells were then exposed to 0.4% ethanol (control cells—upper row) or 0.4% ethanol containing 50 μM N-AcO-AAF (lower row) for 1 hr in serum-free medium. HU was present during the last 20 min of the exposure to stop normal replication. The cells were given fresh medium containing 15% serum, HU, and BrdU and allowed 3 hr to incorporate [^{3}H]-TdR (○). The DNA was extracted and centrifuged to equilibrium in alkaline CsCl gradients, (A) normal cells, (B) reband of the major peak in (A), (C) XP2BE cells, (D) XP4BE, (E) reband of the major peak in (D), (F) XP12BE. The [^{14}C] label locates the unreplicated parental DNA strands at density 1.700 g/cm^3. Centrifugation is from right to left.   (From Ref. 26).

XP4BE and that of normal cells is 1.8 for UV, 1.2–1.7 for aromatic amide carcinogens and 1.3–1.5 for hydrocarbons. For XP2BE, the ratio is 4.0 and 1.8–2.3 for aromatic amides and 2–3 for hydrocarbons.

Physicochemical Evidence of DNA Repair

The ability of these strains to carry out excision repair of DNA following exposure to N-AcO-AAF was determined (*26*) using incorporation of tritiated thymidine ([³H]-TdR) into pre-existing parental strands of DNA as a measure of excision repair (*29, 30*). Figure 6 compares the incorporation of [³H]-TdR into pre-existing [¹⁴C]-labeled (light density) parental strand of the DNA of untreated control cells (upper row) and of cells exposed to 50 μm N-AcO-AAF for 1 hr (lower row). As can be seen, a substantial amount of incorporation of [³H]-TdR into unreplicated (light) parental strands took place when nomal (A) and XP4BE cells (D) were allowed to incubate in the presence of bromodeoxyuridine (BrdU), hydroxyurea (HU) and [³H]-TdR for several hours following attack by N-AcO-AAF. This incorporation persisted even after rebanding in a second gradient (B) and (E). Such incorporation represents DNA repair, since any DNA replication which took place in spite of the HU block would be density labeled by the BrdU. In contrast, the XP12BE and XP2BE cells did not exhibit detectible levels of incorporation during the incubation period although, given sufficient time, cells from XP2BE might have been expected to carry out at least some DNA repair (*10*).

Effect of Excision Repair on the Frequency of Mutations Induced in Human Cells by UV Light

Having found that human cells excise lesions in DNA caused by these 2 classes of carcinogens by processes similar to those used to repair UV damage, we undertook an extensive investigation of the effect of DNA repair on the *frequency of mutations* induced in human cells by such carcinogenic agents—both physical and chemical. First we compared the frequency of mutations induced by UV radiation in normal fibroblasts with that observed in an excision repair-deficient classical XP strain (*27, 31*). The genetic marker chosen for these mutagenicity studies is resistance to 8-azaguanine. The procedures and methods employed have been detailed elsewhere (*23–27, 31, 36, 37*). In summary, for each dose 1–2 × 10⁶ cells are plated into *ca.* 120 individual dishes and allowed 10–12 hr to attach. The medium is removed, the cells rinsed, irradiated, given fresh culture medium, and incubated for sufficient time to undergo at least 3 cell divisions before being exposed to selection medium containing 2×10^{-5} M azaguanine. This expression period, in which the induced mutation is fixed and the normal gene product involved in metabolizing azaguanine diluted out, is critical, varies with the dose, and must be determined empirically (*cf.* Ref. *36*). Accompanying each mutagenicity experiment is a cytotoxicity experiment to provide information on the number of viable cells surviving and a reconstruction experiment to determine the efficiency of recovery of mutants (*cf.* Refs. *23, 24*).

Figure 7 compares the frequency of mutations induced in normal cells with that

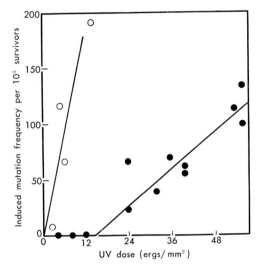

FIG. 7.   Frequency of mutations to azaguanine resistance induced in normal cells and exci-sion-defective XP cells as a function of the dose of UV radiation administered. Lines are cal-culated by the method of least squares. (From Ref. *31*). See Refs. *23* and *24* for details on the method used for quantitating.   ● NF ; ○ XP2BE.

induced in the classical XP2BE, as a function of the dose of UV. It is clear that the XP cells are much more sensitive to the mutagenic action of UV than are normal cells. The latter do not exhibit induced mutations at low doses for which their survival is 100%, whereas the XP cells show high frequencies even at very low doses. The slopes of these induced mutation curves are approximately mirror images of their respective survival curves given in Fig. 3. For example, in Fig. 3 the UV dose (in ergs/mm²) which results in a survival of 37% is *ca.* 5 for XP2BE; *ca.* 35 for NF. From Fig. 7, we see that such doses yield respectively *ca.* 90 induced mutations per 10^5 survivors in XP2BE and *ca.* 80 per 10^5 in the normal cells. For a particular survival level, the normal cells have been exposed to a higher dose and have carried out extensive excision of UV dimers. Nevertheless, they must not have introduced errors (*i.e.*, mutations) into their DNA by means of this repair process since they fail to exhibit a higher mutation frequency than the XP cells which have not been carrying on the process. When the mutation frequencies for the 2 strains are ex-amined as a function of the cytotoxic effect of the radiation (*i.e.*, as a function of the % survival) as shown in Fig. 8, they are found within experimental error to be equal. A preliminary study of the frequency of mutations induced by UV in XP-12BE, a strain which does not excise UV lesions at all (*10*), indicates that although a much lower dose of UV (2–3 ergs/mm²) is required to bring the survival down to 37%, nevertheless at that survival level, the frequency of the mutations is approxi-mately equal to that of NF and XP2BE (data not shown, *cf.* Refs. *27*, *31*). Such results provide evidence that the excision repair of UV damage to DNA is essentially an error-free process and that the cytotoxic and mutagenic effects of exposure to UV result from lesions which cells have failed to excise.

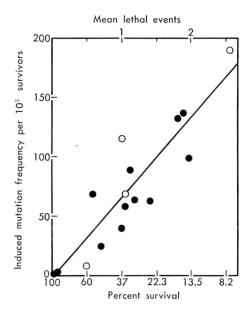

FIG. 8.   Frequency of mutations induced by UV in normal and in excision-defective XP cells as a function of the lethal effect of the UV (*i.e.*, of the % survival of the cloning ability of the cells). The data is from Figs. 3 and 7. Be the Poisson Distribution Function, if 37% of the population survives, the average number of lethal events per cell is one. A survival of 13.5% corresponds to 2 mean lethal events ; 5% survival, three mean lethal hits, *etc.*   (From Ref. *31*). ● NF ; ○ XP2BE.

Effect of Excision Repair on the Frequency of Mutations Induced in Human Cells by Chemical Carcinogens

Similar comparative studies on the induced mutation frequency were undertaken using "K-region" epoxides of carcinogenic polycyclic hydrocarbons as the DNA-damaging agent. The results were similar to those found with UV (*27, 28*). As summarized in Fig. 9, when the frequency of mutations induced in the normal cells is compared with that of XP2BE cells as a function of % survival, they are found to be essentially equal. From Fig. 4, it can be seen that, to achieve equal survival levels in the 2 strains, doses differing by a factor of 2–3 must be administered. The normal cells receive a higher dose and carry on excision repair. Nevertheless, the frequency of induced mutations in the NF at a particular survival level is not higher than in the XP2BE cells. Furthermore, the mutation frequency observed at each cytotoxic level is approximately the same for all 3 chemicals even though *ca.* 10-fold differences in doses are used to achieve equal cytotoxicity. These results support our previous conclusion that it is not the excision process which introduces mutations, but rather, the unexcised damage remaining in the DNA.

We are currently investigating the cytotoxic and mutagenic effect of 2-(2-furyl)-3-(5-nitro-2-furyl) acrylamide (AF-2) in various XP strains and in normal cells. Our preliminary findings show that this chemical is mutagenic, causes greater

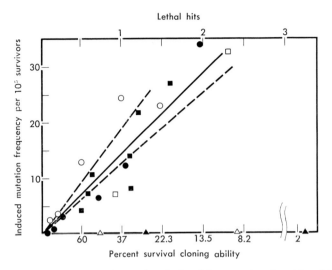

FIG. 9. Frequency of mutations induced in normal and excision-defective XP cells as a function of the lethal effect of the "K-region" epoxides of three carcinogenic hydrocarbons. (From Ref. 27). NF: ● BP-4, 5-oxide ; ■ DMBA-5, 6-oxide ; ▲ BA-5, 6-oxide. XP: ○ BP 4, 5-oxide ; □ DMBA-5, 6-oxide ; △ BA-5, 6-oxide.

cytotoxicity in the XP2BE cells than in NF, and induces a correspondingly greater frequency of mutations in the XP cells than in the normal cells.

Origin of the Mutations

Since the mutation data on human cells that we have reported here demonstrate that at least the majority of the mutations do not result from excision repair, the question arises as to what mechanism is responsible. The hypothesis which best explains our data is that, for a given survival level, approximately the same number of unexcised lesions remain in the DNA at the time of some critical event. It seems likely that DNA synthesis is this critical event and that subsequent processes used by the cells to survive unexcised lesions are ultimately responsible. In bacteria, such postreplication processes have been demonstrated to introduce mutations (*32–35*).

Frequency of Mutations Induced in XP Variants by UV Light

Since XP variant patients are as equally subject to multiple carcinomas of the skin caused by exposure to sunlight as classical XP patients, it was of great interest to determine whether cells from these patients would exhibit frequencies of UV-induced mutations higher than those observed in normal cells. If a correlation exists between carcinogenicity and mutagenicity, then such a greater susceptibility to UV-induced mutations is predicted. As can be seen in Fig. 10, XP4BE exhibits a significantly higher frequency of mutations per dose of UV than normal cells in spite of the fact that, after UV irradiation, both populations of cells possess approximately the same number of unexcised dimers in their DNA at any particular

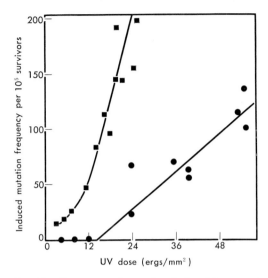

Fig. 10.   Frequency of mutations induced in normal cells and in an XP variant as a function of the dose of UV administered. (From Ref. *36*). Lines are calculated by the method of least squares. ● NF ; ■ XP4BE.

time (*16*). (We find similar increased frequencies with a hydrocarbon epoxide as the DNA-damaging agent.) Such results would be expected if the cell cycle in the variant were shorter than normal so that the interval between UV irradiation and DNA synthesis were shorter and, therefore, less time were available for excision. However, we have determined that the length of the cell cycle in the variant is not different from that of normal cells. The fact that the variant cells exhibit a much higher frequency of mutations than do normal cells suggests that one or more of their mechanisms for handling unexcised dimers is less faithful than that of normal cells (*36*).

Lehmann *et al.* (*16*) have presented evidence that cells from such variants exhibit a significantly lower than normal rate of postreplication repair, *viz.*, of converting initially low molecular weight DNA, synthesized following UV radiation, into high molecular weight DNA equal in size to that found in unirradiated cells. We find similar results with UV (*27*) and with chemical carcinogens. However, since the newly-synthesized low molecular weight DNA attains the same size as that from unirradiated cells long before the next round of DNA synthesis, it is not obvious that this difference in rate of "gap-filling" should be responsible for introducing mutations at a higher frequency than in normal cells. However, caffeine is reported by Lehmann *et al.* (*16*) to prevent gap-filling in XP variants, but not in normal human cells. If incomplete or unfaithful "gap-filling" plays a role in the production of the cytotoxic and mutagenic effects of UV radiation in these variants, one would expect to observe an increase in cytotoxicity and mutagenicity if caffeine were present during repair. We have found that, indeed, caffeine dramatically increases the cytotoxic (*25*) and mutagenic effects (*37*) of UV in XP4BE (see Fig. 11).

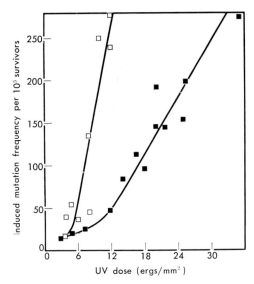

FIG. 11.   Frequency of mutations induced by UV in variant XP4BE with caffeine (0.75 mM) present or absent during the expression time. (*cf.* Ref. *37* for details).   Caffeine: ■ 0.0 mM ; □ 0.7 mM.   (From Ref. *37*).

Regardless of the explanation of the increased UV mutagenicity we observe in these cells, the fact that the cells of both classical and variant XP patients show elevated UV-induced mutation frequencies and both types of patients exhibit increased susceptibility to skin cancer strengthens the correlation between mutagenicity and carcinogenicity.

ACKNOWLEDGMENTS

The generous cooperation of Dr. Peter Sims and Dr. Philip Grover of the Chester Beatty Research Institute, Institute of Cancer Research, Royal Cancer Hospital, London, who supplied and characterized the "K-region" hydrocarbon epoxides, is gratefully acknowledged. This work was supported by U.S. Public Health Grants from the National Cancer Institute CA 13058 and CA 14680, by Research Contract NO1-CP-33226 and by an Institutional Grant to the Michigan Cancer Foundation by the United Foundation of Greater Detroit.

REFERENCES

1.   Boveri, T.   The Origin of Malignant Tumors, Williams and Wilkins Co., Baltimore, 1929.

2.   Miller, J. A. and Miller, E. C. Metabolic activation of carcinogenic aromatic amines and amides *via* N-hydroxylation and N-hydroxyesterification and its relationship to ultimate carcinogens as electrophilic reactants. *In ;* E. D. Bergmann and B. Pullman (eds.), The Jerusalem Symposia on Quantum Chemistry and Biochemistry. Physico-Chemical Mechanisms of Carcinogens, vol. I, pp. 237–261, Israel Acad. Sci. Human., Jerusalem, 1969.

3.   Maher, V. M., Miller, E. C., Miller, J. A., and Szybalski, W.   Mutations and de-

creases in density of transforming DNA produced by derivatives of the carcinogens 2-acetylaminofluorene and N-methyl-4-aminoazobenzene. Mol. Pharmacol., *4*: 411–426, 1968.

4. Maher, V. M., Miller, J. A., Miller, E. C., and Summers, W. C. Mutations and loss of transforming activity of *Bacillus subtilis* DNA after reaction with esters of carcinogenic N-hydroxy aromatic amides. Cancer Res., *30*: 1473–1480, 1970.

5. Maher, V. M. and Reuter, M. Mutations and loss of transforming activity of DNA caused by the O-glucuronide conjugate of the carcinogen N-hydroxy-2-aminofluorene. Mutat. Res., *21*: 63–71, 1973.

6. Lesko, S. A., Jr., Hoffman, H. G., Ts'o, P. O. P., and Maher, V. M. Interaction and linkage of polycyclic hydrocarbons to nucleic acids. *In;* Progress in Molecular and Subcelluar Biology, vol. 2, pp. 347–370, Springer-Verlag, Heidelberg, 1971.

7. Maher, V. M., Lesko, S. A., Jr., Straat, P. A., and T'so, P. O. P. Mutagenic action, loss of transforming activity, and inhibition of deoxyribonucleic acid template activity *in vitro* caused by chemical linkage of carcinogenic polycyclic hydrocarbons to deoxyribonucleic acid. J. Bacteriol., *108*: 202–212, 1971.

8. Maher, V. M., Douville, D., Tomura, T., and Van Lancker, J. L. Mutagenicity of reactive derivatives of carcinogenic hydrocarbons: Evidence of repair. Mutat. Res., *23*: 113–128, 1974.

9. Cleaver, J. E. Defective repair replication of DNA in xeroderma pigmentosum. Nature, *218*: 652–656, 1969.

10. Robbins, J. H., Kraemer, K. H., Lutzner, M. A., Festoff, B. W., and Coon, H. G. Xeroderma pigmentosum—An inherited disease with sun sensitivity, multiple cutaneous neoplasms, and abnormal DNA repair. Ann. Intern. Med., *80*: 221–248, 1974.

11. Cleaver, J. E. Xeroderma pigmentosum: A human disease in which an initial stage of DNA repair is defective. Proc. Natl. Acad. Sci. U.S., *63*: 428–435, 1969.

12. Cleaver, J. E. Repair processes for photochemical damage in mammalian cells. *In;* J. T. Lett, H. Adler, and M. Xelle (eds.), Advances in Radiation Biology, vol. 4, pp. 1–75, Academic Press, New York, 1974.

13. Burk, P. G., Lutzner, M. A., Clarke, D. D., and Robbins, J. H. Ultraviolet-stimulated thymidine incorporation in xeroderma pigmentosum lymphocytes. J. Lab. Clin. Med., *77*: 759–767, 1971.

14. Kleijer, W. J., de Weerd-Kastelein, E. A., Sluyter, M. L., Keijzer, W., de Wit, J., and Bootsma, D. UV-induced DNA repair synthesis in cells of patients with different forms of xeroderma pigmentosum and of heterozygotes. Mutat. Res., *20*: 417–428, 1973.

15. Lehmann, A. R. Postreplication repair of DNA in UV-irradiated mammalian cells. *In;* P. C. Hanawalt and R. B. Setlow (eds.), Molecular Mechanisms for Repair of DNA (ICN-UCLA Symposium 1974), vol. B, pp. 617–623, Plenum Press, New York, 1975.

16. Lehmann, A. R., Kirk-Bell, S., Arlett, C. F., Paterson, M. C., Lohman, P. H. M., de Weerd-Kastelein, E. A., and Bootsma, D. Xeroderma pigmentosum cells with normal levels of excision repair have a defect in DNA synthesis after UV irradiation. Proc. Natl. Acad. Sci. U.S., *72*: 219–223, 1975.

17. Buhl, S. N., Stillmann, R. M., Setlow, R. B., and Regan, J. D. DNA chain elongation and joining in normal and xeroderma pigmentosum cells after ultraviolet irradiation. Biophys. J., *12*: 1183–1191, 1972.

18. Buhl, S. N., Stillmann, R. M., Setlow, R. B., and Regan, J. D. Steps in DNA chain

elongation and joining after ultraviolet irradiation of human cells. Int. J. Radiat. Biol., *22*: 417–423, 1972.

19.   Lehmann, A. R.   Postreplication repair of DNA in mammalian cells, Life Sci., *15*: 2005–2156, 1975.

20.   Cleaver, J. E.   Xeroderma pigmentosum: Variants with normal DNA repair and normal sensitivity to ultraviolet light. J. Invest. Dermatol., *58*: 124–128, 1972.

21.   De Weerd-Kastelein, E. A., Keijzer, W., and Bootsma, D.   Genetic heterogeneity of xeroderma pigmentosum demonstrated by somatic cell hybridization. Nature New Biol., *238*: 80–83, 1972.

22.   Kraemer, K. H., Coon, H. G., Petinga, R. A., Barrett, S. F., Rahe, A. E., and Robbins, H. H.   Genetic heterogeneity in xeroderma pigmentosum. Complementation groups and their relationship to DNA repair rates. Proc. Natl. Acad. Sci. U.S., *72*: 59–63, 1975.

23.   Maher, V. M. and Wessel, J. E.   Mutations to azaguanine resistance induced in cultured diploid human fibroblasts by the carcinogen, N-acetoxy-2-acetylaminofluorene. Mutat. Res., *28*: 277–284, 1975.

24.   Albertini, R. J. and DeMars, R.   Somatic cell mutation detection and quantification of X-ray-induced mutation in cultured, diploid human fibroblasts. Mutat. Res., *18*: 199–224, 1973.

25.   Maher, V. M., Ouellette, L. M., Mittlestat, M., and McCormick J. J.   Synergistic effect of caffeine on the cytotoxicity of ultraviolet irradiation and of hydrocarbon epoxides in strains of xeroderma pigmentosum. Nature, *258*: 760–763, 1975.

26.   Maher, V. M., Birch, N., Otto, J. R., and McCormick, J. J.   Cytotoxicity of carcinogenic aromatic amides in normal and xeroderma pigmentosum fibroblasts with different DNA repair capabilities. J. Natl. Cancer Inst., *54*: 1287–1294, 1975.

27.   Maher, V. M. and McCormick, J. J.   Effect of DNA repair on the cytotoxicity and mutagenicity of UV irradiation and of chemical carcinogens in normal and xeroderma pigmentosum cells. *In;* J. M. Yuhas, R. W. Tennant, and J. B. Regan (eds.), Biology of Radiation Carcinogenesis, pp. 129–145, Raven Press, New York,1976.

28.   Maher, V. M., McCormick, J. J., Grover, P. L., and Sims, P.   Effect of DNA repair on the cytotoxicity and mutagenicity of polycyclic hydrocarbon derivatives in normal and xeroderma pigmentosum human fibroblasts. Submitted to Mutat. Res.

29.   McCormick, J. J., Marks, C., and Rusch, H. P.   DNA repair after ultraviolet irradiation in synchronous plasmodium of *Physarum polycephalum.* Biochim. Biophys. Acta, *287*: 246–255, 1972.

30.   Cleaver, J. E.   DNA repair with purines and pyrimidines in radiation—and carcinogen—damaged normal and xeroderma pigmentosum human cells. Cancer Res., *33*: 362–369, 1973.

31.   Maher, V. M., Curren, R. D., and McCormick, J. J.   Effect of DNA excision repair on the frequency of mutations induced in normal and xeroderma pigmentosum fibroblasts by ultraviolet radiation. Submitted to Proc. Natl. Acad. Sci. U.S.

32.   Rupp, W. D. and Howard-Flanders, P.   Discontinuities in an excision-defective strain of *Escherichia coli* following ultraviolet irradiation. J. Mol. Biol., *31*: 291–304, 1968.

33.   Witkin, E. M. and George, D. L. Ultraviolet mutagenesis in *pol*A and *uvr*A *pol*A derivatives of *Escherichia coli* B/r. Evidence for an inducible error-prone repair system. Genetics, *73* (Suppl.): 91–108, 1973.

34.   Kondo, S.   Evidence that mutations are induced by errors in repair and replication. Genetics, *73* (Suppl.): 109–122, 1973.

35. Kondo, S. DNA repair and evolutionary considerations. Adv. Biophys., *7*: 91–162, 1975.

36. Maher, V. M., Ouellette, L. M., Curren, R. D., and McCormick, J. J. Frequency of ultraviolet light-induced mutations is higher in xeroderma pigmentosum variant cells than in normal human cells. Nature, *261*: 593–595, 1976.

37. Maher, V. M., Ouellette, L. M., Curren, R. D,. and McCormick, J. J. Caffeine enhancement of the cytotoxic and mutagenic effects of UV-radiation in xeroderma pigmentosum variant. Biochem. Biophys. Res. Commun., *71*: 228– 234, 1976.

Discussion of Paper of Drs. Maher et al.

DR. KURODA: Human diploid cells have a limited life span. It is necessary to use cells at an early phase. What did you employ in your experiments?

DR. MAHER: We used cells from the 5th–6th up to about the 18th passage. This is because we want high cloning efficiency for our comparative studies.

DR. FARBER: Your findings are very exciting and may help us to decide ultimately what type of DNA modification may be involved in the biological effects of carcinogens in cells. Do you have any data on methylating or ethylating agents such as methyl methanesulfonate (MMS), N-methylnitrosourea (MNU), ethyl methane-sulfonate (EMS), N-ethylnitrosourea (ENU), *etc.*?

DR. MAHER: We have not studied the methylating agents yet. However, we are very interested especially in ENU because of all that is now known about the mode of action of ENU.

As for MMS or N-methyl-N'-nitro-N-nitrosoguanidine (MNNG), these compounds do not produce different survival curves for the XP cell strains compared to normal cells. That means, these compounds do not cause distortions in DNA which are similar to UV-induced distortions lesions and so will be repaired equally by both strains. We have deliberately concentrated on the carcinogens which are like UV in their action on DNA.

DR. KONDO: Does caffeine reduce the UV survival of your XP variant cells? Does caffeine affect normal cells? How about the caffeine effect on type-A XP?

DR. MAHER: We have shown that caffeine reduces the survival of XP variants after exposure to UV in a dose-dependent manner. It does not have such a syn-ergistic effect on normal cells. It has an intermediate effect on the UV survival curves of XP12BE from group A which is clearly different from its effect on normal cells but not as dramatic as in the variants (Nature, *258*: 760–763, 1975).

DR. RAJEWSKY: Dr. Maher, is it known whether a threshold amount of DNA lesions exists, below which the repair enzyme system would not be "switched on," so that very low number lesions might "sneak through" unexcised?

DR. MAHER: I cannot say for sure whether there is a UV threshold. It appears from our survival data, that as few as 1–2 ergs/mm² of UV radiation will clearly lower the survival of excision minus XP cells from group A, which probably do not excise at all. Since the normal cells have 100% survival up to 15 ergs/mm² dose, I would suggest that they begin excising as low as 1 erg. However, 1 erg/mm² causes about 6,000 dimers in the DNA of a human cell so this is not a threshold dose after all.

Clearly at the opposite end of the spectrum, too great a dose will saturate the excision repair enzyme system.

DR. BOOTSMA: Do you have any evidence of an influence of an extension of the time between treatment of the xeroderma variants and their first DNA replication on the frequency of mutations and on cell survival? By an extension of this time interval "variant" cells might have more time available for the action of the excision repair mechanism.

DR. MAHER: Yes, we have some data which bear on this point. We approached the problem by the use of synchronized cultures. If we shortened the time between the irradiation and the onset of replication in these variants, the survival of the cells was lowered. These data indicate that they did not have as much time to excise and so were forced into trying to replicate past unexcised dimers. This resulted in a greater lethal effect of the UV lesions.

DR. TANOOKA: Have you performed experiments with caffeine only?

DR. MAHER: Yes, for every caffeine experiment, we must have a control population of $1–2 \times 10^6$ cells without caffeine and a second one with caffeine alone in the absence of UV radiation. We observed a slight (2-fold) effect (contrasted with 40- to 50-fold results with UV ±caffeine) in two or three of these many experiments. However, this was not found in the other experiments so we have not considered these data a real indication of induction of mutations by 0.75 mM caffeine in human XP variant cells.

DR. TAKEBE: From your data, are you implying that "variants" are defective in excision repair to some extent? R. Day has shown, using host-cell reactivation (HCR) of UV-irradiated adenovirus, that "variants" were reduced in excision repair. Will you support it?

DR. MAHER: Yes, I am implying that there may indeed be something wrong with the excision repair process in the XP variants. Dr. McCormick and our colleagues in the Foundation are actively examining this question at this moment because we have several indications that all is not normal. Clearly from unscheduled DNA synthesis, data taken alone certainly indicate a 100% rate of excision. Also Lohmann's *et al.* (Proc. Natl. Acad. Sci. U.S., *72*: 219–223, 1975) dimer excision appears normal using endonuclease-sensitive sites as the assay. Nevertheless, the biological data indicate otherwise, and they cannot be explained simply on the basis of a slower rate of postreplication "gap-filling."

DR. WEISBURGER: In your population of cells from normal individuals, have you noted a different sensitivity in regard to age of donor?

DR. MAHER: No, we find no age dependence in our normal cells. We have tested 16-year-old persons and newborns. Others (Epstein *et al.*) have shown there is no correlation between age and excision repair capacity.

DR. FUJIWARA: You used 0.7 mM caffeine. Does such a low concentration have any effects on either postreplication repair or normal replication, especially in variant XP?

DR. MAHER: We have used 0.75 mM and 1.5 mM for mutation studies and a whole series of doses of caffeine for survival studies. They do have an effect on UV survival curves and UV-mutation frequencies. However, we have not been able to confirm Dr. Lehmann's effect of 1.5 mM (3 μg/ml) caffeine on the prevention of the eventual return of small molecular weight DNA to large molecular weight DNA after 7–8 hr. We are investigating this further.

DR. KADA: Does your system work for all the known intercalating frameshift mutagens?

DR. MAHER: I showed mutation data on UV, N-acetoxy-2-acetylaminofluorene and 3 hydrocarbon epoxides. We have no further experiments with other compounds. However, hydrocarbon epoxides have actually been shown to act as frame shifters. Please see Ames *et al.* (Science, *176*: 47–49, 1972) for mutations by BP-epoxides.

FUNDAMENTALS IN CANCER PREVENTION, P. N. MAGEE ET AL. (EDS.),
UNIV. OF TOKYO PRESS, TOKYO / UNIV. PARK PRESS, BALTIMORE, PP. 383–395, 1976

Genetic Complementation Tests of Japanese Xeroderma Pigmentosum Patients, and Their Skin Cancers and DNA Repair Characteristics

Hiraku Takebe

Department of Fundamental Radiology, Faculty of Medicine, Osaka University, Osaka, Japan

Abstract: Forty-two xeroderma pigmentosum (XP) patients in Japan were examined for their clinical characteristics and the DNA repair of their cells. Results are summarized as follows. (1) More than a half of the patients (23/42) were children under 13 years of age. (2) The youngest patients with skin cancers were 5 years old, and a total of 22 patients developed skin cancers, mostly on the face. (3) Genetic complementation tests were performed on 21 cell strains from the patients; 19 belonging to group A, 1 to D, and 1 to E. (4) There were several XP cells with nearly normal levels of unscheduled DNA synthesis, one of them was found to be a "variant." These results were considerably different from those in Europe and the United States where the frequency of patients belonging to group A was lower than in Japan. Cells having 70–100% repair replication were tested for host-cell reactivation (HCR) of UV-irradiated herpes simplex virus and all tested showed reduced HCR capacity, supporting Day's results with adenovirus.

Prevention of skin cancers in the "low-repair" group who usually develop cancers in teens might be extremely difficult. But decisive diagnosis by repair tests as early as at several months after birth followed by proper care against sun exposure could prevent the cancer development. On the other hand patients with partial repair capacities in their cells, more than 50% of normal cells, developed XP symptoms and skin cancers later than the "low-repair" group, and the malignant development could be prevented by proper care against sun exposure since most of the patients in this group should have been diagnosed as XP by repair tests far before onset of skin cancer. Based on the frequency of XP at birth in Japan, the mutation rate from normal allele to the recessive XP gene(s) is estimated to be 10^{-6}–10^{-5}.

Xeroderma pigmentosum (XP) is a rare hereditary disease attributed to autosomal recessive gene(s). The frequency of XP at birth in Japan has been estimated as approximately 1/23,000 for the children of marriages other than first cousins and 1/2,200 for the children of first cousin marriage (24). XP has been well known as a disease which will eventually develop into skin cancers in almost all cases. We surveyed clinical and DNA repair characteristics of 42 XP patients in Japan. More than a half of the patients were under 10 years of age. DNA repair tests on the cells of these young patients revealed all of them belonged to one group with no or little DNA repair activity.

At least 6 genetically different groups or types of XP's have been found in Europe and the U.S.A. (11, 12, 20, 26). We have so far found 4 of them in Japan and the relative frequencies of these groups were considerably different from those in Europe and the U.S.A. In this paper, DNA repair and genetic complementation tests on the cells of XP patients in Japan will be presented, with emphasis on some unique characteristics in comparison with XP's in other countries.

XP Patients in Japan

Table 1 summarizes DNA repair characteristics in terms of relative amount of unscheduled DNA synthesis (UDS) after UV irradiation of the cells derived from XP patients, and the clinical information on the patients. More than a half of the patients belonged to a group which showed no or very little UDS, less than 5% of normal level (will be referred to as "low-repair" group in the following sections). As expected, consanguineous marriages in parents or grandparents of the patients were involved in approximately a half of the patients. Incidence of first cousin marriage among parents of XP patients in Japan has been estimated as 0.40 based on Kawakami's data on 382 cases in 252 sibships (23). Of 37 sibships in Table 1, 11 were the outcome of first cousin marriage, 7 were the outcome of consanguineous marriage of a degree other than first cousin, 1 was the result of consanguineous marriage the degree of which was not stated, in 14 sibships the parents were not consanguineous, and no information was available for 3 cases. Although the number of sibships in this study may be too small to make an accurate estimate, 11 first cousin marriages in 37 cases were fewer than expected. Detailed information on these patients has been and will be published elsewhere (1, 32).

TABLE 1. Clinical Characteristics and DNA Repair of XP Patients in Japan

UDS after UV (% of normal)	Number of patients	Consanguineous marriage (parents and grand-parents of sibships)			Skin cancer		Mental retardation (other neurological abnormalities)		
		Yes	No	Unknown	Yes	No	Yes	No	Unknown
<5	25	8	10	4	9	16	12 (7)	0	13
5–10	1	1	0	0	1	0	0	1	0
25–50	7	5	1	0	7	0	2	5	0
70<	9	5	3	0	5	4	0	7	2
Total	42	19	14	4	22	20	14 (7)	13	15

Skin cancers

Skin cancers were found in more than a half of the patients. Since most of

TABLE 2. Age Distribution and DNA Repair of XP Patients in Japan

UDS after UV (% of normal)	Number of patients	Ages				
		0–9	10–19	20–29	30–39	40<
<5	25 (9)	19 (3)	5 (5)	1 (1)	0	0
5–10	1 (1)	0	1 (1)	0	0	0
25–50	7 (7)	0	1 (1)	2 (2)	2 (2)	2 (2)
70≦	9 (5)	0	1	3 (2)	2 (1)	3 (2)
Total	42 (22)	19 (3)	8 (7)	6 (5)	4 (3)	5 (4)

Numbers in parenthesis are number of patients with skin cancer.

the patients without cancers were children under 10 years, as shown in Table 2, the frequency of patients without cancers during their lifetime should be very small. There were 4 older patients without cancers, all of whom belonged to a group with nearly normal levels of UDS. All patients in the "low-repair" group may develop skin cancers by the age of around 12, since all of 6 patients at 12 years or older in that group had skin cancers. The youngest patients with skin cancers were 5 years old and the oldest was 78. Out of 13 patients with cancers having partial or nearly normal levels of UDS activities in their cells, 5 patients were known to have had the onset of the cancers around the age of 20. If XP patients survive without developing skin cancers until they are over 20 years old, the chance of later development of skin cancer would be small.

Neurological abnormalities

Mental retardation and other neurological abnormalities such as walking difficulties due to Achilles-tendon shortening and hearing difficulties have been known often to accompany XP (26). All of the XP patients over 5 years of age belonging to the "low-repair" group showed some degree of mental retardation. Younger patients, 5 years old or younger, in the same group were difficult to evaluate mentally, and, therefore, were listed as unknown for the mental retardation in Table 1. No mental information was available for 2 "unknown" patients in high UDS group.

Neurological abnormalities other than mental retardation (typical characteristics of de Sanctis-Cacchione syndrome) were found in 7 patients, all of whom belonged to the "low-repair" group as indicated in parenthesis in Table 1. Since these abnormalities have been described to appear at the age of around 10 (26), other young patients in the "low-repair" group may develop these abnormalities later.

Ages of XP patients

Ages of XP patients when they were examined for repair may not reflect the time of onset or degree of symptoms, and also may depend on the medical systems in different countries. Considerable difference, however, was noted between the age distribution of XP patients in Japan and that in Europe and the U.S.A. Most of the patients in Japan were recorded at the first visit to the dermatology clinics

TABLE 3.   Age Distribution and DNA Repair of XP Patients in Europe and the U.S.A.

UDS after UV (% of normal)	Number of patients	Ages				
		0–9	10–19	20–29	30–39	40<
<7	16	11	1	3	1	0
10–25	16	2	7	5	0	2
25–50	6	0	3	3	0	0
50–75	3	0	0	1	1	1
80≦	5	0	0	2	2	1
Total	46	13	11	14	4	4

Compiled from literatures. For detailed information, see Ref *32*.

of university hospitals. Since pediatricians in Japan usually receive patients predominantly with diseases of internal medicine, and were not involved in this survey except for a few cases, we assume the ages of the patients were not selected for younger ages.

The age distribution of XP patients in Europe and the U.S.A. compiled from the literature are shown in Table 3 for the purpose of comparison with Table 2. Although the classification of the levels of UDS is slightly different, there were fewer apparent "low-repair" patients and more older patients than their counterparts in Japan. Since the information concerning skin cancers was not available in many cases, it is not listed in Table 3. An extensive survey of skin cancers at the first visit to dermatology clinics of 41 university hospitals in Japan has been performed by Miyaji (*22*), including 158 cases of XP. The age distribution in Table 1 quite resembled that in Miyaji's survey, in which approximately a half (80/158) of the patients were under 10 years old. Another survey of 46 XP patients by El-Hefnawi and Smith (*13*) in Egypt may be regarded as in-between Europe-U.S.A. and Japan, with the age distribution of 0–9, 15 patients; 10–19, 19 patients; 20–29, 8 patients; 30–38, 4 patients, and no patients over 38. Unfortunately no repair data have been available for those patients. Factors other than DNA repair, such as UV fluence over the regions where patients lived, may also influence the age distribution.

Genetic Complementation Groups of XP in Japan

Results of genetic complementation tests are summarized in Table 4, in comparison with those in Europe and the U.S.A. (*7*). "Suspects" are those not tested for complementation groups. They were assigned to each group depending on the amount of UDS relative to the normal level: A, less than 2%; C, 10–25%, without neurological abnormalities; D, 25–55%; E, 50–60% and "variants," more than 80%. There were several cases which could be assigned to either of 2 neighboring groups, such as the one having UDS of 50%, which are listed in-between 2 columns. Since the only group E cells so far identified in Japan, XP5SE, had UDS of 70% and it is often difficult to determine small differences, all cell lines having UDS of 80% or more were listed as "suspects" in-between group E and the "variants"

TABLE 4.   Genetic Groups of XP Patients in Japan

Area	Complementation groups						"Variants"	Total
	A	B	C	D	E			
Japan	19	0	0	1	1		1	22
(Suspects)	(6)		(1)	(3)	(3)	(7)		(20)
Eastern	5	0	0	1	1		0	7
(Suspects)	(2)			(3)	(2)	(5)		(12)
Western	14	0	0	0	0		1	15
(Suspects)	(4)		(1)		(1)	(2)		(8)
Europe and the U.S.A.	9	1	12	3	2		4	31

Eastern and western areas of Japan were divided by a line between Tokyo and Nagoya.

except for one sure "variant," XP5OS, which was found to have low postreplication repair activity (Fujiwara, personal communication) by the method similar to that used by Lehmann et al. (21). Three distinct points were noted: there were many As, no Cs except 1 "suspect," and different group spectra between eastern and western Japan. The high incidence of patients belonging to group A may account for the high ratio of young XP patients in Japan. Apparently, repair deficiency and the clinical development is closely related, as suggested by Bootsma et al. (3), at least in group A patients. All of 19 patients in 0–9 age group (Table 2) belonged to group A (including 3 "suspects"). All of 7 patients with combined neurological abnormalities (de Sanctis-Cacchione syndrome) were identified to belong to group A, as expected from the original definition of the group (11).

Lack of patients belonging to group C, which is the most frequent in Europe and the U.S.A., is surprising. The gene distribution may differ among races, as is known for ABO blood groups. The difference between eastern and western halves of Japan could be due to the small number of patients examined, although many dermatologists agreed with our data as a possible explanation for why they had observed more moderate cases in northeastern Japan, like Sendai, than in western areas, like Osaka. Another possible cause of such difference in clinical observation in 2 areas is the difference in the influence of ultraviolet light from the sun, which is responsible for the development of XP symptoms (2).

DNA Repair in Normal and XP Cells

Unscheduled DNA synthesis

Since the discovery of DNA repair deficiency in XP (4), measurement by autoradiography of UDS after UV irradiation has been widely used as an indication of DNA repair levels. As shown in Tables 1 and 2, UDS may be used as a reliable source for both diagnosis and prognosis of the patients, especially when UDS is found to be none or low. On the other hand, for the cases having UDS of more than 50% or nearly normal level, decisive diagnosis should depend on additional repair tests.

Colony-forming ability

For colony formation in unestablished cell lines such as XP cells, low plating efficiency may affect the reliability and reproducibility of the data to a considerable extent. Such a disadvantage, however, was overcome when the difference of sensitivity between two cell lines was large (*29*), or by enhancing the plating efficiency with the use of transformed cells (*30*). An XP cell line with a normal level of UDS, XP3KO, has been shown to have UV sensitivity higher than normal but lower than group A cells for colony formation (*14*). A "variant" cell line, XP5SO, was found to have the same UV sensitivity as normal cells (Tanaka, personal communication), as reported by Cleaver previously (*5*). Since colony-forming ability has been regarded as one of the most important characteristics of DNA repair in microorganisms, the usefulness of it in comparing the DNA repair of XP cells should be reevaluated despite its technical difficulty.

Host-cell reactivation (HCR) of UV-inactivated virus

Figure 1 shows the survival curves of herpes simplex virus type I after UV irradiation, assayed for plaque-forming units by normal and various XP cells (*31*). The levels of UDS and the complementation groups, if known, of the cells are shown in Table 5, with the D_0 values of initial parts of the curves. D_0 values of 5 other XP cell lines derived from American patients are also shown in Table 5. The difference in D_0 values, or difference in HCR ability should reflect the DNA repair activity of the excision-resynthesis type as in the case with bacteria. XP cell lines may be classified into two groups depending on HCR. One group consists

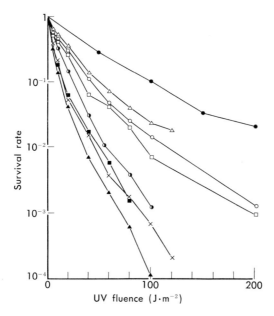

FIG. 1.   Survival curves for UV-irradiated herpes simplex virus in normal and XP cells. ● normal ; △ 10SE ; ○ 13OS ; □ 3KO ; ◖ 1160 ; × 15OS ; ■ 9OS ; ▲ 2OS. KO, Kobe; OS, Osaka; SE, Sendai.

TABLE 5. D_0 Values of UV-survival Curves of Herpes Simplex Virus in Fig. 1

Cell lines	Compl. groups	UDS (%)	D_0 (J/m²)
Normal		100	38
XP10SE		100	18
XP13OS		80	13
XP3KO		100	12
1160	D	25–55	7.5
XP9OS	A	<2	5.5
XP15OS		<2	5
1166	C	15–25	
1170	C	15–25	
1199	B	3–7	4–6
1200	D	25–55	
1223	A	<2	
XP2OS	A	<2	4

Description of Japanese XP cell lines were after proposal by Cleaver *et al.* (*6*).

of cell lines having D_0 values less than 8 J/m², with second components or lower halves of the curves with D_0's of around 10 J/m². XP cells belonging to complementation groups of A, B, C, and D were all in this group. The second group has D_0 values of 12 to 18 J/m², with second components of around 25 J/m². All of 3 cell lines so far tested in the second group have UDS of nearly normal level. Since the difference between the cells belonging to the second group and normal cells is very clear, we believe HCR should be the most reliable method to determine XP. These results generally agree with those reported by Day (*8–10*) using adenovirus.

Excision of pyrimidine dimers from DNA after UV irradiation and chemical DNA damage

Measurement of excision of pyrimidine dimers from DNA after UV irradiation is a direct proof of excision-resynthesis type of repair. In Fig. 2, 3 XP cell lines with partial or nearly normal levels of UDS are compared for the excision of thymine dimers after UV irradiation. Previously XP2OS, a group A cell line, had

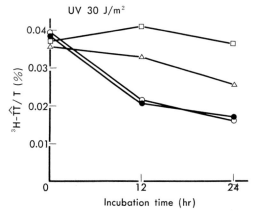

FIG. 2. Changes of thymine dimers in different cells in acid insoluble fraction of UV-irradiated cells during post-UV incubation. □ 1160(D) ; △ XP13OS ; ○ XP3KO ; ● normal.

been shown to lack excision completely (*30*). Line 1160, a group D from an American patient, may also lack excision of the dimers, while 2 other lines, XP13OS with 80% UDS and XP3KO with a normal level of UDS, showed some or normal levels of excision. Although the accuracy of the measurement may not be sufficient to tell the exact differences in excision, the idea that group D cells may have no or very little excision of the dimers may be supported by the levels of HCR similar to group A cells, as shown in Table 5, and by the fact that another group D cell line, 1200 (also in Table 5), showed no excision by similar experiments (Takebe, unpublished). These data, along with results with HCR, suggest that the presence of partial UDS may not necessarily mean partial existence of excision repair. To identify levels of excision repair, however, measurement of HCR activity should be far more dependable than the measurement of dimer excision.

Ikenaga *et al.* (*16*) have found that a similar type of excision of DNA damage caused by a carcinogen, 4-nitroquinoline 1-oxide (4NQO), was present in normal human cells but not present in XP2OS(SV) cells, a SV40-transformed subline of group A cell line. These results at the molecular level support the finding by Takebe *et al.* (*29*) that colony-forming ability of XP cells (XP1OS), a group A "suspect" was more sensitive to 4NQO than normal cells. A similar relationship between 4NQO sensitivity of colony-forming ability and mutation induction (*19*), and excision of 4NQO damage has been reported by Kondo and Kato (*18*), and Ikenaga *et al.* (*15*) in *Escherichia coli*. Such similarity between *E. coli uvrA*⁻ and human XP has been proposed as another indication of common mechanisms of the excision-resynthesis type of DNA repair between *E. coli* and human cells (*16, 29*). Different levels of photoreactivating enzyme activity in different groups of XP (*27, 28*) could play another important role, provided it functions in human skin.

DNA repair tests and prevention of skin cancer for XP patients

Patients with no or little UDS capacity after UV exposure of their cells develop XP symptoms and skin cancers early in their life, and the prevention of skin cancers should be extremely difficult. We have, however, one case, XP8OS belonging to group A, who was diagnosed as XP at 5 months old and has been kept indoors since then, for more than 2 years. The XP symptoms on the skin have been very light and there is little sign of worsening skin lesions (see Photos). Although we do not know whether neurological abnormalities may also be prevented, we certainly have hope of preventing skin cancer and will continue the observation throughout her life. Another possible way to reduce the number of "low-repair" patients is prenatal diagnosis followed by abortion of the homozygous embryo. The first successful case on XP has been reported recently (*25*). Since the screening of "low-repair" patients should be possible when they are less than 2 years old, as far as Japanese patients are concerned, the chance of preventing a second XP patient in the same sibship by prenatal diagnosis may be very good.

For the patients with partial or nearly normal DNA repair activity in their cells, it is important to have decisive diagnosis as early as possible. For that purpose, measurement of UDS followed by HCR tests should give dermatologists, noticing subtle skin lesions, decisive data before such lesions can be identified by further clinical observations only, and, in many cases, plenty of time before the possible onset of skin cancers so that necessary treatment and care can be taken in advance to prevent cancer.

Mutation Rate of XP Gene(s)

If we assume that "low-repair" patients will not have children but others will reproduce normally, and that the frequency of XP has not been changing for generations, we may estimate the mutation rate of new XP gene(s) from the normal allele according to Komai's formula (17), $u \simeq sfq$, where u is the mutation rate, s is the adaptability of the mutant gene, f is the coefficient of inbreeding in the population, and q is a frequency of the recessive gene. The maximum estimate may be obtained as $u \simeq 10^{-5}$ based on $s=0.0032$ (according to Komai) and $q=0.007$. This is a comparable value to some of the rather frequent genetic diseases of auto-somal recessive type. True values of s and f might be much lower and the mutation rate may be between 10^{-6} and 10^{-5}.

ACKNOWLEDGMENTS

The author thanks the coauthors of reference 32, in which most of the data referred to in this paper were presented. This work was supported in part by a Grant-in-Aid for Cancer Research from the Ministry of Education, Science and Culture, Japan, and by the Subsidy for Cancer Research from the Ministry of Health, Japan.

REFERENCES

1. Akiba, H., Kato, T., Nakano, H., and Seiji, M.   Defective DNA repair replication in xeroderma pigmentosum fibroblasts and DNA repair of somatic cell hybrids after UV irradiation. Tohoku J. Exp. Med., *117*: 1–14, 1975.
2. Blum, H. F.   Carcinogenesis by Ultraviolet Light. Princeton University Press, Princeton, New Jersey, 1959.
3. Bootsma, D., Mulder, M. P., Pot, F., and Cohen, J. A.   Different inherited levels of DNA repair replication in xeroderma pigmentosum cell strains after exposure to ultraviolet irradiation. Mutat. Res., *9*: 507–516, 1970.
4. Cleaver, J. E.   Defective repair replication of DNA in xeroderma pigmentosum. Nature, *218*: 652–656, 1968.
5. Cleaver, J. E.   Xeroderma pigmentosum: Variants with normal DNA repair and normal sensitivity to ultraviolet light. J. Invest. Dermatol., *58*: 124–128, 1972.
6. Cleaver, J. E., Bootsma, D., and Friedlberg, E.   Human diseases with genetically altered DNA repair processes. Genetics, *79* (Suppl.): 215–225, 1975.
7. Cleaver, J. E. and Bootsma, D.   Xeroderma pigmentosum—Biochemical and genetic characteristics. Annu. Rev. Genet., *9*: 19–38, 1975.
8. Day, R. S., III.   Cellular reactivation of ultraviolet-irradiated human adenovirus 2 in normal and xeroderma pigmentosum fibroblasts. Photochem. Photobiol., *19*: 9–13, 1974.
9. Day, R. S., III.   Studies on repair of adenovirus 2 by human fibroblasts using normal, xeroderma pigmentosum, and xeroderma pigmentosum heterozygous strains. Cancer Res., *34*: 1965–1970, 1974.

10. Day, R. S., III. Xeroderma pigmentosum variants have decreased repair of ultra-violet-damaged DNA. Nature, *253*: 748–749, 1975.

11. De Weerd-Kastelein, E. A., Keijzer, W., and Bootsma, D. Genetic heterogeneity of xeroderma pigmentosum demonstrated by somatic cell hybridization. Nature New Biol., *238*: 80–83, 1972.

12. De Weerd-Kastelein, E. A., Keijzer, W., and Bootsma, D. A third complementation group in xeroderma pigmentosum. Mutat. Res., *22*: 87–91, 1974.

13. El-Hefnawi, H. and Smith S. M. Xeroderma pigmentosum. A brief report on its genetic linkage with ABO blood groups in the United Arab Republic. Brit. J. Dermatol., *77*: 35–41, 1965.

14. Fujiwara, Y., Tatsumi, M., Ichihashi, M., Higashikawa, T., Takebe, H., and Tanaka, K. DNA mechanisms repair in mammalian cells. XII. Replicative repair in human cells and its abnormality in variant xeroderma pigmentosum. J. Radiat. Res., *17*: 30, 1976 (Abstr.).

15. Ikenaga, M., Ichikawa-Ryo, H., and Kondo, S. The major cause of inactivation and mutation by 4-nitroquinoline 1-oxide in *Escherichia coli*: Excisable 4NQO-purine adducts. J. Mol. Biol., *92*: 341–356, 1975.

16. Ikenaga, M., Ishii, Y., Tada, M., Kakunaga, T., Takebe, H., and Kondo, S. Excision repair of 4-nitroquinoline-1-oxide damage responsible for killing, mutation and cancer. *In;* P. C. Hanawalt and R. B. Setlow (eds.), Molecular Mechanisms for the Repair of DNA, pp. 763–771, Plenum Press, New York, 1975.

17. Komai, T. Human Genetics. Baifukan, Tokyo, 1966 (in Japanese).

18. Kondo, S. and Kato, T. Photoreactivation of mutation and killing in *Escherichia coli*. Adv. Biol. Med. Phys., *12*: 283–298, 1968.

19. Kondo, S., Ichikawa, H., Iwo, K., and Kato, T. Base-change mutagenesis and prophage induction in strains of *Escherichia coli* with different DNA repair capacities. Genetics, *66*: 187–217, 1970.

20. Kraemer, K. H., Coon, H. G., Petinga, R. A., Barrett, S. F., Rahe, A. E., and Robbins, J H. Genetic heterogenecity in xeroderma pigmentosum: Complementation groups and their relationship to DNA repair rates. Proc. Natl. Acad. Sci. U. S., *72*: 59–63, 1975.

21. Lehmann, A. R., Kirk-Bell, S., Arlett, C. F., Paterson, M. C., Lohman, P. H., de Weerd-Kastelein, E. A., and Bootsma, D. Xeroderma pigmentosum cells with normal levels of excision repair have a defect in DNA synthesis after UV-irradiation. Proc. Natl. Acad. Sci. U.S., *72*: 219–223, 1975.

22. Miyaji, T. Skin cancers in Japan: A nationwide 5-year survey, 1956–1960. Natl. Cancer Inst. Monogr., *10*: 55–70, 1962.

23. Neel, J. V., Kodani, M., Brewer, R., and Anderson, R. C. The incidence of consanguineous matings in Japan with remarks on the estimation of comparative gene frequencies and the expected rate of appearance of induced recessive mutations. Am. J. Hum. Genet., *1*: 156–178, 1949.

24. Ohkura, K. Human Society and Genetics, Sekai Hoken Tsushinsha, Osaka, 1975 (in Japanese).

25. Ramsey, C. A., Coltart, T. M., Blunt, S., Pawsey, S. A., and Giannelli, F. Prenatal diagnosis of xeroderma pigmentosum. Report of the first successful case. Lancet, *ii*: 1109–1112, 1975.

26. Robbins, J. H., Kraemer, K. H., Lutzner, M. A., Festoff, B. W., and Coon, H. G.

Xeroderma pigmentosum. An inherited disease with sun sensitivity, multiple cutaneous neoplasmas, and abnormal DNA repair. Ann. Intern. Med., *80*: 221–248, 1974.

27. Sutherland, B. M., Rice, M., and Wagner, E. K.   Xeroderma pigmentosum cells contain low levels of photoreactivating enzyme. Proc. Natl. Acad. Sci. U.S., *72*: 103–107, 1975.

28. Sutherland, B. M. and Oliver, R.   Low levels of photoreactivating enzymes in xeroderma pigmentosum variants. Nature, *257*: 132–134, 1975.

29. Takebe, H., Furuyama, J., Miki, Y., and Kondo, S.   High sensitivity of xeroderma pigmentosum cells to the carcinogen 4-nitroquinoline-1-oxide. Mutat. Res., *15*: 98–100, 1972.

30. Takebe, H., Nii, S., Ishii, M. I., and Utsumi, H.   Comparative studies of host-cell reactivation, colony forming ability and excision repair after UV irradiation of xeroderma pigmentosum, normal human and some other mammalian cells. Mutat. Res., *25*: 383–390, 1974.

31. Takebe, H.   Decreased host-cell reactivation of UV irradiated herpes simplex virus and lack of excision repair in xeroderma pigmentosum cells belonging to different genetic groups. Unpublished.

32. Takebe, H., Miki, Y., Kozuka, T., Furuyama, J., Tanaka, K., Sasaki, M. S., Fujiwara, Y., and Akiba, H.   DNA repair characteristics and skin cancer in xeroderma pigmentosum patients in Japan. Cancer Res., unpublished.

EXPLANATION OF PHOTOS

PHOTO 1-A.   XP4OS, 2 years old.

PHOTO 1-B.   XP4OS, taken 2.5 years after 1-A. Note extensive development of skin lesions since the patient did not receive proper care.

PHOTO 2-A.   XP8OS, 5 months old, she spent a few hours outdoors for the first time since she was born.

PHOTO 2-B.   XP8OS, 1 month after 2-A. Skin changes were almost completely recovered after keeping her indoors for 1 month.

PHOTO 2-C.   XP8OS, 2 years after 2-B.   She has been kept indoors all the time. To protect the skin of her face from sun light, "cover mark" (UV-absorbing cosmetic) was applied topically.

PHOTO 2-D.   XP8OS, she stayed outdoors for 40 min on a June day, for the first time in 2 years since 2-A. Note high sensitivity of her skin for the erythema due to such short exposure to sun light.

Both patients in these photographs were identified to belong to the complementation group A. Photographs are by courtesy of Drs. T. Kozuka (1-A), M. Shimasaki (1-B), and A. Nishioka (2-A, B, C, and D).

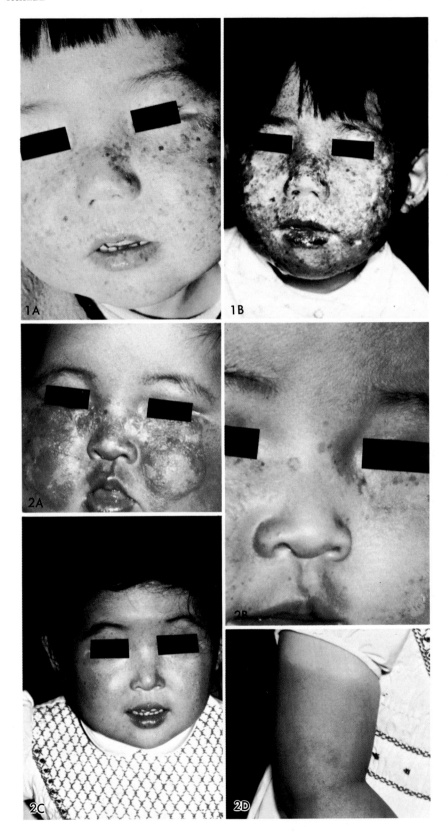

Discussion of Paper of Dr. Takebe

Dr. Bootsma: 1.   I am very excited by the fact that you have found a second case in the complementation group E. a) Did you find normal levels of DNA repair in the case you got complementation? b) Have you identified the hybrid character of the binuclear cells? c) Did you apply the herpes simplex repair system on these E group cells?

2.   I am intrigued by the finding that addition of a UV-endonuclease from bacteriophage T4 to Sendai virus-treated XP cells restores the genetic defects of the cells. Do you have any information about the mode of uptake of the enzyme, in which degradation of the enzyme is prevented? Can you inform us about the duration of the restoration of the enzyme activity after addition of the bacteriophage enzyme?

Dr. Takebe: 1.   a) Yes, in this particular case, the levels of the binuclear cells were clearly at normal levels. b) The group E cells, XP5SE, had an unscheduled DNA synthesis level of 70% of normal. Therefore, it was very difficult to distinguish them. The average number of grains per nucleus was approximately 100 for normal level so that the level of 70% was clearly distinguishable. c) No, we have not. It is now in progress using both XP2RO and XP5SE.

2.   The work has been done by Tanaka *et al.* (K. Tanaka, M. Sekiguchi, and Y. Okada, Proc. Natl. Acad. Sci. U.S., *72*: 4071–4075, 1975).

FUNDAMENTALS IN CANCER PREVENTION, P. N. MAGEE ET AL. (EDS.),
UNIV. OF TOKYO PRESS, TOKYO / UNIV. PARK PRESS, BALTIMORE, PP. 397–408, 1976

Genetic Aspects of DNA Repair Mechanisms in Mammalian Cells

D. Bootsma

Department of Cell Biology and Genetics, Erasmus University, Rotterdam, The Netherlands

Abstract: Progress in the field of somatic cell genetics has stimulated the genetic analysis of inherited disorders in man. The isolation and cultivation of cell strains from patients suffering from a genetic disease has provided suitable mutant cells grown *in vitro*, whereas cell fusion techniques enabled the formation of recombinant genomes which could be used for complementation analysis as well as localization of genes on chromosomes. The application of these techniques in the study of DNA repair in mammalian cells has been hampered because of the paucity of information dealing with the enzymology of DNA repair in these eukaryotic organisms. DNA repair mutants could be obtained from patients suffering from the genetic skin disease xeroderma pigmentosum. Cell fusion techniques have indicated that in this syndrome at least 5 different mutations, all affecting an excision repair mechanism, are present. Evidence is presented that also in the genetic disorders ataxia telangiectasia and Cockayne's syndrome a defect in DNA repair mechanisms is the cause of the disease.

For the localization of genes interspecific cell hybrids are required in which one can differentiate between the homologous gene products of the parental cells. Evidence is presented that these differences can be observed in chick-human hybrid cells even in terms of DNA repair. The relevance of these observations regarding the localization of genes involved in DNA repair will be discussed.

The isolation of mutants being defective in the repair of damaged DNA in microbial systems and the genetic analysis of these mutants have made an important contribution to the elucidation of the mechanisms of DNA repair in these prokaryotic organisms. By the use of *in vitro* cultivated eukaryotic cells comparable approaches became available for the study of the genetic basis of DNA repair mechanisms in mammalian cells including those of man. The techniques have been developed in the last 10 years in the field of somatic cell genetics and mainly concern the formation of new combinations of genomes by means of cell fusion.

Cultures of skin fibroblasts obtained from patients suffering from a genetic disease have in many cases provided mutant cell strains that could be used in these somatic cell genetic studies. In this presentation I will briefly discuss several aspects of these investigations concerning the repair of damaged DNA in human cells. In these studies a relationship between defective DNA repair and carcinogenesis became apparent, mainly as a result of the study of the genetic skin disease xeroderma pigmentosum (XP).

Isolation of DNA Repair Mutants

The best-known class of DNA repair mutants in man has been derived from patients having the genetic skin disease XP. These patients suffer from an intolerance of the skin and eyes to sunlight: abnormal pigmentation with freckling, actinic hyperkeratosis and skin malignancies. Some of these patients show neurological abnormalities in addition to the skin lesions. In 1968 Cleaver detected decreased levels of DNA repair replication and unscheduled DNA synthesis (UDS) in cultivated cells of these patients following exposure to ultraviolet light (UVL) (1). Cleaver (2) and others have shown that these cells are highly UVL-sensitive in terms of cell survival. Moreover, these cells were also deficient in the repair of UVL-exposed viruses (3–7).

Recently Sutherland et al. (8) presented evidence for an impaired photo-reactivation system in XP patients.

In addition to these patients, apparently having a defect in excision repair as well as in photoreactivation, another group of XP patients has been discovered having normal levels of excision repair in their cells. Lehmann et al. (9) has presented evidence that in cells of these XP variants a postreplication repair mechanism is impaired.

Several other genetic diseases have been suggested as being the result of a DNA repair defect. Two of these syndromes will be discussed here: Cockayne's syndrome and ataxia telangiectasia (AT) (Louis-Bar syndrome).

At the annual meeting of the American Society of Human Genetics at Baltimore, October 1975, Chu (10) presented his data indicating a DNA repair defect in cells from two patients with Cockayne's syndrome. This syndrome is an autosomal recessive disease. Amongst the clinical symptoms are dwarfism, prematurely aged appearance, mental retardation, microcephaly and skin hypersensitivity to sunlight. These patients normally do not have a predisposition for skin cancer.

Chu studied cells from two patients and found lower survival following UVL exposure and decreased levels of repair DNA synthesis. A correlation seems to exist between the residual level of UDS (varying from 30% to subnormal levels) and the severity of the symptoms. These data are preliminary and need further confirmation. However, another interesting case of Cockayne's syndrome should be mentioned in this respect. This patient has been described by Robbins et al. (11). The patient is a woman suffering from XP as well as Cockayne's syndrome (XP11BE, complementation group B). Instead of suffering from two independent mutations, which seems very unlikely, this patient might represent a variant form of Cockayne's syndrome having skin tumors in addition to the other characteristic symptoms of Cockayne's syndrome.

The third syndrome that I will mention in this context is AT. AT patients show telangiectasia of the conjunctiva and skin and cerebellar ataxia. Sinopulmonary infections, immunologic deficiencies, mental deficiency, progressive neurologic deterioration, and a predisposition to malignancies are also features of this syndrome. It is an autosomal recessive disorder. The areas with the greatest exposure to the sun are the most affected. An enhanced level of spontaneous chromosome aberrations (12), increased sensitivity to X-rays after radiotherapy (see Ref. 13) and increased chromosome aberrations induced by ionizing radiation in leucocyte cultures (14) have also been reported. Very recently Taylor et al. (15) found a low survival following exposure to gamma rays of cells from 8 different ataxia patients. Moreover, Paterson et al. (16) presented evidence that AT cells are deficient in excision repair of gamma ray-induced base lesions in their DNA.

Several other disorders have been added to the list of genetic diseases in which defective DNA repair might play a role. In 1973 Epstein et al. (17) claimed a defect in the rejoining of X-ray induced single-strand breaks in the DNA of cells from progeria patients. Enzyme studies (18) and immunological investigations (18, 19) of cells from patients suffering from these syndromes with accelerated ageing have indicated that during growth of the cells in culture changes in enzyme activity and HL-A expression occurs. These observations and the reported influence of culture conditions on progeria's DNA rejoining kinetics (20, 21) indicate that the repair phenomenon is not the primary genetic defect in these progeric disorders.

Recently Sasaki (22) presented evidence for a specific defect in the repair of prechromosome aberration lesions induced by difunctional mitomycin in cells from patients with Fanconi's anemia. Again it has to be shown that the repair phenomenon is the primary genetic defect in this autosomal recessive disease.

Another disorder that has been mentioned in this respect is Bloom's syndrome. However, so far there is no direct evidence for a relationship between a defect in a DNA repair mechanism and the high frequency of sister-chromatid exchanges seen in Bloom's cells (23).

Complementation Analysis

The development of techniques for the fusion of mammalian cells *in vitro* has provided new tools for the study of genetic diseases in man. Either spontaneously or mediated by treatment with fusion-stimulating agents, like inactivated Sendai virus, bi- and multinucleated cells can be obtained. A fraction of these cells will contain the genomes of the two parental individuals. In 1972 de Weerd-Kastelein et al. (24) demonstrated the applicability of these hybrid cells in the genetic analysis of defective DNA repair in XP. Following the fusion of cells from different XP patients, in some combinations normal DNA repair (UDS) was observed after UVL exposure of the hybrid cells. These results indicated the presence of different complementary mutations in these patients. A cooperative study of the Rotterdam group and Robbins and coworkers at Bethesda, N.I.H., has now resolved the pres-

TABLE 1.   XP Cell Strains Characterized by Complementation Analysis

Complementation group	Cell strain[a]	UDS % of control	Neurological defects[b]	References[c]
A	XPKMSF	0	+	*11, 26*
	XPPKSF	0	+	*27*
	XP17SF	<5	+	*27, 28*
	XP1LO	<5	−	*25, 26*
	XP4LO	<5	+	*27*
	XP8LO	36	?	*29*
	XP12BE	<2	+	*11, 25, 26*
	XP12RO	<5	+	*24, 27*
	XP25RO	<5	+	*25, 27, 28*
	XP26RO	<5	+	*27*
	XP6PR	<5	+	*29*
	XP7PR	<5	+	*29*
	XP2OS	<2	+	*30*
	XP8OS	<2	?	*30*
	XP9OS	<2	+	*30*
B	XP11BE	3–7	+	*11, 25, 26*
C	XP12SF	10–15	−	*27*
	XP1BE	15–25	−	*11, 25, 26*
	XP2BE	15–25	−	*11, 25, 26*
	XP3BE	15–25	−	*11, 26*
	XP8BE	15–25	−	*26*
	XP10BE	10–20	−	*11, 26*
	XP14BE	15–25	−	*11*
	XP4RO	25	−	*24, 25, 27, 28*
	XP5RO	25	−	*29*
	XP6RO	31	−	*29*
	XP7RO	28	−	*29*
	XP9RO	10–15	−	*24, 27*
	XP16RO	5–10	−	*24, 27, 28*
	XP20RO	10–15	−	*27*
	XP21RO	10–21	−	*27*
	XP1TE	15	−	*29*
D	XP5BE	25–55	+	*11, 25, 26*
	XP6BE	25–55	+	*11, 25, 26*
	XP7BE	25–55	+	*11, 26*
	XP2NE	25	+	*27*
	XP3NE	25	+	*27*
E	XP2RO	40–60	−	*31*
	XP3RO	40–60	−	*31*
	XP5SE	70	−	*30*

a) The proposed standardization of nomenclature of XP strains (*32*) is used throughout. SF, San Francisco (J. E. Cleaver); LO, London (J. M. Parrington); B E, Bethesda (J. H. Robbins) RO, Rotterdam (E.A. de Weerd-Kastelein); PR, Pavia-Roma (A. Falaschi); OS, Osaka (H. Takebe); TE, Tehran (P. Sabour); NE, New Castle (J. E. Cleaver, J. M. Parrington); SE, Sendai (*via* H. Takebe).   b) As shown by Robbins *et al.* (*11*) many XP patients suffer from neurological abnormalities of different types. A few of them have all the abnormalities characteristic for the De Sanctis Cacchione syndrome, many others have one or more of its neurological components. A careful neurological screening of all the XP patients listed here is not available, therefore the indicated absence (−) in this column has to be taken with some doubt.   c) Only references are given which present complementation data.

ence of 5 different complementation groups in the excision repair-deficient XP syndrome (25). In Table 1 the cell strains have been tabulated that were assigned to one of the complementation groups by means of cell fusion. In the past it was suggested that cells from patients with the skin lesions only and cells from patients having neurological defects in addition to the skin lesions were assigned to different complementation groups. So far patients with neurological defects of different types (11) have not been found in complementation group C and E (Table 1). Recently Kraemer *et al.* (26) demonstrated that the cells from patient XP1LO fit in complementation group A. Neurological abnormalities have so far not been detected in this patient (32). This observation clearly indicates that one has to be cautious in assigning patients to a complementation group only on the basis of the clinical symptoms. Even more dangerous is the assignment of cell strains to a complementation group on the basis of the residual level of UDS. Figure 1 shows the result of a complementation experiment in which we tried to characterize an XP strain obtained from J. M. Parrington at London, the XP8LO. Cells of this patient have a residual level of UDS of about 30% of the control cells. Fusion of

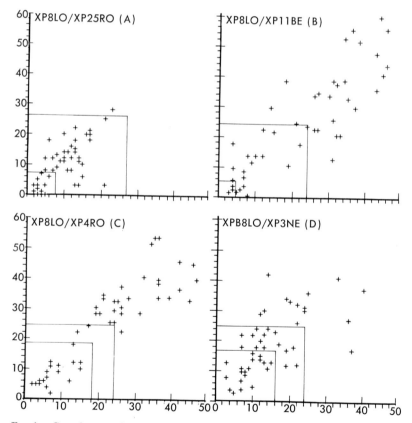

FIG. 1.   Complementation analysis with the XP8LO strain. Each point represents one binuclear cell, determined by the number of grains over each of both nuclei (one nucleus on the ordinate and one on the abscissa). The squares indicate the areas enclosing the grain numbers found over parental nuclei with 95% tolerance limits. For further explanation, see text.

these cells with cells belonging to the B, C, and D groups (and also with the E group, which is not indicated in the figure) resulted in complementation. In these fusions normal levels of UDS were observed in the nuclei of a relatively large fraction of the binuclear cells. Only the fusion with the XP25RO cells did not result in restoration of repair activity, indicating that this strain belongs to complementation group A. This strain represents the first exception in group A, all the other A group strains studied so far have very low or negligible levels of UDS (Table 1).

Very recently K. Jaspers and E. A. de Weerd-Kastelein started a complementation analysis of the XP variants in collaboration with A. R. Lehmann, University of Sussex, England. A system was developed in which they could demonstrate the correction of the defect in the variant cell following fusion with normal human fibroblasts. Fusions between different XP-variant cells are in progress.

Mapping Genes on Human Chromosomes

In the last few years impressive progress has been made in the localization of genes on human chromosomes by using interspecific cell hybrids (*33*). Proliferating mononuclear human-mouse and human-Chinese hamster cell hybrids lose preferentially human chromosomes. If the homologous gene products of both parental cells can be distinguished one can correlate the loss of a chromosome with the loss of one or more phenotypes coded by genes located on that chromosome. The built-in differences in amino-acid composition of homologous enzymes of different species has been extensively used in these studies to separate the parental gene products in the hybrid cells. A paucity of information dealing with the enzymology of DNA repair in mammalian cells has hampered the application of hybridization techniques in mapping repair genes. For these studies we will be dependent on the recognition of the parental physiological parameters of DNA repair (like UDS) in hybrid cells, if differences in these functions do exist. The many rather unknown steps between the primary gene products involved and the physiological parameter of DNA repair make these studies very complicated.

A difference in the mechanisms of DNA repair following UVL exposure of different eukaryotic organisms has been described by Paterson *et al.* (*34*). Exposure of embryonic chick cells as well as human fibroblasts results in DNA repair replication as measured by autoradiography and density gradients. In human cells the UDS is accompanied by a loss of one well-known class of UV photoproducts, the cyclobutane pyrimidine dimers. Therefore it seems likely that in human cells at least a fraction of the UDS is the result of the excision of these dimers. By applying an *in vitro* enzymatic assay (*35*), the UV endo test, Paterson *et al.* (*34*) could demonstrate that in embryonic chick cells dimer excisions did not occur. It appears that embryonic chick cells primarily rely on enzymatic photoreactivation, a process which is very active in these cells. The repair DNA synthesis seen in these chick cells is probably the result of excision of another as yet unidentified photochemical defect. In human-embryonic chick heterokaryons it was shown that the photoreactivating system of the chick and an excision repair enzyme from the human nuclei act on UV-damaged DNA in the foreign nuclei (*36*). Complementary studies

TABLE 2.   UDS in Human Fibroblast-Chick Erythrocyte Heterokaryons Following 270 erg/mm² UV Exposure

Hybrid binuclear cells	Nucleus	Days between fusion and UV exposure	Grains per nucleus
XP25RO/chicken	XP25RO	1	7.6±0.8
		4	19.2±1.8
		8	50.3±2.5
	Chicken	1	0.6±0.1
		4	5.8±0.7
		8	19.5±1.0
Control/chicken	Control	1	—
		4	59.8±3.7
		8	64.6±4.5
	Chicken	1	—
		4	16.7±1.3
		8	28.7±1.9

Mononuclear parental cells	Days between fusion and UV exposure	Grains per nucleus
XP25	8	1.5±0.2
Control	8	62.4±3.3

using UDS as parameter for DNA repair were carried out by E. A. de Weerd-Kastelein, W. Keijzer, and P. Rainaldi in our institute. Preliminary results of these investigations are presented in Table 2. Normal human fibroblasts and fibroblasts from an A group XP cell strain (XP25RO) were fused with embryonic chick erythrocytes. In the heterokaryons formed the genetically inactive chick nucleus is reactivated as a result of interaction with the human genome (37). On morphological grounds the chick nucleus can easily be distinguished from the human counterpart in the hybrid binucleated cells. The cells were exposed to UVL 1, 4, and 8 days after fusion and the UDS performed by the chick and the human nucleus was determined separately. It can be seen in Table 2 that even in the combination of an XP nucleus and a chick nucleus in one hybrid cell considerable levels of UDS were performed by the XP nucleus. In XP as well as chick nuclei the UDS increases by increasing the time between cell fusion and UVL exposure, indicating a dependency on the rate of reactivation of the chick nucleus.

The UDS seen in the XP nucleus could be the result of the chicken repair system acting on nondimer lesions in the XP DNA. Alternatively one might postulate the occurrence of complementation between defective human repair and the nondimer excision repair system of the chick resulting in the excision of dimers from the XP DNA. In order to differentiate between both possibilities two approaches can be followed. Firstly the UDS can be studied under conditions of photoreactivation of the dimers by using the chick photoreactivating system. Decreased levels of UDS following photoreactivation would indicate the occurrence of complementation between XP and chick. Secondly by using the UV endo test of Paterson et al. (35) the fate of the dimers in the XP nuclei could be monitored. A constant level of dimers in the presence of UDS would suggest the action of the chick repair system in the xeroderma nucleus. Experiments along these lines by using the chick erythrocyte-human heterokaryons are in progress. Evidence that in chick-XP heterokaryons complementation does not occur has been described by Paterson et al. (37). In these experiments XP cells were fused with embryonic chick fibroblasts and the UV endo test was applied on multikaryotic cell populations. The number of UVL-induced dimers in the XP nuclei remained constant within the first 24 hr following cell fusion and UVL exposure. In these experiments using chick fibroblasts as parental cells UDS has not been measured, however, the results presented in Table 2 and obtained with embryonic chick erythrocytes do suggest that in these chick-XP hybrids UDS is performed by the XP nuclei. If this holds true for chick fibroblasts than the conclusion that complementation does not occur seems to be valid.

It is well known that chick-human hybrid systems cannot be used for gene mapping because in all cases studied so far the chick chromosomes were lost instead of the human chromosomes. In recent experiments Lohman presented evidence that also in Chinese hamster cells a nondimer excision repair process is active (P.H.M. Lohman, personal communication). If so, one might expect that the dimer excision in proliferating mononucleated Chinese hamster-human hybrids will be dependent on the presence or absence of human genes involved in the excision repair process. This would enable a genetic analysis of the human excision repair process including the mapping of genes involved. Moreover "backcrosses" of these interspecific cell hybrids with XP cells of different complementation groups could then contribute to the characterization of the mutations involved in these groups.

It is obvious that a genetic analysis of DNA repair in human cells, including the localization of genes involved, is still in a very primitive state. The experiments are elaborate, complicated and often difficult to interpret. It is clear that the isolation, purification, and characterization of the enzymes involved in DNA repair in mammalian cells will be a prerequisite for the ultimate elucidation of the genetic basis of DNA repair.

REFERENCES

1. Cleaver, J. E.   Defective repair of DNA in xeroderma pigmentosum. Nature, *218*: 652–656, 1968.
2. Cleaver, J. E.   DNA repair and radiation sensitivity in human (xeroderma pigmentosum) cells. Int. J. Rad. Biol., *18*: 557–565, 1970.
3. Rabson, A. S., Tyrrell, S. A., and Legallais, F. Y.   Growth of ultraviolet-damaged herpesvirus in xeroderma pigmentosum cells. Proc. Soc. Exp. Biol. Med., *132*: 802–806, 1969.
4. Lytle, C. D., Aaronson, S. A., and Harvey, E.   Host-cell reactivation in mammalian cells. II. Survival by herpes simplex virus and vaccinia virus in normal human and xeroderma pigmentosum cells.   Int. J. Rad. Biol., *22*: 159–165, 1972.
5. Aaronson, S. A. and Lytle, C. D.   Decreased host cell reactivation of irradiated SV40 virus in xeroderma pigmentosum. Nature, *228*: 359–361, 1970.
6. Day, R. S., III. Cellular reactivation of ultraviolet-irradiated human adenovirus

2 in normal and xeroderma pigmentosum fibroblasts. Photochem. Photobiol., *19*: 9–13, 1974.

7. Abrahams, P. J. and van der Eb, A. J. Host-cell reactivation of ultraviolet-irradiated SV40 DNA in five complementation groups of xeroderma pigmentosum. Submitted to Mutat. Res.

8. Sutherland, B. M., Rice, M., and Wagner, E. K. Xeroderma pigmentosum cells contain low levels of photoreactivating enzyme. Proc. Natl. Acad. Sci. U.S., *72*: 103–107, 1975.

9. Lehmann, A. R., Kirk-Bell, S., Arlett, C. F., Paterson, M. C., Lohman, P. H. M., de Weerd-Kastelein, E. A., and Bootsma, D. Xeroderma pigmentosum cells with normal levels of excision repair have a defect in DNA synthesis after UV-irradiation. Proc. Natl. Acad. Sci. U.S., *72*: 219–223, 1975.

10. Chu, E. H. Y., Schmickel, R. D., Wade, M. H., Chang, C. C., and Trosko, J. E. Ultraviolet light sensitivity and defect in DNA repair in fibroblasts derived from two patients with Cockayne syndrome. Am. J. Hum. Genet., *27*: 26A, 1975.

11. Robbins, J. H., Kraemer, K. H., Lutzner, M. A., Festoff, B. W., and Coon, H. G. Xeroderma pigmentosum: An inherited disease with sun sensitivity, multiple cutaneous neoplasma, and abnormal DNA repair. Ann. Inern. Med., *80*: 221–248, 1974.

12. Harnden, D. G. Ataxia Telangiectasia syndrome: cytogenetic and cancer aspects. *In;* J. German (ed.), Chromosomes and Cancer, pp. 619–636, Wiley, New York 1974.

13. Cunliffe, P. N., Mann, J. R., Cameron, A. H., Roberts, K. D., and Ward, H. W. C. Radiosensitivity in Ataxia-Telangiectasia. Brit. J. Radiol., *48*: 374–376, 1975.

14. Higurashi, M. and Conen, P. E. *In vitro* chromosomal radiosensitivity in "chromosomal breakage syndromes." Cancer, *32*: 380–383, 1973.

15. Taylor, A. M. R., Harnden, D. G., Arlett, C. F., Harcourt, S. A., Lehmann, A. R., Stevens, S., and Bridges, B. A. Ataxia Telangiectasia: A human mutation with abnormal radiation sensitivity. Nature, *258*: 427–429, 1975.

16. Paterson, M. C., Smith, B. P., Lohman, P. H. M., Anderson, A. K., and Fishman, L. Defective excision repair of gamma ray-damaged DNA in human (Ataxia Telangiectasia) fibroblasts. Submitted to Nature.

17. Epstein, J., Williams, J. R., and Little, J. B. Deficient DNA repair in human progeroid cells. Proc. Natl. Acad. Sci. U.S., *70*: 977–981, 1973.

18. Goldstein, S. and Singal, D. P. Alteration of fibroblast gene products *in vitro* from a subject with Werner's syndrome. Nature, *251*: 719–721, 1974.

19. Singal, D. P. and Goldstein, S. Absence of detectable HL-A antigens on cultured fibroblasts in progeria. J. Clin. Invest., *52*: 2259–2263, 1973.

20. Epstein, J., Williams, J. R., and Little, J. B. Rate of DNA repair in progeric and normal human fibroblasts. Biochem. Biophys. Res. Commun., *59*: 850–857, 1974.

21. Regan, J. D. and Setlow, R. B. DNA repair in human progeroid cells. Biochem. Biophys. Res. Commun., *59*: 858–864, 1974.

22. Sasaki, M. S. Is Fanconi's anaemia defective in a process essential to the repair of DNA cross links? Nature, *257*: 501–503, 1975.

23. Chaganti, R. S. K., Schonberg, S., and German, J. A many-fold increase in sister chromatid exchanges in Bloom's syndrome lymphocytes. Proc. Natl. Acad. Sci. U.S., *71*: 4508–4512, 1974.

24. De Weerd-Kastelein, E. A., Keijzer, W., and Bootsma, D. Genetic heterogeneity of xeroderma pigmentosum demonstrated by somatic cell hybridization. Nature New Biol., *238*: 80–83, 1972.

25. Kraemer, K. H., de Weerd-Kastelein, E. A., Robbins, J. H., Keijzer, W., Barrett, S. F., Petinga, R. A., and Bootsma, D. Five complementation groups in xeroderma pigmentosum. Mutat. Res., *33*: 327–340, 1975.

26. Kraemer, K. H., Coon, H. G., Petinga, R. A., Barrett, S. F., Rahe, A. F., and Robbins, J. H. Genetic heterogeneity in xeroderma pigmentosum; complementation groups and their relationship to DNA repair rates. Proc. Natl. Acad. Sci. U.S., *72*: 59–63, 1975.

27. De Weerd-Kastelein, E. A. Genetic heterogeneity in xeroderma pigmentosum. Thesis Erasmus University, Rotterdam, 1974.

28. De Weerd-Kastelein, E. A., Kleijer, W. J., Sluyter, M. L., and Keijzer, W. Repair replication in heterokaryons derived from different repair-deficient xeroderma pigmentosum strains. Mutat. Res., *19*: 237–243, 1973.

29. De Weerd-Kastelein, E. A., Keijzer, W., and Bootsma, D. Unpublished.

30. Takebe, H. Genetic complementation tests of Japanese xeroderma pigmentosum patients and their characteristics of repair and skin cancer. This volume, pp. 383–395.

31. De Weerd-Kastelein, E. A., Keijzer, W., and Bootsma, D. A third complementation group in xeroderma pigmentosum. Mutat. Res., *22*: 87–91, 1974.

32. Smithers, D. W. and Wood, J. H. Xeroderma pigmentosum. An attempt at cancer prophylaxis. The Lancet, May 10: 945–946, 1952.

33. Rotterdam Conference (1974): Second International Workshop on Human Gene Mapping. Birth Defects; Original Article Series, XI, 3, The National Foundation, New York, 1975.

34. Paterson, M. C., Lohman, P. H. M., de Weerd-Kastelein, E. A., and Westerveld, A. Photoreactivation and excision repair of ultraviolet radiation-injured DNA in primary embryonic chick cells. Biophys. J., *14*: 454–466, 1974.

35. Paterson, M. C., Lohman, P. H. M., and Sluyter ,M. L. Use of a UV endonuclease from *Micrococcus luteus* to monitor the progress of DNA repair in UV-irradiated human cells. Mutat. Res., *19*: 245–256, 1973.

36. Paterson, M. C., Lohman, P. H. M., Westerveld, A., and Sluyter, M. L. DNA repair in human-embryonic chick heterokaryons. Ability of each species to aid the other in the removal of ultraviolet-induced damage. Biophys. J., *14*: 835–845, 1974.

37. Ringertz, N. R., Carlsson, S. A., Ege, T., and Bolund, L. Detection of human and chick nuclear antigens in nuclei of chick erythrocytes during reactivation in heterokaryons with HeLa cells. Proc. Natl. Acad. Sci. U.S., *68*: 3228–3232, 1971.

Discussion of Paper of Dr. Bootsma

DR. TAKEBE: Sometimes the levels of unscheduled DNA synthesis (UDS) in the fused cells reach some intermediate levels. How do you deal with these cases? (1) Cases with levels between normal and the higher levels of fused cells? (2) Cases with the same levels as the higher level of two cells?

DR. BOOTSMA: We consider a UDS level as indicative for complementation, if we find the level of UDS which is found in normal cells tested in the same experiment. In a case where you find a level of UDS comparable with the level found in the parental cells having the highest residual UDS, we think that this is not indicative for complementation. This situation can be explained by assuming that the defective enzyme of this parental origin is also dealing with lesion in the genome of the other parent in the hybridization.

DR. IKENAGA: I would like to ask you about the unknown photoproduct you mentioned in the case of UDS in chicken cells. So far as I am aware, UV product other than pyrimidine dimers is Varghese and Wang's product (PO-T, sometimes called P_2B). Dr. J. Jagger (Univ. Texas) and I measured the yield of P_2B, and found that P_2B yield is only about 10% of the pyrimidine dimer yield at moderate UV dose (less than $100 J/m^2$). Therefore, I think P_2B alone cannot account for the relatively large amount of UDS in chicken cells. Do you have any idea about the unknown product?

DR. BOOTSMA: We have as yet no data clarifying the origin of this lesion in chicken cells.

DR. KURODA: (1) How long a time after cell fusion did you detect UDS in your binucleated cells?

(2) Five complementation groups of XP cells may correspond to different steps or different subunits of repair enzymes in the repair process. Is there a possibility of finding new additional groups of complementation repair?

DR. BOOTSMA: (1) We were able to demonstrate complementation within 6 hr after cell fusion. In fact, such short time intervals have been used by Dr. Paterson and Dr. Lohman in their experiments on the excision of dimers with their UV-endonuclease test system in hybrid cell populations.

(2)   The number of complementation groups has not been extended to more than 5, inspite of the increasing number of patients that have been investigated. Regarding the gene products involved in these mutations one has to consider many possibilities: these mutations might affect the same enzymatic step by impairing the structure of (the subunits of) the enzyme as well as by affecting the control systems of its synthesis. They might also be involved in the synthesis of as yet hypothetical proteins that could play a role in helping the excision repair mechanism to reach the damaged mammalian DNA. Alternatively, one can postulate that the repair enzyme in mammalian cells act in a coordinated way, for instance as "subunits" of a repair "complex." In that case a defect in a later step of the repair process will show up as a defect in the first step of DNA repair, because it will render the whole complex inactive.

DR. OKADA: Do you know in what chromosomes some of these genes are located?

DR. BOOTSMA: No, if the Chinese hamster repair system is different from the human repair, we will be able to use our collection of Chinese hamster-human hybrids to answer your question. Work in this direction is now in progress.

FUNDAMENTALS IN CANCER PREVENTION, P. N. MAGEE ET AL. (EDS.),
UNIV. OF TOKYO PRESS, TOKYO / UNIV. PARK PRESS, BALTIMORE, PP. 409–416, 1976

Photoreactivation in Normal and Xeroderma Cells

Betsy M. Sutherland

Department of Molecular Biology and Biochemistry, University of California, Irvine, California, U.S.A.

Abstract: Cells can repair damage induced in their DNA by ultraviolet light. Most cells contain at least three such repair pathways: excision repair, postreplication repair, and photoreactivation. We find that although fibroblasts—and other cells—from normal humans contain rather high levels of photoreactivating enzyme (PRE), cells from patients with xeroderma pigmentosum contain lowered PRE levels. These low enzyme levels seem to be heritable in a fashion consistent with P the gene for normal PRE, and p that for defective enzyme: all normal individuals we examined were either PP or Pp, and all xeroderma patients were either Pp or pp. We propose that the total resistance of an individual to the environmental burden of damage to his DNA may be evaluated by determining his total repair capacity—the sum of his capacity for excision repair, postreplication repair and photoreactivation. The development and testing of such a repair index may allow the identification of individuals with low repair capacity and thus, perhaps, of increased probability of induction of cancer.

Ultraviolet light (UV) in the wavelength range 220–300 nm produces death and mutations in procaryotes (*1*) and causes skin cancer in man (*2*). Although UV induces a variety of chemical modifications in cells, a major cause of biological damage is the cyclobutyl pyrimidine dimer (or cyclobutadipyrimidine), produced by covalent addition at the 5- and 6-positions of two adjacent pyrimidines on the same DNA strand (*3*). Cells can repair such damage to their DNA: most cells have at least three paths for removing, reversing or bypassing such damage (*1*). In excision repair and postreplication repair, not only dimers but also other types of damage are removed (or bypassed). Photoreactivation stands out in sharp contrast to the other repair pathways. First, the only substrate for this mode of repair is the dimer (*4*); second, the dimer is not removed nor is it ignored, but instead is reversed into two monomeric pyrimidines (*5*); third, light in the wavelength region 300–600 nm is absolutely required for the photolysis event (*6*). The reaction is mediated by a photoreactivating enzyme (PRE), which carrys out its action in a multistep process: the enzyme binds to dimer-containing DNA, presumably at the site of a dimer, to form a stable complex. The enzyme-DNA complex then absorbs a photon, the dimer is broken, and finally the enzyme is released from the DNA. The result of PRE action is the restoration of normal biological activity to the DNA, the disappearance of dimers and the concomitant appearance of pyrimidine monomers.

PRE in Human Cells

Although PRE activity had been found in almost all groups of all phyla, it had been thought to be absent in the placentalia (*7*). However, its otherwise universal distribution led us to suspect that it might be present in placental mammals, but had not been detected for technical reasons. Table 1 shows that although the human PRE is similar to that from *Escherichia coli* in pH optimum, isoelectric point, molecular weight and metal requirement, it differs dramatically in ionic strength optimum (*8*) and action spectrum (*9*). We have also shown that the enzyme does not exist in the same activity in all human cells: although the enzyme is present at rather high specific activities in polymorphonuclear cells and in monocytes, its activity in erythrocytes, lymphocytes, and also in serum is very low (*10*). It is also present in bone marrow (which contains immature, noncirculating polymorphonuclear cells and monocytes) (*10*). The enzyme is present in cultured murine and

TABLE 1. Properties of the *E. coli* and Human PRE

	E. coli	*H. sapiens*
pH optimum	7.2	7.2
Metal requirement	None	None
μ optimum	0.18	0.05
Isoelectric pH	~5	5.4
Molecular weight	~42,500	~40,000
Action spectrum		
Peak	360 nm	400 nm
Red edge	~500 nm	>577 nm

TABLE 2. Repair Capacities of Normal, Xeroderma, and Progeroid Cells

Cell line	Description	UDS	PRE activity (% of normal)
HESM	Normal embryonic	100	100
El San	8 yr. normal	100	112
Le San	33 yr. normal	100	107
XP12BE (Jay Tim)	7 yr. xeroderma A	<2	36
XP-1LO	32 yr. xeroderma A	<2	20
XP7BE (TeKo)	11 yr. xeroderma	25–55	8
XP4BE (WoMec)	Xeroderma	100	11
XP13BE (PeHay)	Xeroderma	100	9
1277 (KeHe)	Progeroid	—	88

human cells and its production is rather independent of the age of the donor, passage number of the cells, or growth rate of the cells (*10, 11*).

Since the enzyme is present at reasonably high levels in cultured fibroblasts from normal humans, we thought it important to examine the specific activity in cells derived from individuals with xeroderma pigmentosum, the hereditary propensity to sunlight-induced skin cancer. Table 2 points out some of the conclusions of this work (*11*): (1) the specific activity of the normal cells was not dependent on the age of the donor, (2) the level of PRE is lower in both xeroderma and xeroderma variant (individuals with all clinical signs of xeroderma although normal in unscheduled synthesis) cells than in normal cells, (3) the level of PRE is not the same for all members of a complementation group for unscheduled DNA synthesis (UDS), (4) PRE activity is not directly correlated with the level of UDS (note that XP12BE with 36% of the normal PRE level has only about 2% of normal UDS level, while XP7BE has only 8% of the normal PRE level and 25–55% of the normal UDS capacity), and (5) cells from individuals with other syndromes (*e.g.*, progeria) do not show decreased levels of PRE (*12*). These data imply a connection between the level of DNA repair enzymes, in specific, the PRE, and the propensity for sunlight-induced skin cancer.

Photoreactivation in Human Cells

If such a correlation exists, we would expect, first, that the biochemical measurements we make of PRE levels would be reflected in the biological repair capacity of the cells. We have thus examined the rates of photoreactivation of pyrimidine dimers in xeroderma cells containing similar excision capacity but differing in PRE levels. XP12BE with 36% of the normal PRE level photoreactivated about 70% of the cellular dimers in a 30 min exposure to photoreactivating light, while XPSG, with about 13% of the normal enzyme level, removed only about 20% of the dimers in the same time. Thus the rate of photoreactivation of dimers in the cell seems directly related to the level of PRE available for that repair (*13*). If the cellular dimer photoreactivation we observe is indeed dependent on the PRE we measure *in vitro*, the action spectrum for the photoreactivation of dimers should agree with that measured for the isolated enzyme. The peak of the action spectrum for the enzyme is about 400 nm, and the range extends from 300 nm to 600 nm (*13*). We have also measured the action spectrum for dimer photoreactivation in intact normal and xeroderma cells: the peak and range for cellular photoreactivation are approximately 400 nm and 300–600 nm, respectively, in good agreement with that found for the isolated enzyme (*13*).

Inheritance of the Gene for Photoreactivation

If the low level of PRE found in the XP cells is a true characteristic of the individual and not only of the cells in culture, we might find that the low enzyme levels are transmitted from parent to offspring. We have thus examined the level of PRE in members of a family (*14*) with normal parents, one normal child and

TABLE 3.   PRE Activity in 6 Members of One Family

Cell line		PRE activity (% of normal)
HESM	Normal embryonic human	100
BeAr	Father	100
CeAr	Mother	34
EmAr	Normal son	119
JaAr (XP2BE)	Xeroderma son	46
PeAr (XP8BE)	Xeroderma son[a]	50
GeAr (XP9BE)	Xeroderma son[a]	32

[a] Identical twins.

5 xeroderma children. Table 3 shows that although cells of the father contain the normal level of enzyme, the mother has only 34% of the normal activity. Although the normal son has a high level of PRE, the 3 xeroderma sons have 28, 45, and 50% of the normal level. If we represent the normal gene for photoreactivating enzyme by P, and a defective one by p, then the father and the normal son would be PP, and the mother and xeroderma children Pp.

How can we test this hypothesis? The ideal method would be the examination of large numbers of families with members afflicted with xeroderma pigmentosum to determine the PRE levels in their cells. However, cells of no other large family groups are readily available (e.g., in the American Type Culture Collection) and this method is thus currently unavailable. We thus devised a test for examining our hypothesis of heritability of PRE levels with the limited number of cell lines available. If the level of PRE in a cell line is indeed determined genetically, we can use parent-child pairs of cell lines in which the child is a xeroderma pigmentosum patient with very low levels of PRE activity. These individuals would thus be pp in our scheme; their parents might be Pp or pp, but should never be completely normal for PRE (PP). We have found 3 pairs of parent-xeroderma child suitable for use in this test; that is, the level of PRE in the children was <20% of normal. Table 4 shows the results of these tests: for each child with a very low level of PRE (presumably pp), the parent had an intermediate level of enzyme and thus could be designated Pp. We found that none of these parents had normal enzyme levels (PP), thus indicating that our data are consistent with the inheritance of PRE levels. Although it is genetically possible, we also found no normal parents with very low PRE levels (pp); we speculate that such a defect might change the phenotype of the individual from "normal" to "xeroderma" or to one of skin cancer of lesser severity.

TABLE 4.   PRE Levels in Parent-Child Pairs

Child			Parent	
XP7BE	(TeKo)	11	ReKo	41
XP11BE	(PoCo)	18	MoCo	73
XP4BE	(WoMec)	11	WinMec	36

DNA Repair and Skin Cancer

How can we use these data—and those rapidly accumulating from other laboratories—to evaluate the role of DNA repair in cancer prevention and to identify individuals at risk of induction of cancer? In evaluating the relationship between DNA repair and skin cancer, we have noticed three points. (1) CeAr is clinically normal although she possesses only 34% of the normal PRE level (14); she does have, however, the normal level of UDS (14). Thus it seems that a deficiency in DNA repair does not *necessarily* lead to the induction of skin cancer by sunlight. (2) Xeroderma variants, who have all the clinical signs of xeroderma, have normal levels of excision repair. They are, however, deficient (most <10% of normal) in both PRE and in postreplication repair. Thus the presence of one intact pathway—in this case, excision repair—dose not guarantee immunity from induction of skin cancer. (3) In our examination of parent-child pairs, we found no normal parents with a pp (very low PRE levels) genotype, although they might have been expected since the child was selected for its pp genotype (very low PRE level). Perhaps the pp genotype might confer a "subnormal" phenotype on the individual, and he or she would not have been selected in our normal parent-xeroderma child pairs.

We thus propose that the total repair capacity, rather than the presence or absence of one repair pathway, is a better biological index of cellular resistance to injury (15). Clearly, excision competence alone is not adequate to confer resistance to skin cancer—the xeroderma variants would then be normal. On the other hand, a deficiency in one repair path (*e.g.*, photoreactivation) does not necessarily confer susceptibility to sunlight-induced skin cancer—both CeAr and all the parents, ReKo, MoCo, and WinMec, would then be xerodermoid. We propose that a rough approximation of total repair capacity be made by simply summing the repair capacity for each individual repair path. Thus a completely repair-proficient individual would be rated 100 for excision, 100 for postreplication repair and 100 for photoreactivation, to total 300. The xeroderma pigmentosum variant, XP4BE (WoMec) with 100% excision ability, 32% postreplication repair (16) and 11% PRE level, would have a total repair capacity of 143. In this scheme, a weighting factor of 1 was applied to each pathway; that is, they were assumed to be equally important. This is doubtless an oversimplification, although assignment of weighting factors of 10 to excision repair led to the prediction that xeroderma variants should be normal, and 10 to postreplication repair or photoreactivation to the prediction that CeAr should be xerodermoid rather than normal.

The total repair capacity gives an estimate of the ability of a cell to withstand damage to its DNA. The net outcome depends, however, not only on the repair capacity, but also on the amount of damage which must be repaired—the environmental burden. This environmental factor is a complex function of life style, latitude of residence, skin pigmentation and a myriad of other such factors. We might ask if the relative values of the environmental burden and repair capacity really play a decisive role in determining the induction of skin cancer. A striking case is that of PeAr and GeAr (XP8BE and XP9BE, respectively), twin boys whose older brother

JaAr has classical xeroderma pigmentosum, and who show deficiencies in both UDS and PRE activity (15). These boys have been kept out of sunlight and in their early teens showed little or no sunlight-type induced abnormalities (14). Clearly, although their repair capacity is low, it is adequate for the (lowered) burden of their restricted regime.

REFERENCES

1. Setlow, R. B.   Molecular changes responsible for ultraviolet inactivation of the biological activity of DNA. *In;* C. Pavan (ed.), Mammalian Cytogenetic and Related Problems in Radiobiology, pp. 291–307, Pergamon Press, New York, 1964.

2. Epstein, J. H.   Ultraviolet carcinogenesis.   *In;* A. C. Giese (ed.), Photophysiology: Current Topics in Photobiology and Photochemistry, vol. 5, pp. 235–273, Academic Press, New York, 1970.

3. Setlow, R. B.   Cyclobutane-type pyrimidine dimers in polynucleotides. Science, *153*: 379–386, 1966.

4. Setlow, R. B. and Setlow, J. K.   Evidence that ultraviolet-induced thymine dimers in DNA cause biological damage. Proc. Natl. Acad. Sci. U.S., *48*: 1250–1257, 1962.

5. Setlow, R. B., Carrier, W. L., and Bollum, F. J.   Pyrimidine dimers in UV-irradiated poly dI: dC. Proc. Natl. Acad. Sci. U.S., *53*: 1111–1118, 1965.

6. Rupert, C. S.   Photoenzymatic repair of ultraviolet damage in DNA. I. Kinetics of the reaction. J. Gen. Physiol., *45*: 703–724, 1962.

7. Cook, J. S.   Photoreactivation in animal cells. *In;* A. C. Giese (ed.), Photophysiology: Current Topics in Photobiology and Photochemistry, vol. 5, pp. 191–233, Academic Press, New York, 1970.

8. Sutherland, B. M.   Photoreactivating enzyme from human leukocytes. Nature, *248*: 109–112, 1974.

9. Sutherland, J. C. and Sutherland, B. M.   Human photoreactivating enzyme: Action spectrum and safelight conditions. Biophys. J., *15*: 435–440, 1975.

10. Sutherland, B. M., Runge, P., and Sutherland, J. C.   DNA photoreactivating enzyme from placental mammals: Origin and characteristics. Biochemistry, *13*: 4710–4715, 1975.

11. Sutherland, B. M. and Wagner, E. K.   Xeroderma pigmentosum cells contain low levels of photoreactivating enzyme. Proc. Natl. Acad. Sci. U.S., *72*: 103–107, 1975.

12. Sutherland, B. M. and Oliver, R. Unpublished.

13. Sutherland, B. M., Oliver, R., Fuselier, C. O., and Sutherland, J. C.   Photoreactivation of pyrimidine dimers in the DNA of normal and xeroderma pigmentosum cells. Biochemistry, 1975, in press.

14. Robbins, J. H., Kraemer, K. H., Lutzner, M. A., Festoff, M. D., and Coon, H. G.   Xeroderma pigmentosum: An inherited disease with sun sensitivity, multiple cutaneous neoplasms and abnormal DNA repair. Ann. Intern. Med., *80*: 221–248, 1974.

15. Sutherland, B. M. and Oliver, R.   Low photoreactivating enzyme levels in xeroderma pigmentosum ' variants.' Nature, *257*: 132–134, 1975.

16. Lehmann, A. R., Kirk-Bell, S., Artlet, C. F., Paterson, M. C., Lohman, P. H. M., Weerd-Kastelein, E. A., and Bootsma, D.   Xeroderma pigmentosum cells with normal levels of excision repair have a defect in DNA synthesis after UV-irradiation. Proc. Natl. Acad. Sci. U.S., *72*: 219–223, 1975.

Discussion of Paper of Dr. Sutherland

DR. SUGIMURA: I noticed, in your slide, some difference in the action spectra between *Escherichia coli* and *Homo sapiens* enzymes. What caused this difference? Amino acid composition?

DR. SUTHERLAND: We do not know yet. We know that the *E. coli* enzyme contains an apoprotein and a cofactor. The human enzyme might contain a different cofactor and a similar apoprotein to the *E. coli* enzyme, or it might contain the same cofactor in a different protein environment.

DR. BOOTSMA: We already discussed many aspects of the finding of defective photoreactivation (PR) in xeroderma pigmentosum (XP). If the PR defect and the excision repair defect are the result of independent genetic events, this most probably will show up in complementation experiments. In combinations XP genomes, where normal excision repair is restored by means of complementation, the PR defect needs not to be restored if this defect is the result of a mutation in the same gene in all XP patients studied so far.

DR. MAHER: Did you obtain the values you showed in your last slide for the size of DNA after UV irradiation from your own work or from the literature?

DR. SUTHERLAND: From Dr. Lohmann's data (Proc. Natl. Acad. Sci. U.S., *72*: 219, 1975).

DR. MAHER: Dr. McCormick and I find similar results with XP4BE. We assay the size of DNA by a 1-hr pulse of tritiated thymidine immediately after irradiation, without allowing for 1 hr before giving the pulse. We see significantly smaller DNA in the variant XP4BE than in the normal cell immediately after the pulse. This is a significant difference between these cell strains.

DR. LIEBERMAN: Have you thought about contacting Dr. Takebe to obtain both parents from some XP patients who live in the greater Osaka area? This would make your familial studies easier than the use of the Bethesda series.

DR. SUTHERLAND: I would be very indebted to Dr. Takebe for any cells of family members he could supply.

DR. SATO: Have you checked the activities of photoreactivating enzyme (PRE) in mammalian cells other than human?

DR. SUTHERLAND: Yes, we have examined murine cells and bovine bone marrow and found enzyme in both. Dr. Helga Harm, University of Texas at Dallas has also examined rabbit, bovine, and human leukocytes and has found PRE in all three, using the *Haemophilus influenzae*-transforming DNA assay.

DR. TAKEBE: I wonder if any dermatologist has applied PR to reactivate skin lesions caused by UV or sunlight.

DR. SUTHERLAND: I do not know of any cases.

FUNDAMENTALS IN CANCER PREVENTION, P. N. MAGEE ET AL. (EDS.),
UNIV. OF TOKYO PRESS, TOKYO / UNIV. PARK PRESS, BALTIMORE, PP. 417–429, 1976

Misrepair Model for Mutagenesis and Carcinogenesis

Sohei KONDO

Department of Fundamental Radiology, Faculty of Medicine, Osaka University, Osaka, Japan

Abstract: Evidence for a mutation theory of cancer is presented by reviewing the
work of the members of a cooperative workshop on molecular mechanism of carcinogenesis related to DNA repair. The oncogenic chemical 4-nitroquinoline 1-
oxide (4NQO) mimics UV light. It produces 4NQO-purine adducts on DNA.
The adducts are repaired by excision repair without detectable errors as measured
by mutations in *Escherichia coli* or transformation of mouse cells, and the unexcised
ones are mainly responsible for the mutations and the cell transformation. Caffeine
administered after the 4NQO treatment greatly suppresses not only the mutation
induction in *E. coli* but also the transformation in mouse cells and the tumor induction in mice, probably because of its inhibiting action on error-prone postreplication
repair to convert 4NQO-damaged DNA to mutated DNA. The transformed state
of mouse cells is fully expressed only after the fourth post-4NQO cell division in a
way similar to the delayed appearance of recessive membrane mutations in *E. coli*.
These and other data presented fit the model that cancers are, at least partly,
caused by deletion mutations. Under this hypothesis and from the aspect of DNA
repair, some possible characteristics of cancer mutations are briefly discussed in
relation to a fundamental key for prevention of cancer in mankind.

In 1957, Nakahara *et al.* (*23*) published the first monumental paper on the
carcinogenicity of 4-nitroquinoline 1-oxide (4NQO). In 1961, when I was continuing my work on theoretical physics (*26*) at the National Institute of Genetics,
Misima, as head of a newly built radioisotope laboratory, Dr. C. Auerbach, from
the University of Edinburgh, came as a visiting professor. From her I learned some
fascinating aspects of mutagenesis. In 1963, right after I was given the present
position in Osaka University, I went to the Biology Division, Oak Ridge National
Laboratory, to learn about radiation biology in *Escherichia coli* from Drs. R. B.
Setlow and J. Jagger. I studied the relationship of UV mutagenesis to DNA repair.
The *E. coli* strains and the experimental methods which I used were those generously

417

provided by Dr. E. M. Witkin to Dr. J. Jagger. In 1964 when I returned to Osaka, Prof. H. Endo, Kyushu University, encouraged me to join his cooperative research team to study chemical mutagenesis. Thus I started my work on chemical mutagenesis in *E. coli* with a gift sample of 4NQO from Prof. Endo.

UV Mimetic Effects of 4NQO on E. coli

To my surprise and with beginner's luck, 4NQO turned out to be UV mimetic and still remains the best UV mimetic agent among the more than 20 kinds of mutagens I have tested since 1965. In 1966, I first presented the UV mimetic characteristics of 4NQO damage in relation to the characteristics of UV-induced premutational damage at the 2nd International Biophysics Congress held in Vienna. Two UV-sensitive, excisionless strains Hs30R and Hs30, which we had isolated, respectively, from Witkin's UV-resistant strains H/r30R and H/r30, turned out to be almost equally (*ca.* 30 times) more sensitive to UV and 4NQO than the wild-type parental strains, with respect to both loss of colony-forming ability and mutations to prototrophy (*21*). The results are reproduced in Fig. 1 for the pair of *uvrA⁻* and wild-type strains.

Based on the above-mentioned and other data with various other types of DNA repair-deficient strains we isolated, we (*19, 21*) proposed a hypothesis that 4NQO-induced lesions are repaired by excision repair at almost the same efficiency as UV-induced pyrimidine dimers. However, the proof for this proposal has been only recently obtained by Ikenaga (*7*) after we obtained generous gifts of ³H-labeled 4NQO from Dr. Y. Kawazoe and 4NQO adducts in poly(A) and poly(G) from Dr. M. Tada. As discussed by Tada and Tada (*27*), 4NQO produces at least 4 kinds of adducts; a 4NQO-adenine adduct and three 4NQO-guanine adducts. One of the 4NQO-guanine adducts is somewhat labile and unstable; it releases 4-amino-

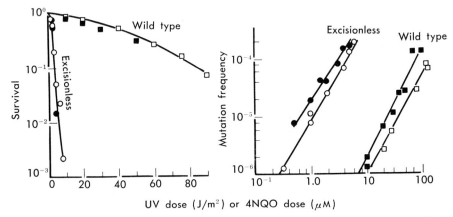

FIG. 1. Fraction of colony formers and frequency of induced mutations in surviving cells of *E. coli* plotted against doses of UV and 4NQO (from Kondo and Kato (*21*)). Mutations scored were reversions to prototrophy (Arg⁻ → Arg⁺). Strains H/r30R (wild type) with B/r-type UV resistance and its excisionless derivative Hs30R (*uvrA⁻*) were used. ○, □: UV. ●, ■: 4NQO.

quinoline 1-oxide (4AQO) upon hydrolysis and disappears slowly from DNA *in vitro*. As shown in Fig. 2, in excisionless strain Hs30R (*uvrA⁻*), 4NQO-purine adducts did not disappear from DNA even after 60-min postincubation of 4NQO-treated cells at 37°C except for a slow disappearance of the unstable, 4AQO-releasing adduct. On the contrary, the yields of 4NQO adducts in the wild type were low even at the zero time of postincubation because excision repair had been already working

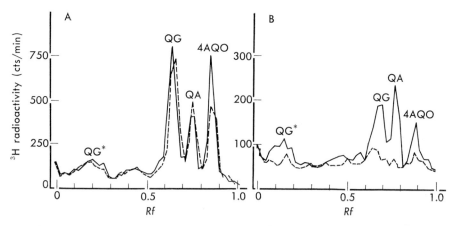

FIG. 2.   Chromatographic patterns of 4NQO products in DNA of *E. coli* strains H/r30 (*uvrA⁺*) and Hs30R (*uvrA⁻*) cells, which were exposed to ³H-labeled 4NQO for 2 hr with and without 60-min postincubation (from Ikenaga *et al.* (7)). QG and QG*, 4NQO-guanine adducts ; QA, 4NQO-adenine adduct ; 4AQO, 4-aminoquinoline 1-oxide released upon hydrolysis from labile and unstable 4NQO-guanine adduct(s).   A) *uvrA⁻* : — 0 ; --- 60 min.   B) *uvrA⁺* : — 0 ; --- 60 min.

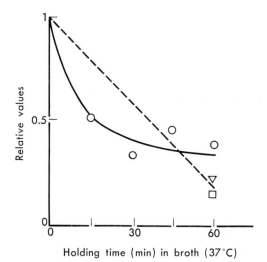

Holding time (min) in broth (37°C)

FIG. 3.   Decrease in 4NQO-induced premutational damage (○ : for Arg⁺ mutations) or 4NQO-purine adducts (▽, □ : from Ikenaga *et al.* (7)) during holding 4NQO-treated cells of *E. coli* strain H/r30R in nutrient broth at 37°C.

during the 2-hour exposure of the cells to 4NQO in phosphate buffer and almost all the adducts disappeared from DNA after 60-min postincubation.

As shown in Fig. 3, the amounts of 4NQO-induced premutational damage in the wild-type cells, which were measured as mutant yields after plating the 4NQO-treated cells on agar medium containing acriflavine to reduce the post-plating excision repair of 4NQO damage, decreased to the level of about 30% during a 60-min postincubation at 37°C and the amounts of 4NQO-purine adducts in DNA of wild-type cells also decreased to the level of about 10% during the 60-min postincubation. From these and other data (7, 19, 21), we can now conclude with confidence that 4NQO treatment of *E. coli* produces 4NQO-purine adducts, which are reparable by the excision repair without detectable mutagenic errors, and that the 4NQO-purine adducts are the major cause of both inactivation and mutation by 4NQO. Furthermore, an estimated number of lesions per lethal hit per haploid genome of the *uvrA⁻ E. coli* strain used was about 100 dimers and about 200 4NQO-purine adducts, respectively, after UV and 4NQO treatments (7). Thus, 4NQO is really UV mimetic except for the nonphotoreparability of 4NQO damage (21).

Basic Idea for Testing Somatic Mutation Theory of Cancer

That cancer may be caused by mutations in somatic cells of multicellular living organisms is one of the oldest theories of cancer. In 1969 when I organized a cooperative research team to study the molecular mechanism of carcinogenesis from the aspect of its relation to DNA repair, I proposed a deletion mutation model (16): the cancerous cells are induced by deletions of some DNA sequences including the sites of some of the many regulatory genes involved in DNA and/or cell replication. Since animal somatic cells usually possess two copies of the wild-type gene for each of the assumed cancer genes, expression of the normal cancerous state is expected to take place only after a multistep process as illustrated in Fig. 4 for the case of four-step mutations.

My idea to test the rather old fashioned somatic mutation theory was to check, step by step, whether the mutagenesis in *E. coli* parallels carcinogenesis in higher animals. Among the 15 members of our cooperative cancer research team, Dr. T. Kakunaga first seriously tested the mutation theory for malignant transformation in cultured cells after he succeeded in isolating a suitable subclone (12) from

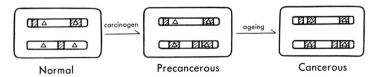

Normal   Precancerous   Cancerous

FIG. 4. "Somatic Deletion Mutation Theory" for carcinogenesis (from Kondo (16)). This imaginary diploid cell has only one pair of homologous chromosomes with double pairs of regulatory genes (△). Deletions (▨) in chromosomes are assumed to occur spontaneously and after carcinogen treatment.

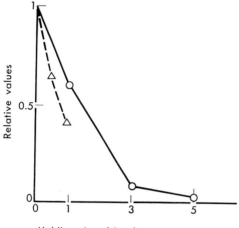

Holding time (days) in confluent state

Fig. 5.   Decrease in 4NQO-induced pretransformational damage ($\bigcirc$: from Kakunaga (14)) and disappearance of 4NQO-purine adducts from DNA ($\triangle$: from Ikenaga et al. (8)) in 4NQO-treated mouse cells during postincubation in a non-DNA-replicating state.

the A31 clone of a BALB/3T3 mouse cell line. He obtained various results which all support the mutation theory of transformation. I will quote a few of his results. The first evidence obtained by Kakunaga (14) is given in Fig. 5. The yields of transformed cells (about 2 transformants per 10^4 treated cells at zero time of holding) diminished with time of holding the 4NQO-treated cells under a non-DNA-replicating condition due to contact inhibition. After being held for indicated times the treated cells were transferred to fresh plates at an inoculum size of about one-30th and incubated for 4 weeks to score transformed foci. The rate of decline of transformation frequency observed by Kakunaga (14) agrees to that of disappearance of 4NQO-purine adducts from DNA of this mouse cell line as shown by a broken line in Fig. 5, which I have quoted from Ikenaga's paper (8). This agreement, together with the parallel data of E. coli in Fig. 3, supports the hypothesis that 4NQO-purine adducts are the major cause of transformation and that they are repaired by an error-free excision repair probably very similar to that in E. coli. It should also be noted that the number of lesions per mouse genome per lethal hit is nearly equal after UV and 4NQO treatments (8). These and other (8) data show that 4NQO is nearly perfectly UV mimetic in its biological effects in human and mouse cells as well as in E. coli.

Misrepair Mutagenesis versus Misrepair Carcinogenesis

There is another type of DNA repair which is supposed to be, at least partially, error-prone. In E. coli, this second type repair is almost completely lost in the recA$^-$ strain (6). The recA$^-$ strain is more UV-sensitive to killing than the excisionless strain (uvrA$^-$) and yet it is unmutable (18, 19, 28), within the limit of the currently used detection method, by 4NQO, UV, X-rays, methyl methanesulfonate,

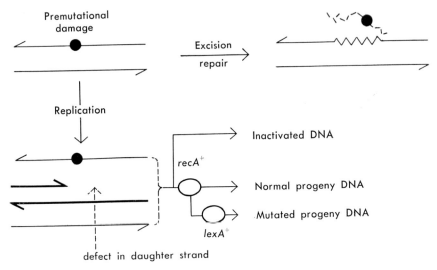

FIG. 6. Models of two types of DNA repair ; error-free excision repair and misrepair mutagenesis *via* error-prone postreplication repair.

mitomycin C and 2-(2-furyl)-3-(5-nitro-2-furyl) acrylic acid amide (AF-2). This means that DNA damage produced by 4NQO (or by other radiomimetic chemicals) is converted to mutated DNA sequences only after the *recA*-gene-dependent system works normally.

Figure 6 shows schematically two types of repair. *E. coli* strains defective at the gene *lexA* (or also named *exrA*) are barely mutable by UV though they are not as sensitive to killing by UV as *recA*⁻ strain (*28*). The *recA*⁻ strains seem to be completely inactivated if they have any unexcised pyrimidine dimers on DNA so that they produce no UV-induced mutants at all. The *recA*⁺-*lexA*⁺ dependent, error-prone repair (Fig. 6) is believed to work usually on defects in daughter strands (see Fig. 6) produced by inhibition of replication opposite the pyrimidine-dimer bearing part of the template DNA strand (*28*). However, we cannot test this misrepair model with mouse cells for no *lexA*⁻- or *recA*⁻-equivalent strains are available. Fortunately, Witkin and Farquharson (*29*) reported that in *E. coli* caffeine posttreatment partially mimics the phenotype of the *lexA*⁻ strain.

Figure 7 compares some essential features of the effects of caffeine on transformation in rodent cells and on mutations in *E. coli*. The transformation frequency produced by 4NQO in mouse cells progressively decreased with increase in caffeine dose administered for 48 hr after 4NQO treatment (*15*). This frequency decline paralleled the diminution of 4NQO-initiated mutagenesis by caffeine in an excisionless strain of *E. coli*. However, Donovan and DiPaolo (*2*) reported that low doses of caffeine enhanced the transformation frequency induced by N-acetoxy-2-fluorenylacetamide (AcAAF) in Syrian hamster cells although caffeine at their highest dose considerably suppressed the transformation (Fig. 7). This bimodal action of caffeine can be simulated by caffeine posttreatment effects on mutations of 4NQO-treated wild-type *E. coli* cells (Fig. 7). From these and other data (*3, 13,*

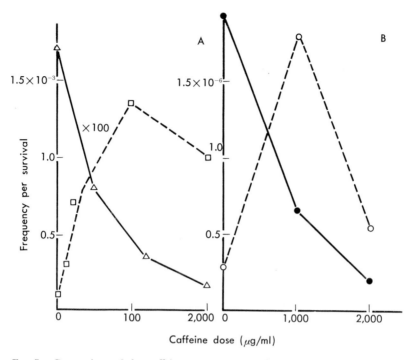

Fig. 7.   Comparison of the caffeine-posttreatment effects on transformation in rodent cells and mutations in *E. coli*. Transformed cells were induced by 4NQO in mouse cells (Kakunaga (*15*)) and by AcAAF in Syrian hamster cells (Donovan and DiPaolo (*2*)). Mutations to prototrophy were induced by 4NQO. 4NQO-treated mouse cells and AcAAF-treated hamster cells were posttreated with caffeine at indicated doses for proper time before seeding on fresh plates to score transformed foci. 4NQO-treated cells of *F. coli* strains H/r30R (wild type) and Hs30 (*uvrB⁻* : excisionless) were plated on semienriched agar plates containing caffeine at indicated concentrations (unpublished).   A : tranformation. B : mutation in *E. coli*. □ hamster ; △ mouse ; ○ wild type ; ● excisionless.

22, 29) we may conclude that caffeine suppresses the error-free repair at low doses and the error-prone repair at high doses in *E. coli* (and possibly also in Donovan-DiPaolo's hamster cell line) but suppresses only the error-prone repair in Kakunaga's mouse cell line.

Since a bacterium usually contains two or more haploid nuclei, at least two cell divisions are needed to yield a homokaryotic mutant bacterium from a heterokaryotic bacterium which has experienced a mutation in one of its nuclei. Furthermore, if the mutation is concerned with such a specific character as cell membrane, the mutant character will appear only after some further cell divisions which enable all the old parts concerned with the character of the cell to be replaced with new mutant material. In fact, as shown in Fig. 8, the full expression of recessive deletion mutations to resistance to colicin B (ColB^R) takes 4 cell generations after UV irradiation (*9*), whereas the expression of dominant mutations from auxotrophy to prototrophy occurs virtually within one cell generation after exposure to 4NQO (see Haas and Doudney (1959) in Ref. *5* for the case of UV). The 4NQO-induced

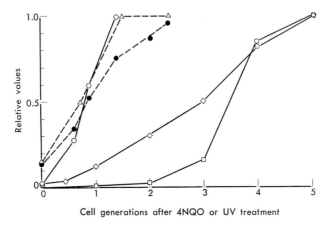

FIG. 8.   Kinetics of fixation of 4NQO-induced premutational damage in *E. coli* (●: unpublished), 4NQO-induced pretransformational damage in mouse cells (△: from Kakunaga (*15*)) and 4NQO-induced pretumorigenic damage in mice (▼ : from Nomura (*25*)) compared with kinetics of expression of 4NQO-induced Arg⁺ mutations (○ : dominant, base-change mutations ; unpublished) and UV-induced ColB^R mutations (◇ : recessive, deletion mutations ; from Ishii and Kondo (*10*)) and expression of 4NQO-induced transformation in mouse cells (□: from Kakunaga (*14*)). — expression ; - - - fixation.

transformation in mouse cells takes 4 cell generations for the full expression as shown by the kinetics curve of its expression (*14*) in Fig. 8. It should be noted that, as shown by two kinetics curves in broken line in Fig. 8, both the premutational damage in *E. coli* and the pretransformational damage in mouse cells were fixed, that is, made insensitive to suppression by caffeine treatment, virtually within the first post-4NQO cell division. These results suggest that fixation of 4NQO-induced pretransformational damage occurs through a mechanism similar to that in 4NQO-induced mutagenesis in *E. coli*, that is, probably *via* errors in postreplication repair of the defects in daughter DNA strands produced by inhibition of replication opposite the 4NQO-purine adducts on old DNA template strands. The delayed appearance of transformed characteristics in mouse cells is compatible with various data (*5*) of the delayed appearance of mutations in bacteria if we assume that transformation in mouse cells is caused by recessive mutations.

The recessive mutation theory fits the fact that malignancy can be suppressed when malignantly transformed cells are fused with nonmalignant cells (*4*). However, the recessive mutation theory must explain how the two homologous wild-type genes presumably coexisting in the diploid genome can be mutated to recessive alleles by a single exposure to carcinogen. A simple explanation for this puzzling problem is to assume that neoplasia-sensitive cells, either in cultured lines or some parts of animal organs, are heterozygous, *i.e.*, possessing wild-type and recessive alleles, or that one of the pair of the genes is being turned off in the sensitive cells. This is the basic problem pertinent to most of the recently reported recessive mutations in cultured mammalian cells.

Very recently, Nomura (*25*) found that the yields of lung tumors induced by a single injection of 4NQO in the ICR mouse strain can also be suppressed to as low as 30% by caffeine administered even 5 days after the 4NQO injection (Fig. 8). Zajdela and Latarjet (*30*) reported that UV-inducible skin cancer in mice can be suppressed by the presence of caffeine.

Some Characteristics of Cancer Mutations

If the somatic mutation theory holds true, then we can predict some characteristics of the mutations responsible for cancer. Compared with 4NQO (*10, 21, 25*), in *E. coli*, AF-2 (a food additive widely used in Japan until 1974) is a strong base-change mutagen (for Arg$^+$ mutations) (*18*) but rather a weak deletion mutagen (for ColB^R mutations) (*20*), and a weak carcinogen in mice (*24*). Similarly, DNA base analogs, *e.g.*, BUdR, are potent mutagens for base-pair substitutions and yet are virtually noncarcinogenic. So it is tempting to assume that, at least for transformation of mouse cells and lung tumors in mice, the 4NQO-induced neoplastic cells are produced *via* induction of deletion mutations in progenitor cells.

Since, roughly speaking, a nearly equal concentration of 4NQO-purine adducts (or pyrimidine dimers) per unit length of DNA is produced at 37% survival dose (D_{37}) of 4NQO (or UV) for both the excisionless strain of *E. coli* and the mouse cell (*7, 8, 17*), the transformation frequency of 2.5×10^{-3} in mouse cells at 0.5 μM of 4NQO (D_{37}) (*12*) corresponds to deletion mutation frequency of 1.5×10^{-4} in the *uvrA*$^-$ strain of *E. coli* at 4 μM of 4NQO (D_{37}) (*10*). If we use the actual concentration of 4NQO adducts per unit DNA length at 37% survival (*7, 8*), the ratio of the target size for transformation in mouse cells to that for ColB^R deletion mutations in *E. coli* becomes about 30 instead of 17 ($=2.5 \times 10^{-3} \div 1.5 \times 10^{-4}$). Since the relative target size for mutation as measured by mutation rate per locus per rad is about 100- to 1,000-fold larger for the mouse than that for ColB^R deletions in *E. coli* (see Ref. *17* for review), the present estimate for the size of the transformation target in the mouse cell is not an unreasonable value.

If we assume the deletion mutation theory of cancer and the generality of misrepair mutagenesis, we may predict from mutagenic efficiency at 37% survival for ColB^R deletion mutations in *E. coli* (*10*) that the order of carcinogenic efficiency at an equal toxicity would be N-methyl-N′-nitro-N-nitrosoguanidine$\simeq$4NQO> UV$\simeq$AF-2>hydroxylamine>X-rays>mitomycin C. However, this prediction may not completely hold true for the error-prone repair responsible for mutagenesis differs in its detailed mechanism between *E. coli* and mammals (*17*).

Induction of leukemia by atomic bomb radiations, which was higher in Hiroshima than in Nagasaki (*11*), is the only reliable, quantitative data for the relationship between carcinogen exposure and cancer in human beings. The higher incidence in Hiroshima can be reasonably explained by the fact that the radiation in Hiroshima was a mixture of fast neutrons and γ-rays in about a one to one ratio whereas the radiation in Nagasaki was made of almost γ-rays alone (*11*). It is well known from laboratory experiments that fast neutrons induce chromosome aberrations in human and other mammalian cells at a higher efficiency than γ-rays (*1*). Therefore, these results also fit the deletion mutation hypothesis that deletions in some parts of DNA of human chromosomes may lead to leukemia.

The above hypothesis implies the following. Most of the lesions induced by ionizing radiations are repaired, but a small fraction of lesions occurring in clusters, which are produced more frequently by fast neutrons than by γ-rays, remain unrepaired. The unrepaired lesions in DNA evoke the assumed misrepair mechanism so that some of the damage-bearing cells are rescued, usually without harmful cytotoxic defects but occasionally with deletion mutations some of which may produce, after a long unknown process, neoplastic cells.

Lastly, we must remember that the cancer induction frequency in mankind (*11*) is much lower than those usually observed with experimental animals. Therefore, a fundamental key for prevention of cancer in human beings may lie in the reason why we often cannot induce cancer in some species or strains of animals. I believe that DNA repair is, at least partly, involved in the suppression of cancer induction in these animals. There is evidence that eukaryotes have more advanced DNA repair than prokaryotes although we are just beginning to understand the difference (*17*).

ACKNOWLEDGMENTS

I wish to express my gratitude to Drs. V. M. Maher and M. W. Liberman for comments during the preparation of the manuscript.   This work was supported by the funds from the Ministry of Education, Science and Culture and from the Ministry of Health and Welfare.

REFERENCES

1. Auxier, J. A. (ed.).   Symposium on Neutrons in Radiobiology, 1969, CONF-691106, Federal Sci. & Tech. Information, National Bur. Standards, Virginia, 1970.
2. Donovan, P. J. and DiPaolo, J. A.   Caffeine enhancement of chemical carcinogen-induced transformation of cultured Syrian hamster cells. Cancer Res., *34*: 2720–2727, 1974.
3. Fujiwara, Y. and Kondo, T.   Caffeine-sensitive repair of ultraviolet-damaged DNA of mouse L cells. Biochem. Biophys. Res. Commun., *47*: 557–564, 1972.
4. Harris, H., Klein, G., Worst, P., and Tachibana, T.   Suppression of malignancy by cell fusion. Nature, *223*: 363–368, 1969.
5. Hayes, W.   The Genetics of Bacteria and Their Viruses. 2nd ed., Wiley, New York, 1969.
6. Howard-Flanders, P.   DNA repair. Annu. Rev. Biochem., *37*: 175–200, 1968.
7. Ikenaga, M., Ichikawa-Ryo, H., and Kondo, S.   The major cause of inactivation and mutation by 4-nitroquinoline 1-oxide in *Escherichia coli*: Excisable 4NQO-purine adducts. J. Mol. Biol., *92*: 341–356, 1975.
8. Ikenaga, M., Ishii, Y., Tada, M., Kakunaga, T., Takebe, H., and Kondo, S.   Excision-repair of 4-nitroquinoline-1-oxide damage responsible for killing, mutation and cancer.   *In;* P. Hanawalt and R. B. Setlow (eds.), Molecular Mechanisms for the Repair of DNA, pp. 763–771, Plenum Press, New York, 1975.
9. Ishii, Y. and Kondo, S.   Spontaneous and radiation-induced deletion mutations in *Escherichia coli* strains with different DNA repair capacities. Mutat. Res., *16*: 13–25, 1972.

10. Ishii, Y. and Kondo, S. Comparative analysis of deletion and base-change mutabilities of *Escherichia coli* B strains differing in DNA repair capacity (*wild-type, uvrA⁻, polA⁻, recA⁻*) by various mutagens. Mutat. Res., *27*: 27–44, 1975.

11. Jablon, S., Fujita, S., Fukushima, K., Ishimaru, T., and Auxier, J. A. RBE of neutrons in Japanese survivors. *In;* Symposium on Neutrons in Radiobiology, 1969, CONF-691106, pp. 547–577, Federal Sci. & Tech. Information, National Bur. Standards, Virginia, 1970.

12. Kakunaga, T. A quantitative system for assay of malignant transformation by chemical carcinogens using a clone derived from BALB/3T3. Int. J. Cancer, *12*: 463–473, 1973.

13. Kakunaga, T. The process of cell transformation initiated by chemical carcinogens. Igaku no Ayumi (The Stride of Medicine), *86*: 746–750, 1973 (in Japanese).

14. Kakunaga, T. Requirement for cell replication in the fixation and expression of the transformed state in mouse cells treated with 4-nitroquinoline 1-oxide. Int. J. Cancer, *14*: 736–742, 1974.

15. Kakunaga, T. Caffeine inhibits cell transformation by 4-nitroquinoline-1-oxide. Nature, *258*: 248–250, 1975.

16. Kondo, S. Errors in genetic information and DNA repair—Classification of possible cause of cancer. Nippon Rinsho (*Japan. J. Clin. Med.*), *29* (Suppl.): 70–75, 1971 (in Japanese).

17. Kondo, S. DNA repair and evolutionary considerations. Adv. Biophys., *7*: 91–162, 1975.

18. Kondo, S. and Ichikawa-Ryo, H. Testing and classification of mutagenicity of furylfuramide in *Escherichia coli*. Japan. J. Genet., *48*: 295–300, 1973.

19. Kondo, S., Ichikawa, H., Iwo, K., and Kato, T. Base-change mutagenesis and prophage induction in strains of *Escherichia coli* with different DNA repair capacities. Genetics, *66*: 187–217, 1970.

20. Kondo, S., Ichikawa-Ryo, H., and Nomura, T. Mutagenesis in bacteria and teratogenesis in mouse by furylfuramide. Mutat. Res., *31*: 263–264, 1975.

21. Kondo, S. and Kato, T. Photoreactivation of mutation and killing in *Escherichia coli*. Adv. Biol. Med. Phys., *12*: 283–298, 1968.

22. Morita, T. and Tada, M. Effects of caffeine on post-replication repair of DNA damaged by 4-hydroxyaminoquinoline 1-oxide in human and mouse cells. Unpublished.

23. Nakahara, W., Fukuoka, F., and Sugimura, T. Carcinogenic action of 4-nitroquinoline-N-oxide. Gann, *48*: 129–137, 1957.

24. Nomura, T. Carcinogenicity of the food additive furylfuramide in foetal and young mice. Nature, *258*: 610–611, 1975.

25. Nomura, T. Diminution of 4-nitroquinoline 1-oxide-initiated tumorigenesis by posttreatment with caffeine in mice. Nature, *260*: 547–549, 1976.

26. Ono, S. and Kondo, S. Molecular theory of surface tension in liquds. *In;* Handbuch der Physik, vol. 10, pp. 134–280, Springer-Verlag, Berlin, 1960.

27. Tada, M. and Tada, M. Metabolic activation of 4-nitroquinoline 1-oxide and its binding to nucleic acid. This volume, pp. 217–228.

28. Witkin, E. M. Ultraviolet-induced mutation and DNA repair. Annu. Rev. Genet., *3*: 525–552, 1969.

29. Witkin, E. M. and Farquharson, E. L. Enhancement and diminution of ultraviolet

light-initiated mutagenesis by post-treatment with caffeine in *Escherichia coli. In;* Ciba Foundation Symposium on Mutation as Cellular Process, pp. 36–49, London, 1969.

30. Zajdela, F. and Latarjet, R.   Effect inhibiteur de la caféine sur l'induction de cancers cutanés par les rayons ultraviolets chez la Souris. Compt. Rend. Acad. Sci., Paris, Série D, *277*: 1073–1076, 1973.

Discussion of Paper of Dr. Kondo

DR. MAHER: Your contribution is extremely valuable because it brings together many of the main points discussed by various speakers at the Symposium. I am sure I did not grasp all of its implications and hope to discuss it with you at length in the next few days. What is the evidence that caffeine is affecting Dr. Kakunaga's BALB/3T3 strain to mimic postreplication repair deficiency?

DR. KONDO: According to Kakunaga's 1975 data, the suppressive effects of caffeine posttreatment are limited mostly to the period of first post-4NQO DNA replication and accompanied by parallel decrease in survival of 4NQO-treated cells.

Closing Remarks

Dr. Peter N. Magee

What I would just like to reflect on is the conversation that took place right at the beginning of the meeting. You may have noticed that I came in with Her Imperial Highness and Dr. Nakahara. I had the honor of being presented to her outside, and of talking to her a little while. The conversation got around to the title of this symposium. Then, I realized how extremely good the English is of Her Imperial Highness and of Dr. Nakahara. What they were discussing was whether this should have been " Fundamentals of Cancer Prevention," as it turned out to be, or " Fundamentals in Cancer Prevention." I expressed the opinion that I thought that " Fundamentals in Cancer Prevention " would be better. I was rather embarrassed when Dr. Nakahara pointed out that I had been the one suggesting " Fundamentals of Cancer Prevention " before. I think you will see what I am getting at when one speaks of fundamentals of a subject. It implies that we know something about it. A textbook on fundamentals of chemistry is about fundamental aspects of chemistry.

When we talk of cancer prevention, we have to realize that we know very little about it except the obvious things that have been discussed, that is, if you want to prevent cancer, to avoid broad exposure to those agents of causes, as far as you can. Beyond that the situation become much more tenuous and if it is fundamentals in cancer prevention, this to me, and I hope to you, implies that what is being discussed is fundamental scientific work that may have bearing on practical aspects of cancer prevention in the future. So, the question that perhaps we should ask ourselves is: have our more basic discussions helped us in our thinking for the future on how we may better prevent cancer?

I really hope they have because when we planned this symposium we had based it on three sessions, the first being modulating the activation and the inactivation of carcinogens. I think we certainly have seen on the experimental side that it is possible to prevent cancer by doing just this—to modulate the activity of an enzyme. A good example is Dr. Wattenberg's example of complete prevention of dimethylhydrazine cancer induction in colon by disulfiram, which probably is based on modulation of the activation enzyme. There have been other examples that we have discussed. Can this sort of work develop in such a way that it can be applied to human subjects? I must confess that at the moment I cannot see exactly how it can be done, but I think we heard enough in the meeting to feel some confidence that, if this work is pursued, it will lead to this sort of approach to cancer prevention. I think that one of the other things to emerge was the great importance of studies on human cells, either *in vitro* or, as Dr. Gelboin pointed out, on that material which is most easily obtained from human being, which, of course, is blood, and one might also say human urine for metabolites.

Then the next session was DNA modification by carcinogens and its repair. I think I tried to indicate, in both of my presentations, that this really is dependent on the acceptance that some sort of change in DNA has got something to do with the causation of cancer. I feel that as the papers were being presented during this meeting, this idea was strengthened. Everybody, it seems to me, has been sympathetic to this view. In the work on Xeroderma we had more evidence which really does seem to indicate that cancer can probably result from some sort of DNA modification. Therefore, all this work we have heard on DNA repair, if we could device methods of modifying it, might be a true way of preventing the evolution cancer, even if the initiation reaction has taken place. This may in fact be unavoidable because there are certain radiations and so on we simply cannot avoid. There may be environmental mutagens we cannot avoid. This is extremely important.

The third topic was blocking the carcinogenic process and characterizing the pre-cancerous state. We have heard some excellent presentations on various aspect of the pre-cancerous state and have had some lively discussion on what it really is, and when it is a nodule or not a nodule, when it is a tumor, and so on. And here again it seems only through fundamental basic research of this kind that we will ever arrive at ways in which the already transformed cells can be controlled, before they actually become overt cancer.

So, I hope you will agree with me, this meeting really has made some contribution to all our thinking aimed at the practical question of prevention of cancer. I hope that sometime, in the not too distant future, another meeting can be held. Dare I even suggest another Princess Takamatsu Symposium the title of which could really be " Fundamentals of Cancer Prevention " rather than " Fundamentals in."

So now I would like on behalf of all of us to thank some of the people here who have done so much to make this such a very pleasant occasion, as well as a stimulating one scientifically. Obviously, I want to thank the other members, the Japanese members, of the organizing committee, that is, Drs. Sugimura, Takayama and Matsushima, and their staffs. Last, but of course, by no means least, we must thank Dr. Nakahara. He was the father of, I believe it is right to say, these Princess Takamatsu Symposia. Without his initial effort and his continued stimulus they could not have occurred at all. So, I just ask you to join with me in thanking our Japanese hosts for their great kindness.